ADVANCES IN

Dermatology

Editor-in-Chief
William D. James, MD

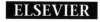

PHILADELPHIA   LONDON   TORONTO   MONTREAL   SYDNEY   TOKYO

VOLUME 22

VOLUME 23

Vice President, Continuity Publishing: John A. Schrefer
Editor: Carla Holloway

Editorial Office:
Elsevier
1600 John F. Kennedy Blvd,
Suite 1800
Philadelphia, PA 19103-2899

International Standard Serial Number: 0882-0880
International Standard Book Number: 1-4160-5178-3
978-1-4160-5178-7

Editor-in-Chief

WILLIAM D. JAMES, MD, Paul R. Gross Professor of Dermatology; Vice Chairman and Residency Program Director, University of Pennsylvania School of Medicine, Philadelphia, Pennsylvania

Associate Editors

CLAY J. COCKERELL, MD, Clinical Professor of Dermatology and Pathology, University of Texas Southwestern Medical Center; Director, Cockerell and Associates, Dermpath Diagnostics, Dallas, Texas

SAM T. HWANG, MD, PhD, Senior Investigator, Dermatology Branch, National Cancer Institute, Bethesda, Maryland*

AMY JO NOPPER, MD, Associate Professor of Pediatrics and Chief, Section of Dermatology, Children's Mercy Hospitals and Clinics, University of Missouri-Kansas City School of Medicine; Kansas City, Missouri

SUZANNE M. OLBRICHT, MD, Associate Professor of Dermatology, Harvard Medical School, Boston; and Chair, Department of Dermatology, Lahey Clinic, Burlington, Massachusetts

---

*Editorial comments were written by Dr. Hwang in his personal capacity and do not necessarily represent the opinions or endorsement of the National Institutes of Health, Department of Health and Human Services, or the Federal Government.

CONTRIBUTORS

JACK L. ARBISER, MD, PhD, Department of Dermatology, Emory University School of Medicine, Georgia

BRIAN L. BAKER, MD, Fellow, Mohs Micrographic Surgery and Cutaneous Oncology, Department of Dermatology, Saint Louis University, Saint Louis, Missouri

CLAY J. COCKERELL, MD, University of Texas Southwestern School of Medicine, Dallas, Texas

KELLY M. CORDORO, MD, Assistant Clinical Professor of Dermatology, Adult and Pediatric Dermatology, University of California, San Francisco, California

ODILE ENJOLRAS, MD, Consultation des Angiomes, Service de Chirurgie Maxillo-Faciale et Chirurgie Plastique, AP-HP, Hopital d'Enfants Armand Trousseau, Paris, France

SCOTT W. FOSKO, MD, Professor and Chairman, Department of Dermatology; Associate Professor, Departments of Otolaryngology, Ophthalmology, and Internal Medicine; Director, Mohs Surgery and Cutaneous Oncology; and Director, Melanoma and Cutaneous Oncology Section, Saint Louis University Cancer Center, Saint Louis, Missouri

LEVI E. FRIED, BA, Department of Dermatology, Emory University School of Medicine, Atlanta, Georgia

JORGE GARCIA-ZUAZAGA, MD, MS, Department of Dermatology, Mohs Micrographic Surgery and Cutaneous Oncology, Lahey Clinic, Harvard Medical School, Burlington, Massachusetts

JOEL M. GELFAND, MD, MSCE, Assistant Professor, Medical Director, Clinical Studies Unit, Department of Dermatology; Associate Scholar, Center for Clinical Epidemiology and Biostatistics, University of Pennsylvania, Philadelphia, Pennsylvania

MARIA HORDINSKY, MD, Professor and Chair, Department of Dermatology, University of Minnesota, Minneapolis

SETH L. MATARASSO, MD, Clinical Professor of Dermatology, University of California School of Medicine, San Francisco, California

LLOYD S. MILLER, MD, PhD, Assistant Professor, Division of Dermatology, Center for Health Sciences, University of California Los Angeles, Los Angeles, California

SUZANNE OLBRICHT, MD, Chair, Department of Dermatology, Lahey Clinic; Associate Professor of Dermatology, Harvard Medical School, Boston, Massachusetts

WILLMAR D. PATINO, MD, Department of Pathology, University of Texas Southwestern Medical Center in Dallas, Dallas, Texas

ARNAUD PICARD, MD, Service de Chirurgie Maxillo-Faciale et Chirurgie Plastique, AP-HP, Hopital d'Enfants Armand Trousseau, Paris, France

STEPHEN K. RICHARDSON, MD, Clinical Assistant Professor of Dermatology, Florida State University College of Medicine/Dermatology Associates of Tallahassee, Tallahassee, Florida.

CARLOS RICOTTI, MD, University of Texas Southwestern School of Medicine, Dallas, Texas

DAWN H. SIEGEL, MD, Assistant Professor, Department of Dermatology and Pediatrics, Oregon Health and Science University, Portland, Oregon

VÉRONIQUE SOUPRE, MD, Service de Chirurgie Maxillo-Faciale et Chirurgie Plastique, AP-HP, Hopital d'Enfants Armand Trousseau, Paris, France

SARAH A. STECHSCHULTE, BA, University of Miami L. Miller School of Medicine, Miami, Florida

JOSEPH SUSA, DO, Clinical Assistant Professor, Department of Dermatology, Division of Dermatopathology, University of Texas Southwestern Medical Center in Dallas, Dallas, Texas

KEVIN C. WANG, MD, PhD, Department of Dermatology, University of California at San Francisco School of Medicine, San Francisco, California

LEE T. ZANE, MD, MAS, Assistant Clinical Professor of Dermatology, Department of Dermatology, University of California at San Francisco School of Medicine, San Francisco; and Vice-President, Clinical Development, Anacor Pharmaceuticals, Palo Alto, California

Botulinum Toxin: Concepts and Use in 2008
By Seth L. Matarasso

The Nose: Principles of Surgical Treatment
By Brian L. Baker and Scott W. Fosko

Cutaneous Squamous Cell Carcinoma
By Jorge Garcia-Zuazaga and Suzanne Olbricht

Epigenetics of Cutaneous Melanoma
By Willmar D. Patino and Joseph Susa

Toll-Like Receptors in Skin
By Lloyd S. Miller

Application of Angiogenesis to Clinical Dermatology
By Levi E. Fried and Jack L. Arbiser

Uncommon Benign Infantile Vascular Tumors
By Odile Enjolras, Véronique Soupre, and Arnaud Picard

Management of Childhood Psoriasis
By Kelly M. Cordoro

Update on the Natural History and Systemic Treatment of Psoriasis

By Stephen K. Richardson and Joel M. Gelfand

Recent Advances in Acne Vulgaris Research: Insights and Clinical Implications

By Kevin C.Wang and Lee T. Zane

Current Concepts: Dermatopathology of Pigmentary Alteration Disorders in the Hispanic Population
By Carlos Ricotti, Sarah A. Stechschulte, and Clay J. Cockerell

Cutaneous Mosaicism: a Molecular and Clinical Review
By Dawn H. Siegel

Advances in Hair Diseases
By Maria Hordinsky

Botulinum Toxin: Concepts and Use in 2008

Seth L. Matarasso, MD

University of California School of Medicine, 490 Post Street, Suite 700, San Francisco, CA 94102, USA

EDITORIAL COMMENTS

Dr. Seth Matarasso is one of dermatology's most experienced practitioners with the use of botulinum toxin. In this article, he discusses the pharmacology of the toxin, the preparation that is available currently (Botox), new preparations that are on the horizon, and indications and contraindications for its use. He outlines technique of injection in each cosmetic area. Most useful are the pearls he gives for proper placement, and the kinds of problems that can arise with misplacement in each site. Such is the state of the art in 2008!

Suzanne Olbricht

L ike many medical innovations, either for therapeutic or for cosmetic purposes, botulinum toxin has an interesting historical chronology. Ironically, the story of the toxin, now the most popular aesthetic procedure for both genders in the United States, originally began when the signs and symptoms of fatal systemic botulism were first reported in 1820. The organism was not correctly identified until approximately 1900 and it was not until 1973 that the profound clinical ramifications of its toxin were first appreciated. Initially used for the treatment of muscular dystonias, botulinum toxin did not receive Food and Drug Administration (FDA) approval for the treatment of strabismus and benign essential blepharospasm until 1989. The cosmetic usefulness of the toxin was appreciated from the observation of patients suffering from ocular dysfunction who were treated with small doses of botulinum toxin injected directly into the periocular muscles. Coincidentally, a simultaneous reduction in surrounding facial wrinkles was noted, which ushered in the next wave of popularity for the agent. Initially met with skepticism because it was labeled a "toxin" and had been intimately associated with untimely demise, the first report documenting the reduction in periocular rhytids following local injections appeared in the dermatology literature in 1992. It was not until 2001 that it was approved by Health Canada and in 2002 "Botox Cosmetic" was

E-mail address: slm_md@msn.com

0882-0880/08/$ – see front matter
doi:10.1016/j.yadr.2008.09.005

approved by the FDA "for the temporary reduction of lines and wrinkles due to the corrugator and supercilii muscles in patients 65 years or younger." Soon thereafter, in 2004, Botox gained FDA approval for axillary hyperhidrosis [1,2].

PHARMACOLOGY

Botulinum toxins are produced by the anaerobic spore-forming bacterium *Clostridium botulinum* and are considered among the most potent biologic substances found in nature. Eight immunologically distinct serotypes are known to exist, designated A, B, C-1, C-2 (which affects vascular permeability rather than nervous tissue), D, E, F, and G. The different subtypes ultimately have the same effect at the neuromuscular junction but they have subtle differences in their molecular weight, biosynthesis, and intracellular site of action [3].

Botox (Allergan, Inc., Irvine, CA), containing serotype A toxin, is currently the only commercially available botulinum toxin. It is supplied in vacuum-sealed, 100-unit vials of lyophilized powder that are shipped on ice and, on receipt, should be kept refrigerated at 4°C. The packet insert that accompanies the product states that the protein in the product is labile and should be stored for no longer than 4 hours after reconstitution, that reconstitution should be atraumatic (without agitation and foam formation), and that the vials are for single use only [4]. The FDA recommends that 2.5 mL of unpreserved sterile normal saline (0.9% sodium chloride) be used to reconstitute the product, yielding a final concentration of 4 units/mL. However, a dilution chart with greater volumes of diluent accompanies the product. Higher dilutions cause a greater tendency for unwanted toxin spread. Similarly, the product is more robust than originally anticipated and can be kept refrigerated in a liquid state for a week or longer without losing its original potency [5]. It has also been reported that injections cause less pain when normal saline containing the preservative benzyl alcohol is used for reconstitution [6].

Botox consists of large protein complexes that include the neurotoxin and other nontoxic proteins. The neurotoxin exerts its effect at the neuromuscular junction by inhibiting release of acetylcholine at the motor neurons at the neuromuscular junction end plate. This results in chemodenervation and a flaccid paralysis of exposed striated skeletal muscles with an onset of approximately 3 to 7 days. With flaccid paralysis of the underlying musculature, the superimposed skin relaxes and clinically, dynamic rhytids are reduced. Muscle function recovers after roughly 120 days through terminal sprouting of motor axons and formation of new motor end plates [7], and dynamic rhytids reappear. Subsequent treatments have a longer duration of effect, attributed to disuse muscle atrophy.

Many other botulinum toxins are undergoing intensive investigation and some have completed phase 3 clinical trials and therefore may soon be available for use. Most of the toxins that are being researched have the same active ingredient, botulinum toxin type A, the most powerful of the toxins. These include Puretox (Mentor Corporation, Santa Barbara, CA, USA), Xeomin (Merz Pharmaceuticals, Frankfort, Germany) Linurase, (Prollenium Technologies, Ontario,

Canada), Chinese toxin (Lanzhou Biologics, Lanzhou, China), and Neuronox (Medytox Inc., South Korea).

All of the pivotal studies of Reloxin (Dysport), the type A toxin that will be distributed by Medics (Scottsdale, AZ), have been completed and FDA approval and availability are expected shortly. Although Reloxin is similar in effect, onset, efficacy, and safety when compared to its predecessor, Botox, the two preparations are distinct and should not be considered interchangeable products. Many of the preliminary studies have suggested that 1 unit of Botox is clinically equivalent to 3 units of Reloxin. In addition to the protein content and potency dissimilarity, the most important difference may be that Reloxin has a smaller total complex molecular weight than Botox. Therefore, it may have the potential for greater diffusion pattern, perhaps exerting its effect on nontargeted muscles [8,9].

Myobloc (Neurobloc), manufactured by Elan Corporation (San Francisco, CA) is the sole agent containing botulinum toxin type B serotype. It is also distinct in that it is available in liquid form and therefore does not require reconstitution with saline. It was approved in the United States in December 2000 for the treatment of cervical dystonia. The conversion ratio was estimated to be 100 units of Myobloc to 1 unit of Botox. It has similar efficacy to Botox with a quicker onset of action but, because of a slightly more acidic pH, it is slightly more painful on injection. The briefer duration of action with quicker reappearance of facial rhytids [10] makes it less useful in the cosmetic arena.

An initial concern with the use of botulinum toxin was that the use of high doses or brief intervals in between injections presented a potential risk for formation of neutralizing antibodies and the lack of clinical response. To date, no good documentation exists that the small amounts that are used to treat facial muscles antibody formation are problematic. However, if immuno-genicity does develop as the use of the toxin increases, other toxin serotypes may be used to impart a clinical change because no cross reactivity occurs.

CONTRAINDICATIONS

Botox is categorized as a class C medication and therefore it is not recommen-ded for women who are pregnant or breast feeding. The primary medical contraindications are those patients who could be allergic to the product and, importantly, those who have a pre-existing neuromuscular disease that could be exacerbated by botulinum toxin, such as myasthenia gravis or amyotrophic lateral sclerosis. Aminoglycoside antibiotics can also potentiate the effect, so lower doses of Botox should be administered to these patients. Patient selection is crucial in optimizing results because a subset of patients may not be psycho-logically prepared for this type of therapy and alternative treatment options should be discussed.

INDICATIONS

Botox is only FDA approved for the treatment of glabellar rhytids and axillary hyperhidrosis; however, its list of other innovative usages is seemingly inexhaustible. In cosmesis, many facial hyperfunctional muscles with superimposed cutaneous dynamic rhytids, both above and below the zygomatic arch, can be treated with small precise injections of the neurotoxin. Pan-facial treatment is often accompanied by other procedures, such as soft tissue augmentation with dermal fillers, resurfacing techniques, and surgical intervention [11]. By way of the anticholinergic effect of botulinum toxin, disorders of apocrine glands have been expanded to include treatment of excess localized and generalized sweat production, palmoplantar and craniofacial sweating, and disease states (Hailey-Hailey disease, Darier's disease, and dyshidrosis). In addition, colored sweat (chromhidrosis), malodorous sweat (bromhidrosis), and aberrant sweat from trauma and surgery (Frey's syndrome) respond well to botulinum toxin [12,13].

Perhaps one of the greatest untapped uses of botulinum toxin is in pain management. It is well established for the treatment of cervical dystonias and migraine headaches, and interest has been growing in such syndromes as post–herpetic neuralgia and temporomandibular joint dysfunction [14,15]. It is also increasingly used increasingly as an adjuvant in facial reconstruction procedures for the minimization of muscle action that can distort wounds and scars.

When addressing newer uses, whether for aesthetic or therapeutic reasons, the physician and the patient must be reminded that indications other than the midline glabellar crease and axillary hyperhidrosis remain off label and are not sanctioned by the FDA.

INJECTION TECHNIQUE AND COMPLICATIONS
Patient preparation is essential for a good outcome. Prior to initiating any facial procedure, it is wise to have a frank discussion with the patient, emphasizing not only the technique and anticipated outcomes but also the potential risks, alternatives, and complications. A consent form detailing this information should be signed by the patient. Preprocedure photographs are always important because it is not atypical for a patient to minimize the magnitude of his/her original facial defect. To adequately photograph and assess the rhytid or document baseline asymmetry, patients should be seated in an upright position with adequate overhead lighting. Ideally, to prevent unwanted bruising from a percutaneous injection, it is helpful for patients to refrain from taking products, either prescription or over-the-counter preparations, that may interfere with platelets or the clotting cascade for 7 to 10 days before their office visit. Although this ambulatory procedure is not considered too uncomfortable, topical anesthetic creams or ice applied to the proposed treatment area not only may decrease any pain but also may alleviate anxiety.

Historically, physicians were instructed to inject the reconstituted Botox solution with a tuberculin syringe and a 30-gauge 0.5-inch needle. However, it has become increasingly popular to use syringes that do not have "dead space" at the needle hub. This type of syringe reduces the unnecessary loss of product. Diabetic syringes not only serve that function but are also preassembled with 32-gauge needles, which may cause less pain on injection. As an added benefit, these syringes have small calibrations that allow for delivery of precise volumes.

There are many individual physician preferences and few absolutes exist when injecting Botox into facial muscles. The amount injected should be based on muscle mass and the degree of hypertrophy. In general, men require more toxin than younger patients and women. The art of the technique is that the sites of injection should always mirror the muscle fiber distribution as the sites and amount injected tend to vary with repeat injections [16].

In the glabella region, the muscles and their expanse can be readily appreciated by having the patient contract the muscles by repeatedly frowning. To ensure proper toxin placement, electromyographic guidance may be helpful. Glabellar frown lines are caused by hyperkinetic movement of three muscle groups: the solitary midline procerus muscle and the medial fibers of the orbicularis oculi (depressor supercilii), which pull the brow inferiorly, and the winged bilateral corrugator supercilii muscle, which moves the brow medially. Because this area is the only one approved by the FDA, it is has been studied extensively and an injection protocol has been established. The treatment sites and doses should be individualized because the muscle mass and location vary based on patient age, gender, and prior treatment. Generally, 35 units of toxin in 5 to 7 aliquots are injected deep into the belly of the muscles. The injection sites include one into the procerus and two into the medial fibers of the orbicularis oculi, and an additional two injections into the corrugator supercilii at their lateral aspect. This later placement is technically crucial. It should be at least 1 cm above the orbital rim and, ideally, it should not cross the midpupillary line. Violating these boundaries could result in unwanted eyelid ptosis [17], which may occur in as many as 2% of patients. With increased experience and improved technique, this incidence has been reduced. If drooping of the eyelid does occur, alpha adrenergic agents placed in the eye stimulate the Mueller's muscle of the upper eyelid and restore it to a normal resting position until the effect of the toxin spontaneously resolves.

Another concern that can arise when the glabellar complex is appropriately immobilized is that patients have a tendency to recruit adjacent intact muscles. The most common is contraction of the horizontal nasalis muscle that can cause fanning "bunny lines" at the radix root of the nose. This muscle is easily weakened by the addition of 2 to 4 units into the belly of the upper nasalis as it traverses the bony dorsum of the nose (Fig. 1).

As opposed to recruitment of neighboring muscles and the appearance of new or worsened dynamic lines, a common source of frustration for patients is that, despite muscle inactivation, residual nondynamic lines persist. These lines are often static and due primarily to actinic change. The patient must be educated that these wrinkles are often not dynamic and they will require other interventions, such as dermal fillers or ablative resurfacing. Bruising, headache, and flu-like symptoms are possible systemic complications, which are usually time limited and treatment, if required, is usually palliative and symptomatic in nature.

The lines that radiate in an arciform pattern from the lateral ocular canthus, the crow's feet, are due solely to the underlying orbicularis oculi muscle

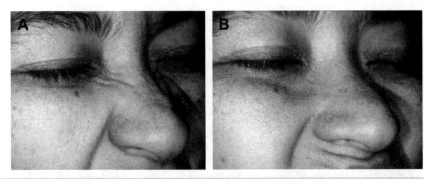

Fig. 1. (A) Intact nasalis muscle without treatment. (B) Following injection of 3 units of Botox in three equal doses, the muscle has minimal contraction, with reduction in the appearance of "bunny lines" across the nasal root.

(Fig. 2), which is a sphincter-like muscle that is responsible for voluntary eyelid closure; therefore, treatment is not designed to achieve complete paralysis, but only muscle paresis. Because the muscle is located directly under the skin with little subcutaneous fat and the vascular plexus is rich, injections can be superficial and made directly into the mass of the muscle. Twelve to 15 units of Botox in three to four equal doses are injected per side. Injections should be 1 cm from the lateral orbital rim and distributed in a fan-like pattern. The superior injection is located at the tail of the eyebrow and the most inferior injection should be well above the zygoma. Placement below the zygomatic arch can result in inactivation of the zygomaticus major muscle and a consequent ipsilateral upper lip droop.

Another common concern when treating in the periocular area is the appearance of a step off, where the lateral fibers of the orbicularis oculi have visibly been reduced but the inferior fibers remain hypertrophic. This can impart or accentuate a pre-existing fullness to the lower eyelid that produces a tired or overweight appearance instead of an improved appearance. This anatomic

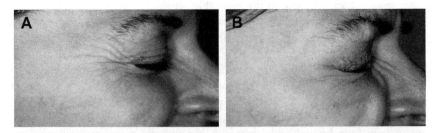

Fig. 2. (A) Lateral view of the crow's feet at maximal muscle contraction prior to treatment with botulinum toxin (B) Following three superficial injections, a total of 12 units per side, of toxin into the orbicularis oculi muscle, the appearance of the crow's feet shows improvement.

and aesthetic discrepancy can be reduced by placing an additional 1 to 2 units subcutaneously in the pretarsal orbicularis oculi in the lower midpupillary line, about 3 mm beneath the ciliary margin. An additional unit injected at the lateral canthus can also be beneficial. This technique reduces the appearance of infraocular fullness and lines, it also widens the eyelid aperture, giving the eye a more annular appearance. It is important to make sure that prior to infraocular injections, the patient has an adequate snap test with good skin recoil. Poor skin elasticity will cause cutaneous redundancy beneath the eyelid. Diplopia, decreased strength of eyelid closure, and an abnormal Schirmer's test have also been reported when treating this area, but these adverse events are infrequent [18–20].

Although horizontal forehead lines are due to one muscle, the frontalis, addressing this muscle can be daunting. This muscle is the sole brow elevator and when treated aggressively with too much toxin, too many injections, or erroneous placement, it can yield an unforgiving result, with brow ptosis, lateral ocular hooding, complete immobility of the upper third of the face, and the inability to be expressive. This risk is irreparable and apparent even to the lay person. Conversely, incomplete treatment of the frontalis muscle, leaving the inferior fibers untreated, can result in isolated brow elevation with a quizzical appearance ("Mr. Spock brow") (Fig. 3). This muscle is a large vertical muscle that inserts superiorly into the galea aponeurotica and inferiorly into the skin of the brow. A total of 10 to 20 units of toxin are divided into multiple injection sites that are distributed in a grid-like pattern across the midbrow and placed 2 to 3 cm above the superior orbital rim [6–8]. By definition, inactivation of this large brow elevator muscle results in a slight, but clinically relevant, brow descent. It is therefore reasonable to simultaneously inject the midline brow depressor (the procerus muscle) with 5 units and an additional 2 units

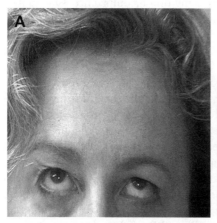
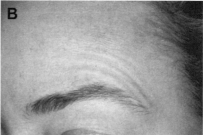

Fig. 3. (A) Brow ptosis (forehead droop) due to excess and inappropriate placement of Botox (B) Incomplete treatment of the frontalis muscle with a resultant quizzical ("Mr. Spock") brow.

in the superior fibers of the orbicularis oculi at the lateral tale of the eyebrow. These fibers are also powerful brow depressors. Treating brow depressor muscles simultaneously with the brow elevator should maintain the brow in a neutral anatomic position [21].

When addressing hyperfunctional muscles in the lower third of the face, below the zygomatic arch, small amounts and precise placement of toxin are required. The primary aim is to weaken the muscle, as opposed to completely inactivating it. Diffusion or improper placement results in cosmetic asymmetry and functional impairment.

The nasolabial fold, extending from the lateral nasal ala to the external oral commissure, has many contributing factors and consequently has innumerable treatment options. Dermal fillers have long been considered a mainstay treatment option. For those folds that are deep and that would require a cost-prohibitive amount of filler, the superior third of the fold can be blunted with Botox, thereby diminishing the total amount of filler required. This blunting can be accomplished by injecting 1 to 2 units of toxin at the nasal pyriform aperture in the nasofacial groove, which weakens the levator labii superioris alaeque nasi muscle. This procedure is not done routinely because patients must be forewarned that not only will this reduce, if present, a gummy smile but, as a normal consequence, it can elongate the upper lip and flatten the cupids bow. It is a technique that should be reserved for motivated patients and for physicians with much experience and intimate knowledge of facial anatomy.

The "lipstick or smoker's lines" that radiate vertically up from the lip can be treated with the plethora of available filling agents or ablative resurfacing procedures. However, these perioral lines are often exaggerated by the purse string action of the orbicularis oris muscle, a sphincter muscle that completely encircles the mouth and is responsible for lip closure and puckering. Treatment is aimed at muscle weakness without inducing oral incompetence. One unit of toxin per quadrant, a total of 4 to 6 units, is placed superficially at the vermillion border of the upper lip either alone or in concert with the lower lip. To avoid flattening and drooping of the lip, treatment of the Cupid's bow and corners of the lip should be avoided. The microparesis that ensues does not eliminate all lines but reduces them while concurrently relaxing muscle action, causing eversion and "pseudoaugmentation" of the lip. For further wrinkle effacement, fillers can be used adjunctively. Some debate exists about which injectable product should be placed first, the filler or the toxin. Theoretically, placing the toxin first can result in spreading on injection of the filler, yielding unwanted complete paralysis of the lip. Ultimately, timing is contingent on physician preference and the end result will be technique dependant. Even with conservative Botox dosing, perioral complications that can arise include an alteration in proprioception, sphincter incompetence and drooling, and an inability to pronounce some consonants (Bs and Ps) [22].

The horizontal crease situated between the middle of the lower lip and the prominence of the chin is the mental crease. This crease is a deeply etched line that is closely tethered to the bony mentum and, as such, is not responsive to resurfacing and only partially amendable to monotherapy with soft tissue dermal fillers. Because part of the cause of the defect is chronic contraction of the underlying mentalis muscle, the line can be ameliorated with botulinum toxin. Placing the toxin directly into the crease weakens the orbicularis oris muscle and results in an incompetent mouth. However, injecting 5 to 10 units of Botox into the belly of the mentalis muscle at the apex of the chin sufficiently weakens it so that the crease is reduced. This technique is also useful for patients who may have a "cobble stone" (peau d'orange) appearance to the chin, due to trauma or a genetic predisposition (Fig. 4). As in any area, residual lines or contour irregularities can be further augmented with a soft tissue filler.

With age, the lateral oral commissure descends and can relay an unwanted negative emotion. This area, the "marionette line," extends from the lateral corner of the mouth down to the lateral chin. Because the underlying cause is dermal atrophy and gravitational changes, this area has traditionally been successfully rebuilt and the oral commissures buttressed up with the more robust cross-linked injectable collagens and the hyaluronans. However, this area is highly mobile and the repetitive movement contributes to rapid breakdown of most semipermanent fillers. Paresis of the contributory muscle, the depressor anguli oris (DAO), which is a lateral lip depressor, aids in lifting the lateral oral commissure, restoring it to a more horizontal position by the unopposed action of the antagonist zygomaticus major muscle. This reduces the total amount of filler that would have been required and with reduced muscle movement, it sustains the effects of soft tissue augmentation. This muscle, also known as the depressor triangularis oris because of its shape, is small and can be difficult to isolate. Improper placement or toxin diffusion can weaken the adjacent lip depressor muscle, the depressor labii, which lies in close proximity. Inadvertently inactivating the depressor labii results in flattening of the lower lip, which can be pronounced on animation (Fig. 5). The location of the DAO can be found either by having the patient clench the large masseter muscle and

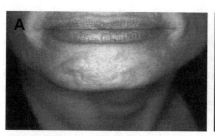 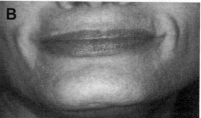

Fig. 4. (A) Frontal view of contraction of the mentalis muscle with a cobblestone appearance. (B) Following 5 units of Botox into the belly of the muscle at the apex of the chin, the contour irregularities are diminished.

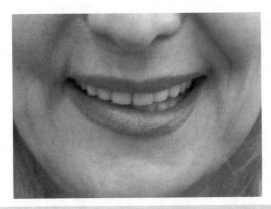

Fig. 5. Inadvertent unilateral paralysis of the depressor labii muscle when attempting to treat the adjacent DAO with Botox.

palpating the DAO, which can be found anterior to that, or by tracing the nasolabial fold down to the chin and locating the DAO posterior to that. Two to 3 units can be placed immediately above the angle of the mandible and 1 cm lateral to the lateral oral commissure. Keeping the injection site lateral and low at the junction of the DAO helps reduce compilations [23].

As patients have become more comfortable with the concept of using a toxin for aesthetic purposes and have become less inclined to undergo surgical procedures with the concomitant risks, the use of neurotoxins below the chin, in the neck and chest, has slowly gained acceptance. Loss of the cervicomental angle from accumulation of subcutaneous fat, cutaneous laxity, or platysmal muscle hypertrophy is often unacceptable to patients. Although not a replacement for surgery, treatment of the platysma muscle, in the properly selected patient, restores a sharper facial profile. Patients who may benefit from chemodenervation of the platysma muscle are those who may have had prior surgical rhytidectomy or submental liposuction and have residual platysmal banding or those who have not had surgery but have apparent platysmal bands with good cervical skin laxity and minimal fat deposition. The platysma muscle originates from the superior fascia of the upper chest and continues superiorly to join the superficial musculoaponeurotic system (SMAS). The posterior fibers blend with the inferior muscles of facial expression, including the DAO, mentalis, risorius, and orbicularis oris. Platysmal bands form when the anterior fibers separate into two discrete vertical bands. It is these anterior bands that are most often treated with Botox. To address the muscle, the patient contracts the muscle, the platysmal bands are grasped by the physician's nondominant hand, and Botox is injected into three to four sites, beginning from the mandible, at 1.0 to 1.5 cm intervals, with 5 units per site. Generally, the two anterior bands can be treated with a total of 20 to 30 units. Doses larger than that can produce weakness of the neck flexor muscles, causing the patient to have difficulty raising his/her head from a lying position. Additionally, because the platysma muscle is close to the larynx and the muscles of deglutition, large doses can also cause dysphagia. Because the two to three horizontal "necklace" lines that encircle the anterior neck are caused by the SMAS attachments in the neck, the treatment protocol for platysmal bands simultaneously can reduce them. However, when these lines are resistant or have been elected to be treated individually, they can be injected with superficial subdermal blebs of 1-unit aliquots spaced at about 2 to 3 cm intervals directly into the line [24].

Often possessing many of the stigmata of chronic photodamage, such as dyschromia and wrinkles, the décolleté of the chest is one of the more difficult areas to improve. Although many of the newer fractionated resurfacing devices have been used with increasing success, it has been reported that treating the underlying pectoralis major muscle with Botox can subtly improve the appearance. Superficially injecting 50 to 75 units of toxin in a "V"-shaped pattern seems to weaken the pectoralis muscle sufficiently and reduce some of the fine lines without compromising the muscular action.

For all sites, much debate is ongoing about postinjection guidelines. Because the toxin is a liquid with the intrinsic ability to diffuse about 1 to 2 cm, patients may be instructed to reduce further migration to untreated muscles by remaining upright with head elevation for 2 to 3 hours and, although the physician may massage the area, patients should be instructed not to manipulate the area for a similar amount of time. Evidence exists that botulinum toxin binds preferentially at activated stimulated muscles; therefore, patients are encouraged to contract the treated musculature for 2 to 3 hours until the toxin has been taken up at the neuromuscular junction.

The only other FDA-approved indication for botulinum toxin is axillary hyperhidrosis. Perhaps not perceived as a physically debilitating condition, excess sweat can have distressing psychologic effects for many patients. Treatments include topical preparations, oral anxiolytics, and surgical sympathectomy but none are as safe, effective, and reproducible as Botox. A preinjection starch iodine test can be used to help delineate the areas to be treated, but the entire axillary vault can be treated with relative impunity. Bruising is one of the few risks in this area. Unlike in other areas, toxin diffusion is encouraged so that the anticholinergic effect will be on a large cross-section. To aid toxin spread, 4 mL of saline can be used to reconstitute the crystallized botulinum. Contingent on the actual size of the total area, between 50 and 100 units of the toxin, divided into 10 to 20 injection sites, can be placed superficially in a targetoid pattern. A similar method is used for other conditions, such as palmar and plantar hyperhidrosis. In these peripheral areas, injections are more painful and, despite cutaneous anesthesia achieved with topical preparations, ice, and counter-stimulation with handheld vibrating tools, nerve blocks are often necessary [25]. Treatment of axillary hyperhidrosis is the one indication for which insurance companies may cover Botox material and office fees. To help defray the costs of the injections, specific codes should be used to document the procedure.

SUMMARY AND FUTURE TRENDS

Botulinum toxin has truly revolutionized the way we analyze and treat the aging face. No longer is an attempt made to eradicate solitary lines with mono-therapy but, instead, multiple injectable products are used simultaneously to shape the senescent face three-dimensionally. Traditionally, only caustic chemical agents were available to diminish static lines and photodamage; now, however, an impressive and growing array of ablative and nonablative tools is available. Similarly, where once only bovine collagen was available for dermal augmentation, now an ever-expanding array of filling agents is at our disposal. The next evolutionary change, which is imminent, will be the introduction of many new chemodenervating neurotoxins. Although the newer toxins, all botulinum toxin serotype A, will have similar chemical properties, they will have various injection techniques, newer indications, and different complication profiles and, as such, they should be viewed as distinct agents with steep learning curves.

Botulinum toxin has been an exemplary illustration of technology keeping pace with patient demand. Harnessing the chemical properties of what was once considered a lethal poison has catapulted it into the most popular aesthetic procedure, with unparalleled patient satisfaction. Botox is now firmly established as a cornerstone of any cosmetic practice, and the future ramifications of newer toxins and the therapeutic and aesthetic indications are conceivably just being appreciated.

References

[1] Scott AB. Development of bolutinum toxin therapy: dermatol clinics. WB Saunders, Philadelphia. 2004;vol.22:p. 131–3.

[2] Erbguth FJ, Naumann M. Historical aspects of botulinum toxin: Justimus Kerner (1786–1862) and the "sausage poison". Neurology 1999;53:1850–3.

[3] Carruthers A, Carruthers J. In: Bolognia J, Jorizzo JL, Rapini RV, Horn T, editors. Botulinum toxin dermatology. London: Mosby, Harcourt Health Sciences; 2003. p. 2439–49.

[4] Botox (botulinum toxin type A) purified neurotoxin complex [Package insert]. Irvine (CA): Allergan Inc.; 2004.

[5] Lizarralde M, Gutierrez SA, Venegas A. Clinical efficacy of botulinum toxin type A reconstituted and refrigerated 1 week before its application in external canthus dynamic lines. Dermatol Surg 2007;33:1328–33.

[6] Alam M, Dover JS, Arndt KA. Pain associated with injection of botulinum A exotoxin reconstituted using isotonic sodium chloride with and without preservative: A double blind randomized controlled trial. Arch Dermatol 2002;138:510–4.

[7] Borodic GE, Ferrante R, Pierce B, et al. Histologic assessment of dose related diffusion and muscle fiber response after therapeutic botulinum A toxin injection. Mov Disord 1994;9:31–9.

[8] Lowe NJ. Botulinum toxin type A for facial rejuvenation. United States and United Kingdom perspectives. Dermatol Surg 1998;24:1216–8.

[9] Durif F. Clinical bioequivalence of the current commercial preparations of botulinum toxin. Eur J Neurol 1995;2:17–8.

[10] Matarasso SL. Comparison of botulinum toxin types A and B: a bilateral double-blind randomized evaluation in the treatment of the canthal rhytids. Dermatol Surg 2003;29:7–13.

[11] Kadunc BV, De Almeida ART, Vanti AA, et al. Botulinum toxin A adjunctive use in manual chemabrasion: controlled long-term study for treatment of upper perioral vertical lines. Dermatol Surg 2007;33:1066–72.

[12] Solish N, Bertucci V, Dansereau A, et al. A comprehensive approach to the recognition, diagnosis, and severity-based treatment of focal hyperhidrosis: recommendations of the Canadian Hyperhidrosis Advisory Committee. Dermatol Surg 2007;33:908–92.

[13] Matarasso SL. Botulinum toxin for the treatment of facial eccrine chromhidrosis. J Am Acad Dermatol 2005;52:89–91.

[14] Blumentfield AM, Dodick DW, Silberstein SD. Botulinum neurotoxin for the treatment of migraine and other primary headache disorders. Dermatol Clin 2004;22:167–75.

[15] Schwartz M, Freund B. Treatment of temporomandibular disorders with botulinum toxin. Clin J Pain 2002;18(Suppl 6):S198–203.

[16] Carruthers J, Fagen S, Matarasso SL. Consensus recommendations on the use of botulinum toxin type A in facial aesthetics. Plast Reconstr Surg 2005;114:1–22.

[17] Carruthers A, Carruthers J, Samireh S. Dose-ranging study of botulinum toxin type A in the treatment of glabellar rhytids in females. Dermatol Surg 2005;31:414–22.

[18] Lowe NJ, Ascher B, Heckmann M, et al. Double-blind, randomized, placebo-controlled, dose-response study of the safety and efficacy of botulinum toxin type A in subjects with crow's feet. Dermatol Surg 2005;31:257–67.

[19] Matarasso SL. Decreased tear expression with an abnormal Schirmer's test following botulinum toxin for the treatment of lateral canthal rhytides. Dermatol Surg 2002;28:149–52.

[20] Matarasso SL, Matarasso A. Treatment guidelines for botulinum toxin type A for the periocular region and a report on partial upper lip ptosis following injections to the lateral canthal rhytid. Plast Reconstr Surg 2001;108:208–14.

[21] Matarasso SL. Complications of botulinum-A exotoxin for hyperfunctional lines. Dermatol Surg 1998;24:1249–54.

[22] Semchyshyn N, Sengelmann RD. Botulinum toxin A treatment of perioral rhytides. Dermatol Surg 2003;29:490–5.

[23] Choe SW, Cho WI, Lee CK, et al. Effects of botulinum toxin type A on contouring of the lower face. Dermatol Surg 2005;31:502–8.

[24] Matarasso A, Matarasso SL, Brandt FS, et al. Botox-A exotoxin for the management of platysmal bands. Plast Reconstr Surg 1999;103:645–52.

[25] Vadoud-Seyedi J. Treatment of plantar hyperhidrosis with botulinum toxin type A. Int J Dermatol 2004;43:969–71.

The Nose: Principles of Surgical Treatment

Brian L. Baker, MD[a,*], Scott W. Fosko, MD[a,b,c,d,e]

[a]Department of Dermatology, Mohs Micrographic Surgery and Cutaneous Oncology, Saint Louis University, 1402 South Grand Boulevard, Saint Louis, MO 63104, USA
[b]Department of Otolaryngology, Saint Louis University, 1402 South Grand Boulevard, Saint Louis, MO 63104, USA
[c]Department of Ophthalmology, Saint Louis University, 1402 South Grand Boulevard, Saint Louis, MO 63104, USA
[d]Department of Internal Medicine, Saint Louis University, 1402 South Grand Boulevard, Saint Louis, MO 63104, USA
[e]Saint Louis University Cancer Center, Saint Louis University, 1402 South Grand Boulevard, Saint Louis, MO 63104, USA

EDITORIAL COMMENT

The nose is a common place for benign or malignant lesions that require biopsy and treatment. Important for the dermatologist is an understanding of anatomic considerations and surgical options. Dr. Baker and Dr. Fosko extensively review the general principles of surgery on the nose, highlighting the preservation of normal function and cosmesis as well as reviewing the literature for cure rates. They supply key examples of common repairs in specific cosmetic subunits. Both novice dermatologists and experienced dermatologic surgeons will find useful concepts for improving their practices in this article.

Suzanne Olbricht

S urgery on the nose is a broad topic that involves all aspects of dermatologic surgery. The nose is an airway, and the flow of air without obstruction must be a primary goal after any procedure. Because much of a person's identity is determined by the appearance of the nose, the need for cosmesis in addition to functionality also is paramount. A normal-appearing nose is defined by the shape, shadows, and positioning of key landmarks such as the tip and alar rim [1]. Patients frequently have unrealistic expectations, and some expect to look the same as they did before developing their pathologic condition. Surgeons are obliged to meet these expectations whenever possible. Doing so requires precise matching of contour, size, color, and texture when performing reconstructions.

*Corresponding author. E-mail address: blbake1@hotmail.com (B.L. Baker).

0882-0880/08/$ – see front matter
doi:10.1016/j.yadr.2008.09.001

This article describes a range of dermatologic surgery procedures and outlines general principles for those beginning their study of the discipline. It briefly reviews nasal anatomy and then discusses the various procedures commonly performed by dermatologists on the nose. The focus is on the management of benign and malignant neoplasms, with reference to recent literature.

ANATOMY

The nose is divided into cosmetic subunits: the root, dorsum, sidewalls, tip, alae, columella, and soft triangles (Fig. 1). The glabella and upper lip triangles, although not technically subunits of the nose, also are critically important in maintaining a natural configuration and appearance. These subunits actually are a complex fusion of planes, convexities, and concavities with their accompanying reflections and shadows [2]. Reconstructions generally should attempt to stay within cosmetic subunits, but in some instances removal of healthy skin is justified to make scars lines fall along junction lines. This situation typically occurs when the defect consumes greater than 50% of the subunit. Repair of defects spanning more than one subunit requires a different approach. In these instances, the use of multiple smaller repairs can preserve boundaries between the subunits [3].

The bony structure of the nose consists of paired nasal bones and frontal processes of the maxilla (Fig. 2). The nasal bones join superiorly to the frontal bone at the nasion and inferiorly with the septal cartilages at the rhinion. Septal cartilage forms the nasal septum interiorly and extends exteriorly as lateral processes that provide the structure for much of the nasal sidewall. The alar cartilage is a U-shaped structure whose medial crura join the septal cartilage to

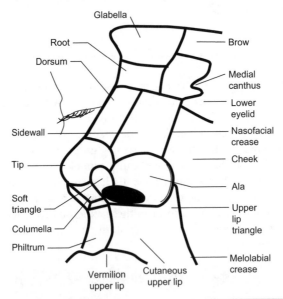

Fig. 1. Cosmetic subunits of the nose.

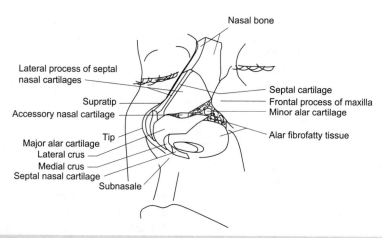

Fig. 2. Bony and cartilaginous structure.

form the columella, and lateral crura define the medial alae. Laterally the alae are not supported by cartilage and contain only fibrous bands admixed with adipose tissue.

The nose is rich with vasculature, and the presence of many anastomoses makes transection of small arteries inconsequential (Fig. 3). Branches of the internal carotid artery include the anterior and posterior ethmoid arteries (via the ophthalmic artery) and the infraorbital artery (via the internal maxillary artery). These branches provide nutritive blood flow to the superior aspects of the nose and glabella. The external carotid artery supplies most of the external nose via the facial artery, which becomes the angular artery superior to the superior labial artery. The angular artery is deep to muscle but may be encountered at the attachment of the ala to the cheek or near the medial canthus.

Veins generally follow the arterial pattern. Direct communication with the cavernous sinus, as well as the lack of valves, makes possible the spread of

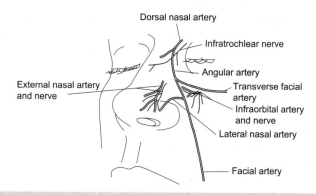

Fig. 3. Vasculature and nerves.

nasal and periorbital infection to the central nervous system. Septic thrombosis of the cavernous sinuses, which almost always was fatal before the antibiotic era, now is rarely encountered. Dermatologists, however, should be observant for fever, ptosis, proptosis, and cranial nerve palsies in the setting of midface infections [4]. The diagnosis can be confirmed with high-resolution CT or MRI.

Lymphatics drain in a posterior and inferior direction toward the retropharyngeal nodes. Some lymph also flows anteriorly to the upper deep cervical nodes and/or submandibular glands. Patients who have any type of skin cancer on the nose, especially squamous cell carcinoma (SCC) and melanoma, should have the parotid gland palpated by bimanual examination in addition to cervical lymph node examination.

Sensation on the nose is provided by branches of the trigeminal nerve (see Fig. 3). The ophthalmic division, V1, divides into the nasociliary branch and the frontal branch. Distally, the nasociliary branch further divides into the anterior ethmoidal nerve, which innervates skin from the rhinion to the tip, and the infratrochlear nerve, which innervates the medial eyelids, nasion, and bony dorsum. The frontal branch of V1 distally becomes the supratrochlear nerve to innervate the skin of the glabella and medial eyelids. The maxillary division, V2, primarily innervates the external nares via the infraorbital nerve. The infraorbital nerve exits the infraorbital foramen in the mid-pupillary line approximately 1 cm below the orbital rim. This palpable landmark is an excellent location for a nerve block when performing lengthy or extensive procedures on the nose. Approximately 2 mL of 1% lidocaine with epinephrine can be injected percutaneously or intraorally along the gingival sulcus above the first canine incisor. Up to 20 minutes may be required for full effect, and additional cutaneous injection may be needed. Less extensive procedures on the nose may be anesthetized by direct infiltration alone. The pain of injection can be minimized by injecting slowly into the subcutis as a 30-gauge needle is being withdrawn [5]. Over 2 to 5 minutes, as the anesthesia is taking effect, a more superficial dermal injection is well tolerated and provides complete anesthesia. Other techniques to minimize discomfort are adding sodium bicarbonate and creating a mechanical distraction by rhythmically pinching the tissue [6,7]. The addition of epinephrine is recommended because of the rich vascular supply. Particular attention should be paid to patients who ooze moderately or heavily. This oozing and the rich vascular supply may contribute to a shorter anesthetic effect than the 1- to 2-hour duration seen in most other sites. Patients seldom complain of postoperative sensory changes after dermatologic surgery on the nose, presumably because sensory nerves are present in the pedicle of most flaps, whether laterally or superiorly based.

Motor innervation of the nose is provided by anastomosing branches of the facial nerve, specifically the temporal, zygomatic, and buccal branches. Nerves generally course from an inferior and lateral direction deep to the muscles of facial expression. The nasalis muscle is divided into transverse and alar parts (Fig. 4). Variations among individuals and good outcomes after transection or removal suggest that its functional significance is minimal. Theoretically,

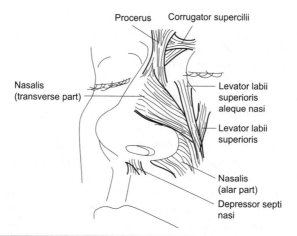

Fig. 4. Musculature.

however, the absence of a functional nasalis could contribute to airway obstruction.

The nasal valve is a critical functional area of the nose and ala and exists at the narrowest portion of the nasal airway. Its trapezoidal borders are the septum, the upper lateral cartilage, and the anterior aspect of the inferior turbinate [8]. Many factors can compromise the function of the valve, and, although the valve is not often visible or of cosmetic concern, improper functioning can be very bothersome to the patient. Patients also may complain of "collapse" of the valve when in a recumbent position. One should monitor visually the configuration of the ala and vestibule preoperatively, intraoperatively, and postoperatively to assess for any immediate changes that need to be addressed. Function also can be assessed by having the patient, in a recumbent position with lips tightly closed, inspire nasally to assess for any immediate airway obstruction. Some edema effects are normal and expected, but they should not be functionally significant. Of note, it is common for a patient to note some palpable intranasal swelling, especially with transposition flaps. This swelling often resolves spontaneously over 2 to 4 months.

The procerus lies in the midline from the superior part of the nasal bones to the skin of the nasal root and acts to pull the brows inferiorly and medially, causing "bunny lines." Injection of botulinum toxin to paralyze this muscle and hence reduce wrinkling has become extremely popular. The two remaining muscles of the nose are the depressor septi nasi and the levator labii superioris alaeque nasi, which pull the septum inferiorly and the upper lip superiorly, respectively.

BIOPSY TECHNIQUES

Biopsies on the nose can be performed in a variety of ways. Anticipation of the clinicopathologic correlation and the extent of tissue required for diagnosis (or sometimes treatment) is essential. Factors to consider when choosing the type of biopsy include the expected depth of the pathologic condition, the breadth of epidermis needed to evaluate lesion architecture, prognostic or staging information, and scarring. Biopsy anywhere on the body can create undesirable cosmetic concerns. The lower third of the nose is especially challenging because the resultant scars can have markedly different contour, color, and texture. Inflammatory conditions restricted to the nose and face generally do not require biopsy for diagnosis, and inflammatory conditions involving other parts of the body should not be biopsied on the face. Therefore this discussion focuses on the biopsy of neoplasms.

Shave biopsies are acceptable for most benign and premalignant lesions as well as non-melanoma skin cancers (NMSC). The biopsy should be deep enough to sample the papillary dermis. Even though normal epidermis averages only 0.05 mm thick, shave biopsies commonly do not sample the dermis enough to allow accurate diagnosis [9]. Good intentions to minimize scarring can lead to diagnoses such as "hyperplastic actinic keratosis, invasive squamous cell carcinoma cannot be ruled out," which may necessitate further surgery and much more significant aesthetic concerns than a slightly deeper initial biopsy would have caused. One type of neoplasm that ideally should not be diagnosed with shave biopsy is invasive melanoma. Accurate determination of Breslow depth, which is important for both staging information and treatment decisions, is not possible when the base of the melanoma is transected. The current staging system is based on depths up to 4 mm, which is thicker than a shave biopsy can be on the nose [10]. These comments should not be understood as implying that the shave technique is inappropriate for all pigmented lesions. Many dermatopathologists prefer the broader tissue sample for thin melanomas and melanoma in situ [11]. Clinically benign compound and dermal nevi probably are managed best by shave biopsy.

Punch biopsies are acceptable for lesions suspicious for melanoma that cannot be excised, and some authorities consider punch biopsies to be superior for NMSC. This technique allows better sampling of neoplasms that involve the reticular dermis, such as infiltrative basal cell carcinomas (BCC). Another condition in which punch biopsies on the nose may be warranted is lentigo maligna or lentigo maligna melanoma, subtypes of melanoma in situ and melanoma, respectively. Multiple "mapping" punch biopsies can help minimize sampling error, evaluate for invasive disease, and assist in delineating the extent of the lesion. Suturing of the biopsy site is helpful to minimize scarring, especially where the sebaceous nature of the nasal tissue is prominent.

The deep shave biopsy, also known as a "scoop" or "saucerization," is used when the intent is to remove the lesion, such as with clinically atypical pigmented lesions. This technique also can be used in special circumstances to remove clinically well-defined NMSC with vertical section evaluation of margins. Special effort must be taken to communicate with the pathologist that a full-margin assessment is needed as opposed to diagnostic sectioning only. One would expect the recurrence rate after "clear" margins to be significantly higher than with Mohs surgery [12].

Incisional biopsy is an acceptable alternative to punch biopsy for lesions such as lentigo maligna and melanoma when their size makes excisional biopsy impractical. Strong evidence exists that incisional biopsy does not adversely affect survival [13]. Unlike punch biopsies, the larger tissue sample allows histologic evaluation of architecture and transition zones.

Excisional biopsy, defined as a fusiform incision into the subcutaneous tissue, is preferred for any lesion suspicious for melanoma. Margins should be limited or absent because the diagnosis is not known. If an excisional biopsy is performed, it is advantageous to leave the wound open, without definitive reconstruction, until the pathology report has been received and any additional plans for excision or further treatment can be accomplished. This approach provides the managing surgeon the full use of viable tissue for the final repair.

NONSURGICAL TREATMENT OF SKIN CANCER

Two topical medications are available for the treatment of superficial BCC and SCC in situ. 5-Fluorouracil (available in 5% and 0.5% creams) is applied once or twice daily for a period of 3 to 12 weeks for superficial BCC. A "good" response is one that involves significant erythema and crusting. The drug may be discontinued once erosion occurs. A recent study of 31 superficial BCC resulted in a histologic cure rate of 90% after an average of 10.5 weeks [14]. This approach can be an excellent alternative to surgery, especially for patients who have cosmetic concerns and when tissue conservation is important. SCC in situ on sun-exposed areas commonly occurs within a background of actinic keratosis, which makes the appropriate surgical margin difficult to determine. Topical therapies offer an added advantage of treating surrounding skin in these cases. Application twice daily for 4 weeks is a commonly used regimen; however, a longer treatment period of 9 weeks reduces the recurrence rate to 8% [15].

A newer medication is imiquimod 5% cream. It was approved by the Food and Drug Administration in 2004 for actinic keratosis and superficial BCC. Treatment of other neoplasms including melanoma in situ, lentiginous subtype, is under investigation. A similar response with erythema, edema, erosions, and crusting is sought, but the application schedule is three to five times per week for 6 to 12 weeks. An Australian study reported an 87.9% histologic clearance rate in 33 superficial BCC treated once daily for 6 weeks [16]. For SCC in situ, a clearance rate of 73% in 15 lesions was reported recently [17]. Repeat biopsy after inflammation has resolved is a good idea to confirm cure. Proper patient selection and close monitoring during treatment are essential for the success of this modality.

DESTRUCTION

Destruction is somewhat of a catchall term encompassing treatment modalities such as cryosurgery, electrodessication, curettage, topical vesicants, topical immunoreagents, intralesional immunoreagents and chemotherapeutic agents, laser ablation, and photodynamic therapy. The underlying principle is that viable tissue is damaged irreversibly so that a skin lesion is sloughed and replaced with regenerated tissue. Another commonality is that margins are not assessed.

This approach is quite acceptable for benign and premalignant skin lesions, because outcomes generally are good even in the setting of recurrence, but patients should be informed in advance of this likelihood.

Actinic keratoses and warts make up 11.5% and 6.7% of dermatology office visits, respectively, making them the third and fifth most common reasons for seeing a dermatologist [18]. More importantly, actinic keratoses are a risk factor for developing SCC, because the average patient who has multiple actinic keratoses has a 6% to 10% risk of developing SCC over 10 years [19]. Studies have reported anywhere from 0.1% to 10% of individual actinic keratoses progress to SCC [20]. Most are managed with cryosurgery, which is the application of liquid nitrogen, but many of the other forms of destruction are acceptable and sometimes are preferred. Side effects of cryosurgery include discomfort upon application, variable recovery periods, and hypopigmented scarring. Note that the terms "cryosurgery" and "cryotherapy" are not synonymous. "Cryotherapy" refers to the application of less-damaging agents, such as carbon dioxide, in the treatment of acne [21].

Seborrheic keratosis can appear anywhere on the body, including the nose, during adulthood. Curettage is arguably the best destructive modality for removing such a lesion because of superior depth control and minimal pigmentary disturbance. Large lesions may require local anesthesia, but smaller lesions often can be removed in limited numbers with less pain than caused by injection of the anesthetic. A bendable razor blade can also allow a very delicate superficial removal with an excellent cosmetic result.

NMSC can be managed in a number of ways, including destruction by electrodessication and curettage. Clinically obvious tumor is removed by shave technique and sent for histopathologic evaluation. Then the base is lightly curetted to define better the extent of the lesion. The area is electrodessicated to destroy microscopic cancer cells on the margin, and the sequence is repeated one or two more times. This method results in a 5-year recurrence rate of 17.5% for BCC on high-risk sites including the nose, paranasal areas, nasolabial groove, ear, chin, mandibular, perioral, and periocular areas [22]. In comparison, a 5-year recurrence rate of 8.6% was seen on the neck, trunk, and extremities [22]. Cure rates as high as 96.3% have been reported for primary SCC, probably relating to careful case selection [23]. In general, the literature reports lower recurrence rates than studies of the surgical margin would suggest. This discrepancy may result from the inflammatory response invoked by electrodessication [24]. Data specific to the nose are less plentiful, but most dermatologists would agree that recurrence is more common at this site. Whether the greater rate of recurrence results from anatomic considerations, from less aggressive technique, or from both is unknown. One study found that all subtypes of BCC on the nose were at high risk for extensive subclinical spread [25]. Relative to the cheek, tumors on the tip, bridge, and ala were 2.8, 2.4, and 2.3 times more likely, respectively, to require three or more stages of Mohs surgery. Even more concerning was that basosquamous and morpheaform BCC on the nose were 7.2 and 6.9 times, respectively, more likely to have extensive subclinical spread than nodular BCC on the cheek. Other negative prognostic factors for SCC include diameter greater than 2 cm; depth greater than 4 mm; tumor involving bone, muscle, or nerve; location on ear or lip; tumor arising in scar; immunocompromise; and absence of inflammation [23]. The potential for regional metastasis always should be considered for large SCC of the skin [26]. Therefore cure rates are greatly affected by various clinical and pathologic features, and careful case selection is important when using destructive treatment modalities.

EXCISION

Excision is defined as removal of a lesion, including margins, through the full thickness of the dermis [21]. Small BCC and SCC on the upper two thirds of the nose can be managed properly in this way when the skin is mobile and amenable to primary closure. Five-year recurrence rates are 10% and 8.1% for primary BCC and SCC, respectively, and are 17.6% and 23.3% for recurrent BCC and SCC, respectively [23,27,28]. A margin of 4 mm will remove BCC smaller than 2 cm completely in 98% of cases, whereas a margin of 2 mm completely removes only 75% [29]. The nose is considered a high-risk site for SCC, and therefore margins of 6 mm are recommended to achieve complete removal in 95% [30]. Even the smallest tumors on the lower third of the nose result in significant defects once a margin is removed. Biopsy specimens may be sent for frozen or permanent vertical sectioning. Flaps after vertical-section histopathologic evaluation should be performed with caution because the precise location of residual tumor is difficult or impossible to identify, and options for a second reconstructive procedure may become more limited.

For melanoma and melanoma in situ, wide local excision remains the treatment of choice. A margin of 5 mm is recommended for melanoma in situ, and margins of 1 cm and 2 cm are recommended for melanomas of Breslow depths up to 1 mm and greater than or equal to 2 mm, respectively [13]. The recommendation for melanomas of a Breslow depth of 1 to 2 mm is less well defined. Specimens typically are sent for vertical section evaluation, although some dermatologic surgeons recommend paraffin-embedded tangential sections. This approach has been referred to as a "slow Mohs" or "modified Mohs" technique [31]. It is especially helpful in the management of lentigo maligna and lentigo maligna melanoma, where it has been well documented that a 5-mm margin often is insufficient for complete tumor removal and highlights the reason for the high local recurrence rate of these melanoma subtypes [31,32]. Areas of central, clinically obvious tumor or scar can be sectioned separately in a vertical fashion to avoid compromise of the diagnosis or depth measurement and to provide full tumor prognostic information. Although frozen-section histopathology can be less reliable for detecting tumor melanocytes, many dermatologic surgeons advocate traditional Mohs surgery in the management of melanoma and melanoma in situ [32,33]. Local recurrence rates, metastasis rates, and disease-specific survival rates have been reported to be equal to or superior to historical controls [32].

MOHS SURGERY

Mohs surgery is indicated for NMSC of any size on the nose for the purpose of tissue conservation and because it is considered a high-risk anatomic site. Other indications that may or may not apply are tumor recurrence, aggressive histologic subtype (micronodular, morpheaform, infiltrative), and ill-defined clinical features [34]. Perineural invasion is probably more common than once thought and occurs with equal frequency on the ear, nose, and forehead [35]. It is reported to occur in 10.2% of BCCs that require more than one stage of Mohs surgery [35]. Tumors with perineural involvement may be managed adequately by Mohs surgery without adjuvant radiation therapy [35].

Clinically obvious tumor may or may not be removed by sharp debulking or by curettage. Then a margin of 1 to 3 mm is incised circumferentially around the lesion into the subcutaneous tissue. Colored ink and surgical nicks on the specimen and surrounding skin are used to map precisely and remove any residual tumor cells in subsequent stages. Some Mohs surgeons employ a technique whereby only a very thin layer of remaining dermis is removed and evaluated. This technique offers the benefit of rapid and aesthetically pleasing healing by second intention but may have a slightly higher false-negative rate because of "skip" areas extending down follicles and/or tumor cells residing deep to the biopsy scar.

Five-year cure rates are 99% and 96.9% for primary BCC and SCC, respectively, and are 94.4% and 90% for recurrent BCC and SCC, respectively [23,27,28]. Although Mohs surgery offers a higher cure rate for these types of cancer, other modalities also offer reasonable cure rates and may be appropriate in some cases.

RECONSTRUCTION

The subject of nasal reconstruction is exceedingly complex and is addressed in detail in several excellent texts. In general, the lower third of the nose is more sebaceous and less mobile than the upper two thirds. This consideration is very important when choosing a reconstructive modality, because symmetry of free margins must be maintained, and nasal inspiration must be unobstructed. Identifying and working within cosmetic subunits is another point of emphasis. Placing suture lines at the junction of cosmetic subunits leads consistently to aesthetically acceptable outcomes. Most surgeons agree that a plane of undermining just superficial to the periosteum or perichondrium helps minimize bleeding and allows more evenly distributed scar contraction. An approach that sometimes is helpful is to close circular defects with an initial buried suture and then to excise redundant tissue as it declares itself. Apical angles of 60° are adequate to dissipate raised tissue cones in most areas of the body, but more acute angles often are necessary on the nose. Achieving the desired result for nasal reconstruction requires meticulous design and execution, especially with regard to redundant or bulky tissue. The authors have found that if the desired result is not evident immediately postoperatively, the changes are unlikely to improve with time and probably will require revision at some point.

The following sections highlight a commonly used reconstructive option for each of the cosmetic subunits (see Fig. 1).

Glabella

Primary closure in a vertical to slightly oblique orientation generally is preferred for smaller defects in the glabella. As mentioned earlier, the skin of the upper two thirds of the nose is less sebaceous and quite mobile. Scar lines may be placed within relaxed skin tension lines, but care should be taken to avoid exaggerating a rhytid or "crowding" the eyebrows in this area. Primary closures on the lower parts of the nose sometimes can be successful but may lead to flaring of the nostrils or indentation of the side profile, even in experienced hands.

The rhombic transposition flap is another excellent choice for defects occurring in the glabella and nasal root (Fig. 5). A reserve of mobile skin typically is present in the glabella and lower forehead, and scar lines can be camouflaged easily within rhytides in most patients. The first leg of the flap should be placed within an existing rhytid if possible, and the second leg is extended approximately 60° from the first so that closure of the secondary defect is not problematic. After elevation of the flap and undermining, the key suture is placed to close the secondary defect, and the flap is transposed into the primary defect. Undermining in the subcutaneous fat generally is not dangerous because motor nerves are not present and the vasculature is rich with anastomoses.

Medial canthus

The best reconstruction in concave areas such as the medial canthus and alar crease is often no reconstruction [36]. Second intention healing can be extremely successful, especially when the wound is not too deep. Deep wounds are more likely to form hypertrophic scars and contract against free margins. In the medial canthus area, defects that extend disproportionately superior

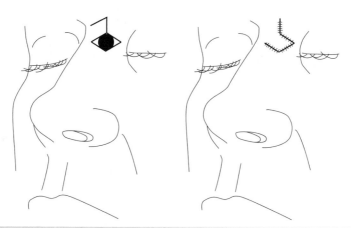

Fig. 5. Rhombic flap: nasal root.

or inferior to the canthus are more prone to cause ectropion. The best defect for second intention healing is one that has equal components superior and inferior to the angle of the canthus. Wound care instructions should include petrolatum ointment with or without a bandage. Prophylactic antibiotics generally are not indicated. Possible adverse effects include webbing, blunting, ectropion, and depressed scars.

Upper sidewall and nasal dorsum

The mobility and sebaceous quality of the skin in the upper sidewall and nasal dorsum vary widely among individuals, and primary closure may or may not be feasible. A good approach is to undermine the skin surrounding the defect in a submuscular plane before making a commitment to a specific closure. A key stitch can be placed centrally to judge the effects on free margins and overall contour, including the side profile. If any undesirable consequences occur, the stitch can be removed and repositioned with a different tension vector. If satisfactory, redundant tissue cones (dog ears) should be removed aggressively within relaxed skin tension lines because improvement with time is rarely seen. Buried sutures should be placed from the subcutaneous tissue to the middle to deep dermis to achieve adequate support and eversion. Superficial sutures provide finishing touches by correcting uneven wound edges and maximizing eversion without sacrificing epidermal approximation. Primary closures can be converted easily to full-thickness skin grafts (FTSG) using Burow's triangles of redundant tissue as the donor (Fig. 6) [37]. Other defects in these subunits may be repaired best with a local flap.

Lower sidewall and perialar regions

Defects on the lower sidewall and supra-alar areas typically are not amenable to primary closure because of the thick sebaceous skin that lies inferior. FTSGs, although simple to perform, often have poor matching of contour and texture.

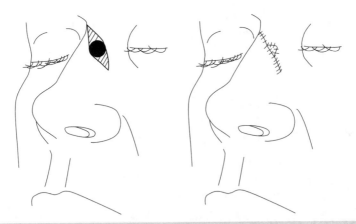

Fig. 6. Burow's full-thickness skin graft: nasal dorsum.

For these reasons, random-pattern flaps are preferred. A favorite of many dermatologic surgeons is the Burow's advancement flap (Fig. 7). (Removing the inferior tissue cone in a more curved or arching fashion has been described as a "crescentic advancement flap.") The simple design allows placement of scar lines into cosmetic junctions while respecting the upper triangle of the lip and nasal junction [38]. The procedure is begun by undermining the full circumference of the defect and making a short incision within or just superior to the alar crease. The flap then is elevated, and the incision is lengthened down the nasolabial crease until movement is adequate to close the primary defect with a buried suture. This technique creates redundant tissue superior and inferior to the suture. A narrow triangle or crescent of skin is removed inferolaterally so that the secondary defect can be closed without redundancy. Superiorly, a cone of redundant skin is removed in standard fashion. Depending on the thickness of the skin in this area, the medial leg of the superior dog ear may be incised earlier in the procedure to assist with tissue undermining and flap movement. Buried and superficial sutures are placed as previously described. The beauty of this flap is the hiding of scar lines within cosmetic junctions, the preservation of the upper lip triangle, and the avoidance of geometric patterns.

Supratip
The bilobed flap is a workhorse flap for defects up to 1.5 cm on the lower one third of the nose (Fig. 8). The design allows skin of matching texture to be transposed into the primary defect and at the same time redirects tension from vertical to horizontal by tapping into a reservoir of skin not immediately adjacent to the defect. Closure of the more mobile superior tissue allows closure of the primary defect in a more oblique fashion that minimizes vertical tension on the alar free margin. Although technically classified as a transposition flap, a combination of transposition and rotation movements are involved. The bilobed flap can be thought of as a flap within a dorsal nasal rotation flap.

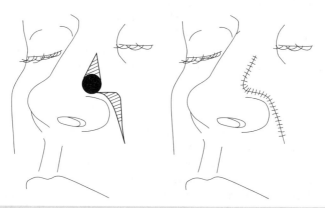

Fig. 7. Burow's advancement flap: lower sidewall.

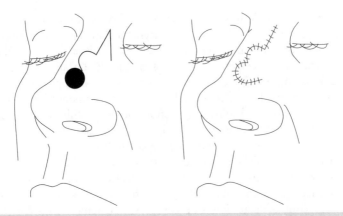

Fig. 8. Bilobed flap: supratip.

When the technique first was described, a 180° arc of rotation was used. Later modifications require only a 90° to 100° arc of rotation [39]. The first step is to imagine the flap's vascular pedicle, which is based laterally more often than medially. Two lobes approximately equal to the primary defect in size are designed along the nasal sidewall. Undermining should be done in a submuscular plane directly above the perichondrium or periosteum even when wound closure tension does not require undermining. This approach provides a well-vascularized flap and distributes scar contraction more evenly throughout the undermined area. Traditionally, a key buried stitch is placed to close the tertiary defect, but one of the authors of this article (SWF) often finds that the flap can be positioned more optimally with initial delicate suturing of the primary lobe. Buried stitches also should be used sparingly to approximate and evert wound edges throughout the flap. Simple interrupted or horizontal mattress sutures then can be used for precise placement of the epidermis. The design is much more complex than a casual observer might suspect. Considerations must include filling the primary and secondary defects, compression of the nasal valve, pulling forces on the lower eyelid, and pulling forces on the alar rim and nasal tip. In general, the tension vector created by primary closure of the tertiary defect should be parallel to the both alar rim and lower eyelid.

Tip

Sometimes both the bilobed flap and vertically oriented primary closure are possible for nasal tip defects. FTSGs can provide equal if not superior results for defects up to 2.5 cm [1]. In some cases additional healthy skin may be removed to place graft margins along the junction lines of cosmetic subunits. Shallow defects may be grafted immediately, but deeper defects often benefit from a delay of 1 to 3 weeks. The conchal bowl can be a good choice of donor site because of similar sebaceous quality as well as ease of healing of the donor site [40]. Burow's wedge grafts of tissue immediately superior often have excellent matching of color and texture, but closure of the donor site can cause problems such as "beaking" or uneven contour from the side profile. Care should be taken to approximate dermis to dermis and epidermis to epidermis at a tension equal to that of uninterrupted skin. Deep defects that have been allowed to granulate should be sharply refreshed to create crisp vertical and undermined wound edges that allow this approximation. FTSGs also are beneficial on the soft triangle and ala to avoid the potential scar contraction seen with second-intention healing. An added benefit of grafting is the ease with which recurrent tumors may be addressed.

Ala

Alar defects must be evaluated for remaining structural support on a case-by-case basis. Wounds of significant depth or proximity to the alar rim may require free cartilage grafts to prevent collapse of the nasal valve or notching of the alar rim (ecnasion) after scar contraction. A simple technique used by the author (SWF) to help avoid compromise of the nasal valve is to place a suture from the belly of the flap into the floor of the defect. FTSGs, nasolabial transposition, and interpolation flaps are common choices for covering the defect with skin. Using a single flap to cover defects that span more than one cosmetic subunit may not result in a normal-appearing nose, and in those cases repairs should attempt to recreate interunit junctions [3]. A technique for repairing defects of the ala and the immediately perialar area is to combine a cheek advancement flap with a Burow's FTSG [41]. Closure of the cheek portion creates redundancy both superiorly and inferiorly that can be used for an FTSG on the alar portion (Fig. 9). The nasolabial transposition flap also can provide an excellent result in reconstructing defects involving the lateral sidewall and ala but has the potential to create excess bulk without a defined alar crease (Fig. 10). In some cases placement of small suspension sutures within the crease may preserve the natural contour [42].

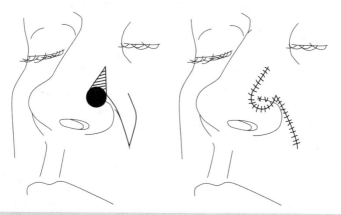

Fig. 9. Nasolabial transposition flap: ala.

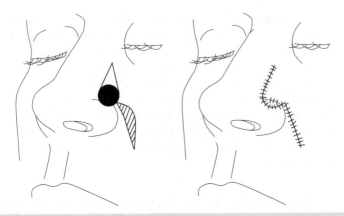

Fig. 10. Crescentic advancement flap with Burow's graft.

SUMMARY

Surgery on the nose is inseparable from the practice of dermatology. Extensive training and experience is required to account for the nose's unique role in determining individuality, its function as an airway, and its predilection for hosting aggressive tumors. This overview of anatomy and general surgical principles provides the novice with a foundation on which to build and the experienced practitioner a review of pertinent literature.

References

[1] Menick FJ, Burget GC. Nasal reconstruction: creating a visual illusion. Plastic and Reconstructive Surgery 1990;6:193–220.
[2] Burget GC, Menick FJ. The subunit principle in nasal reconstruction. Plast Reconstr Surg 1985;76(2):239–47.
[3] Dzubow LM, Zack L. The principle of cosmetic junctions as applied to reconstruction of defects following Mohs surgery. J Dermatol Surg Oncol 1990;16:353–5.
[4] Ebright JR, Pace MT, Niazi AF. Septic thrombosis of the cavernous sinuses. Arch Intern Med 2001;161(22):2671–6.
[5] Arndt KA, Burton C, Noe JM. Minimizing the pain of local anesthesia. Plast Reconstr Surg 1983;72:676–9.
[6] McKay W, Morris R, Mushlin P. Sodium bicarbonate attenuates pain on skin infiltration with lidocaine with or without epinephrine. Anesth Analg 1987;66:572–4.
[7] Fosko SW, Gibney MD, Harrison B. Repetitive pinching of the skin during lidocaine infiltration reduces patient discomfort. J Am Acad Dermatol 1998;39(1):74–8.
[8] Kridel RW, Kelly PE, MacGregor AR. The nasal septum. In: Cummings CW, Flint PW, Haughey BH, et al, editors. Otolaryngology—head & neck surgery. 4th edition. Philadelphia: Mosby; 2005.
[9] Bergstresser PR, Costner MI. Anatomy and physiology. In: Bolognia JL, Jorizzo JL, Rapini RP, editors. Dermatology. 1st edition. Philadelphia: Mosby; 2003. p. 25.
[10] Balch CM, Buzaid AC, Soong SJ, et al. Final version of the American Joint Committee on Cancer Staging System for Cutaneous Melanoma. J Clin Oncol 2001;19(16):3635–48.
[11] Ng PC, Barzilai DA, Ismail SA, et al. Evaluating invasive cutaneous melanoma: is the initial biopsy representative of the final depth? J Am Acad Dermatol 2003;48(3):420–4.

[12] Rapini RP. Comparison of methods for checking surgical margins. J Am Acad Dermatol 1990;23(2 Pt 1):288–94.

[13] Sober AJ, Chuang T, Duvic M, et al. Guidelines of care for primary cutaneous melanoma. J Am Acad Dermatol 2001;45:579–86.

[14] Gross K, Kircik L, Kricorian G. 5% 5-Fluorouracil cream for the treatment of small superficial basal cell carcinoma: efficacy, tolerability, cosmetic outcome, and patient satisfaction. Dermatol Surg 2007;33:433–40.

[15] Sturm HM. Bowen's disease and 5-fluorouracil. J Am Acad Dermatol 1979;16:513–22.

[16] Marks R, Gebauer K, Shumack S, et al. Imiquimod 5% cream in the treatment of superficial basal cell carcinoma: results of a multicenter 6-week dose-response trial. J Am Acad Dermatol 2001;44:807–13.

[17] Patel GK, Goodwin R, Chawla M, et al. Imiquimod 5% cream monotherapy for cutaneous squamous cell carcinoma in situ (Bowen's disease): a randomized, double-blind, placebo-controlled trial. J Am Acad Dermatol 2006;54:1025–32.

[18] Feldman SR, Fleischer AB, McConnell C. Most common dermatologic problems identified by internists, 1990–1994. Arch Intern Med 1998;158:726–30.

[19] Dobson JM, DeSpain J, Hewett JE, et al. Malignant potential of actinic keratoses and the controversy over treatment: a patient-oriented perspective. Arch Dermatol 1991;127:1029–31.

[20] Salasche SJ. Epidemiology of actinic keratoses and squamous cell carcinoma. J Am Acad Dermatol 2000;42:S4–7.

[21] Beebe M, Dalton JA, Espronceda M, et al. CPT 2007 Standard Edition: Current Procedural Terminology. Chicago: American Medical Association Press; 2007.

[22] Silverman MK, Kopf AW, Grin CM, et al. Recurrence rates of treated basal cell carcinomas, part 2: curettage-electrodessication. J Dermatol Surg Oncol 1991;17:720–6.

[23] Rowe DE, Carroll RJ, Day CL, et al. Prognostic factors for local recurrence, metastasis, and survival rates in squamous cell carcinoma of the skin, ear, and lip. Implications for treatment modality selection. J Am Acad Dermatol 1992;26:976–90.

[24] Salasche SJ. Curettage and electrodessication in the treatment of midfacial basal cell epithelioma. J Am Acad Dermatol 1983;8(4):496–503.

[25] Batra RS, Kelley LC. Predictors of extensive subclinical spread in nonmelanoma skin cancer treated with Mohs micrographic surgery. Arch Dermatol 2002;138:1043–51.

[26] Dinehart SM, Pollack SV. Metastases from squamous cell carcinoma of the skin and lip. An analysis of twenty-seven cases. J Am Acad Dermatol 1989;21:241–8.

[27] Rowe DE, Carroll RJ, Day CL, et al. Long-term recurrence rates in previously untreated (primary) basal cell carcinoma: implications for patient follow-up. J Dermatol Surg Oncol 1989;15:315–28.

[28] Rowe DE, Carroll RJ, Day CL, et al. Mohs surgery is the treatment of choice for recurrent (previously treated) basal cell carcinoma. J Dermatol Surg Oncol 1989;15:424–31.

[29] Wolf DJ, Zitelli JA. Surgical margins for basal cell carcinoma. Arch Dermatol 1987;123:340–4.

[30] Brodland DG, Zitelli JA. Surgical margins for excision of primary cutaneous squamous cell carcinoma. J Am Acad Dermatol 1992;27:241–8.

[31] Stonecipher MR, Leshin B, Patrick J, et al. Management of lentigo maligna and lentigo maligna melanoma with paraffin-embedded tangential sections: utility of immunoperoxidase staining and vertical sections. J Am Acad Dermatol 1993;29:589.

[32] Bricca GM, Brodland DG, Ren D, et al. Cutaneous head and neck melanoma treated with Mohs micrographic surgery. J Am Acad Dermatol 2005;52(1):92–100.

[33] Barlow RJ, White CR, Swanson NA. Mohs micrographic surgery using frozen sections alone may be unsuitable for detecting single atypical melanocytes at the margins of melanoma in situ. Br J Dermatol 2002;146(2):290–4.

[34] Drake LA, Dinehart SM, Goltz RW, et al. Guidelines of care for Mohs micrographic surgery. J Am Acad Dermatol 1995;33:271–8.

[35] Ratner D, Lowe L, Johnson TM, et al. Perineural spread of basal cell carcinomas treated with Mohs micrographic surgery. Cancer 2000;88:1605–30.

[36] Zitelli JA. Wound healing by secondary intention. J Am Acad Dermatol 1983;9:407–15.

[37] Robinson JK, Dillig G. The advantages of delayed nasal full-thickness skin grafting after Mohs micrographic surgery. Dermatol Surg 2002;28(9):845–51.

[38] Mellette JR, Harrington AC. Applications of the crescentic advancement flap. J Dermatol Surg Oncol 1991;17(5):447–54.

[39] Zitelli JA. The bilobed flap for nasal reconstruction. Arch Dermatol 1989;125(7):957–9.

[40] Rohrer TE, Dzubow LM. Conchal bowl skin grafting in nasal tip reconstruction: clinical and histologic evaluation. J Am Acad Dermatol 1995;33:476–81.

[41] Levasseur JG, Mellette JR. Techniques for reconstruction of perialar and perialar-nasal ala combined defects. Dermatol Surg 2000;17(5):1019–23.

[42] Zitelli JA. The nasolabial flap as a single-stage procedure. Arch Dermatol 1990;126: 1445–8.

Cutaneous Squamous Cell Carcinoma

Jorge Garcia-Zuazaga, MD, MS[a], Suzanne M. Olbricht, MD[b],*

[a]Department of Dermatology, Mohs Micrographic Surgery and Cutaneous Oncology, Lahey Clinic, Harvard Medical School, 41 Mall Road, Burlington, MA 01805, USA
[b]Department of Dermatology, Lahey Clinic, Harvard Medical School, 41 Mall Road, Burlington, MA 01805, USA

EDITORIAL COMMENT

Dermatologists have been taking care of squamous cell carcinomas (SCCs) of the skin for decades. The incidence has been increasing, with a concomitant increase in morbidity, metastasis, and death. Patients who have received solid organ transplants and other immunosuppressed patients can have massive numbers of SCCs and can be difficult to care for, but tumors in these patients have also given rise to new insights. The authors review this now common tumor with a special emphasis on new information concerning etiology and an evidence-based review of treatment options.

Suzanne Olbricht

P rimary cutaneous SCC is a form of nonmelanoma skin cancer that originates from epithelial keratinocytes or their appendages [1]. This cutaneous malignancy has multiple etiologies: it may arise de novo, as a result of previous exposure to ultraviolet (UV) ionizing radiation or arsenic; within chronic wounds or scars; or from preexisting lesions, such as actinic keratosis, SCC in situ, Bowen's disease (intraepidermal SCC), bowenoid papulosis, or erythroplasia of Queyrat [2,3]. It is locally aggressive and, without treatment, has the potential to metastasize to other parts of the body [3]. This article summarizes the epidemiology and new insights into its pathogenesis and reviews the current treatment modalities for cutaneous SCC.

EPIDEMIOLOGY

SCC is the second most common skin malignancy affecting whites [1,4,5]. In the United States, approximately 200,000 cases of cutaneous SCC occur per year, resulting in approximately 2000 deaths [4,5]. Although the mortality is low, the associated morbidity is significant. Epidemiologic studies report that since the 1960s, the overall incidence of SCC has been increasing annually

*Corresponding author. E-mail address: suzanne.m.olbricht@lahey.org (S.M. Olbricht).

0882-0880/08/$ – see front matter
doi:10.1016/j.yadr.2008.09.007

[1,4,5] Recent data from the Rochester Epidemiologic Study indicate that the incidence of SCC in people younger than 40 years of age is now 3.9 per 100,000 and continues to increase [6]. Furthermore, the age-standardized rate of SCC worldwide has also been increasing over the past decade. Reports from Australia indicate the incidence for SCC as 387 per 100,000 people in 2006 [7]; in Canada, the incidence of nonmelanoma skin cancer, including SCC, has nearly tripled from 1960 to 2000 [8].

Epidemiologic and molecular data point to UV radiation as the most important factor for the development of primary cutaneous SCC [1,3,9]. Moreover, other agents, including host immune response, genetic predisposition [10] (as in epidermodysplasia verruciformis and xeroderma pigmentosa), certain chronic dermatoses, arsenic exposure [1,2], and viral infection [1,3,11], are also likely to be involved in its pathogenesis (Box 1). Individuals with impaired immune function, such as those patients receiving immunosuppressive therapy after solid organ transplantation or those with leukemia and lymphoma, are at increased risk for developing SCC [1,2,10].

There is significant evidence linking SCC with chronic actinic damage. SCC arises more commonly in sun-exposed areas, including the head, neck, and arms, but also occurs on the trunk, buttocks, and other areas [12]. Several population-based studies support the role of sun exposure and geographic latitude in the pathogenesis of SCC. The reported incidence of SCC is higher in tropical regions than in temperate climates, with an annual incidence approaching 1:100 in Australia [12–15]. Regional differences related to latitude have also been noted in the United States [1,2,15–17]. In the Swedish database of familial cohorts, analysis suggested intentional tanning as a contributing factor in the increase in incidence of SCC among the younger generation [18].

Other risk factors for SCC include older age, male gender, Celtic ancestry, oral psoralens, cigarette smoking, coal-tar products, and UV-A photochemotherapy [1,4,5]. Stasis ulcers, osteomyelitic sinuses, scarring processes (eg, lupus

---

Box 1: Factors associated with development of squamous cell carcinoma

Chronic UV exposure

Fitzpatrick skin types I–III

Geographic latitude

Genodermatoses

Human papillomavirus infection

Psoralen–UV-A therapy

Chronic inflammatory conditions

Allogenic transplant recipients

Smoking

Male gender, age >50 years

vulgaris), and vitiligo have been reported to increase the risk for SCC. For these latter conditions, it is unclear if the morphology of the underlying process obscures or delays the diagnosis [1,4,5].

PATHOGENESIS

The development of primary cutaneous SCC is multifactorial, with environmental exposures, occupational exposures, and genetic predisposition playing major roles. This section summarizes recent advances in the knowledge of the pathogenesis of SCC.

Ultraviolet radiation

Sun exposure is commonly believed to be the most common contributor to the development of primary cutaneous SCC [19,20]. UV-B (290–320-nm wavelength) radiation from sunlight is primarily responsible, with UV-A contributing to the likelihood of SCC formation. Several studies have shown that exposure to UV radiation generates specific mutations in the p53 tumor suppressor gene [19–21]. In UV-B–damaged skin, the most frequent mutations are from nucleotide substitutions in the form of C-to-T changes at pyrimidine sites [19,20]. These cyclobutane dimers result in DNA point mutations during keratinocyte replication, leading to abnormal cell function and replication [19–21]. The result of this process leads to aberrant clonal expansion of keratinocytes and manifests itself clinically as SCC in situ and invasive cutaneous SCC [19,20].

UV-A radiation (320–400-nm wavelength) also seems to be important in the pathogenesis of SCC. Molecular studies show that UV-A may act as a tumor promoter by means of activation of the signal transduction molecule protein kinase C [19–22]. In addition, the role of UV-A as a potent modulator of cutaneous immunosuppression by means of the interleukin (IL)-10 pathway of suppressor T cells is currently being studied as a possible contributor to the formation of cutaneous malignancies [19]. The current premise is that UV-B and UV-A work jointly to initiate the cutaneous carcinogenesis cascade: UV-B starts keratinocyte DNA damage by means of clonal expansion of aberrant cells, and UV-A–induced immunosuppression promotes the sequence of cancer formation [19,22].

Human papillomavirus

Human papillomaviruses (HPVs) are increasingly recognized as important human carcinogens. A high prevalence of HPV DNA, particularly in SCC samples of immunosuppressed patients, has renewed interest in a possible etiologic role of HPV in nonmelanoma skin cancer [23]. This family of viruses is characterized into phylogenetic genera α, β, γ, μ, and ν [23]. The oncogenic role of α-HPV has been clearly established in cervical cancers (HPV-16) and other anogenital cancers. In contrast, current evidence suggests that β-HPVs are the main etiologic HPV genus in keratinocyte cancers. It is estimated that up to 90% of nonmelanoma skin cancers from immunocompromised individuals and up to 50% of those from immunocompetent individuals contain DNA from cutaneous β-HPV [24]. Among these β-HPVs are HPV-5 and HPV-8 (epidermodysplasia verruciformis–related) types [24,25].

All HPVs contain genes for the viral proteins E6 and E7. Investigators now are proposing the idea that HPV may play a role in tumor initiation and progression based on initial findings of the behavior of these proteins [23,26]. E6 and E7 viral proteins have been shown to inhibit the tumor suppressor gene products p53 and Rb [23]. In addition, new studies show that E6 and E7 viral proteins may work through alternate (p53-independent) pathways [24]. There is recent evidence that E6 and E7 viral proteins target Bak, a cellular protein involved in signaling apoptosis in the skin in response to UV-B damage [24,25]. In vitro studies show that E6 viral protein may modify cellular response to UV exposure by altering the G_1 phase of the cell cycle and by decreasing DNA repair mechanisms of UV-damaged skin [24,26,27]. Moreover, E6 viral protein seems to alter DNA repair by interacting with single-strand break repair protein XRCC1 to reduce its repair activity [28,29]. Because β-HPVs infect skin cells, they may increase the risk for developing skin cancer by promoting cell division with a concomitant reduction in DNA repair and resistance to UV-induced apoptosis.

From these observations, several researchers have postulated that keratinocyte carcinoma associated with HPV infection may develop through an interaction between UV radiation and HPV types 5 and 8 (epidermodysplasia verruciformis–related types) by altering DNA repair activity [23,24,28]. In 2006, Karagas and colleagues [30] performed a population-based case-control study of 252 patients who had cutaneous SCC, and these investigators used multiplex serology to detect antibodies in plasma samples against 16 HPV types. This study found that risk for SCC was associated with seropositivity to HPV (specifically with the β-HPV types). From this study, these investigators determined that among individual HPV types, SCC risk was specifically associated with HPV-5 and HPV-20. This may indicate that the role of HPV for skin cancer may be more of a "vulnerability factor" that interacts with other exposures and host traits (DNA repair capacity) to increase disease risk [30]. The possible modifying effects of UV radiation and individual susceptibility for HPV-related skin cancers require additional research. In the future, studies may identify new cellular targets for HPV oncoproteins that prove to be relevant to skin cancer, independently or by interaction with UV radiation.

SPECIAL CASES
Organ transplant recipients

SCC is a major cutaneous problem in solid-organ transplant recipients, which is likely potentiated by the use of immunosuppressive medications [31]. Despite the increased incidence of cutaneous SCC and its increased morbidity and mortality in this patient population, there are only a few prospective controlled studies published addressing the treatment of SCC in patients undergoing organ transplantation.

The rate of primary cutaneous SCC in transplant recipients is high, particularly in those with a kidney or heart transplant [31–34]. Although much of the published evidence concerns renal transplant recipients, those who have undergone heart or lung transplantation are also highly susceptible to tumor formation. Interestingly, in contrast to the general population, transplant recipients have SCCs more often than basal cell carcinomas (BCCs).

SCC is up to 65 times as likely to develop in transplant recipients as in age-matched control subjects, with lesions appearing an average of 2 to 4 years after the transplantation and increasing in frequency over time. Also, solid organ transplant recipients usually develop multiple tumors, which can be extremely aggressive. Penn [35] reported in the Cincinnati Tumor Registry that 5.2% of all allogenic renal and cardiac transplant recipients died of skin cancers, with approximately 63% of those deaths secondary to cutaneous SCC.

In 2004, the International Transplant–Skin Cancer Collaborative (ITSCC) published guidelines for the management of SCC in organ transplant recipients [36]. This comprehensive position paper reviewed more than 300 articles relating to SCC in the transplant population and integrated the current basic scientific and clinical research experience to develop criteria to assist in the management of these patients. Several factors were identified that are considered high risk for patients who receive organ transplants [36,37]. Among the most important factors to consider in the initial screening of patients receiving organ transplants include past history of skin cancer or actinic keratosis, Fitzpatrick skin types I through III, past history of sun exposure or multiple sun burns, older age, duration and intensity of immunosuppression, prior history of HPV infection, and evidence of CD4 lymphocytopenia [38,39]. The ITSCC group recommends that extensive pretransplantation patient education about the real risk for developing skin cancer and its associated morbidities be an integral part of the patient evaluation. The focus should be on sun protection, the use of daily effective sunscreen with UV-B and UV-A range, avoidance of tanning beds, and early detection and aggressive surgical and medical treatment [36]. Educational information for patients and providers can be found on the ITSCC Web site [40].

The ITSCC guidelines also recommend consideration of decreasing the level of immunosuppression in cases of rapid development of multiple SCCs. How immunosuppression increases the risk for SCC is not fully known, but in addition to lowering surveillance functions, recent reports suggest a strong association with common viral infections such that the immunosuppression allows the viral-induced disease to degenerate into malignancy [41–43]. Decreasing the immunosuppressive therapy helps to reduce the number of SCCs. There have been reports of decreased skin cancers after weaning of immunosuppressive therapy in patients undergoing organ transplantation [41,42]. This decision must be made in consultation with the patient's multidisciplinary medical team. Further studies are needed to determine how altered immune responses influence the development of SCC.

The use of chemoprophylaxis with oral retinoids has been successful in reducing the growth of skin cancers and premalignant lesions in transplant recipients [44–46]. To date, there are no long-term safety studies on this subject. Each patient should be counseled on the adverse drug reactions and possible side effects of these medications before starting therapy.

Recently, there has been increasing interest in the role of folic acid as a prevention tool for SCC in patients receiving transplants. It has been documented in the medical literature that polymorphisms in the methylene tetrahydrofolate reductase (MTHFR) gene and the vitamin D receptor (VDR) gene have been linked to malignancies. Specifically, in dermatology, MTHFR polymorphisms have been linked to certain thrombophilic disorders [43,47,48]. In 2007, Laing and colleagues [49] evaluated two pathways for genetic associations of SCC that might be modifiable by vitamin supplementation. These researchers looked at these polymorphisms in 367 renal transplant recipients, including 117 with SCC. A significant association with MTHFR polymorphisms was shown in their analysis. No similar relations were found for VDR polymorphisms, however.

Chronic dermatoses and wounds

SCC is more likely to develop in injured or chronically diseased skin, including skin affected by long-standing ulcers, sinus tracts, osteomyelitis, radiation dermatitis, or vaccination scars [2,3]. Tumors arising at these sites may not be identified for years, and if neglected, they carry a substantial risk for metastasis.

Certain chronic inflammatory disorders may also predispose patients to the development of tumors; these disorders include discoid lupus erythematosus, lichen sclerosus, lichen planus, dystrophic epidermolysis bullosa, and cutaneous tuberculosis [1–4]. SCC arising from such damaged skin is more aggressive, with some reports citing 38% metastasis rates [1,2,4,49]. The cause for malignant degeneration at these sites in not clear.

Occupational exposure

Chemical carcinogens have historically been a major cause of primary cutaneous SCC. Arsenic, which was used in various medications in the past and has been found in tainted wine and unprocessed well water in developing countries, can also stimulate carcinogenesis [6,8]. Metal workers and insecticide handlers may also be at risk. Arsenic exposure produces invasive tumors and carcinoma in situ on the skin, whether or not the skin is exposed to the sun, in addition to arsenical keratoses on the palms and soles [6,8,10]. The carcinogenic effects depend on the dose and carry an associated risk for internal cancers.

Polycyclic aromatic hydrocarbons, derived from the combustion and distillation of carbon compounds, such as coal tar, cutting oils, and pitch, may also cause cutaneous SCC [3,6,8]. Occupational exposure to these agents has led to well-recognized malignancies, such as SCC of the scrotum in chimney sweeps as a result of exposure to soot [2,6,8].

Ionizing radiation

Ionizing radiation has also been implicated in the pathogenesis of SCC carcinoma. This type of radiation was used in the 1950s to treat many cutaneous conditions, including hemangiomas, chronic dermatoses, and acne. The risk for SCC is directly related to the cumulative total dose of radiation [4].

HISTOLOGIC AND GENETIC MARKERS

Although primary cutaneous SCCs are frequently easily treatable, they have the ability to reappear locally and even to metastasize, leading to significant morbidity and mortality. As a result, researchers are looking to identify those tumor markers that are more aggressive and require closer follow-up and additional treatments. Only a few molecular markers are known to be associated with progression or prognosis of cutaneous SCC. Recently described proteins whose abnormal expression contributes to a malignant phenotype in SCC are described next.

STAT3

This protein, a known regulator of cell motility, is a member of the signal transducer and activator of transcription (STAT) family [50,51]. The expression of phosphorylated STAT3 has been described to be stronger in poorly differentiated than in well-differentiated SCC. Moreover, the percentage of tumor cells expressing this marker correlated with the depth of tumor invasion and with metastasis formation [50,51].

E-cadherin

This molecule plays an important role in intercellular adhesion and is specifically expressed in epithelial cells and tissues. It is calcium dependent, and its main function is to maintain intercellular connections. Decreased expression of E-cadherin in samples of primary SCC is correlated with the development of regional lymph node metastasis [52]. Furthermore, decreased expression of E-cadherin is more often associated with well-differentiated than with poorly differentiated SCC [52,53]. These observations suggest that E-cadherin might be useful as an indicator for the metastatic potential of certain well-differentiated SCCs [52].

Ets-1

This molecule is a transcription factor regulating the expression of various genes, including matrix metalloproteinases (MMPs) [54]. Recently, it has been suggested that Ets-1 might be important in the pathogenesis of invasive SCC. This may be another helpful marker to distinguish between well-differentiated and poorly differentiated SCC in the future [54,55].

CD44

A cell surface marker, CD44, is a glycoprotein widely distributed in the extracellular matrix [53,56]. In a study by Rodriguez and colleagues [57], it was shown that lymph node metastases of cutaneous SCC of the vulva were immunoreactive for CD44-9v. Also, CD44-10v expression was present in 78% of tumors compared with only 56% of normal epithelium. CD44-10v membrane expression, but not cytoplasmic expression, correlates with disease recurrence [56,57].

CLINICAL PRESENTATION AND DIAGNOSIS

Most SCCS arise on the sun-damaged skin of the head and neck, with fewer lesions arising on the extremities and occasional tumors occurring on the trunk [4]. Early lesions frequently present as a red scaly papules. Later, lesions may form nodules or firm plaques, either of which can ulcerate (Fig. 1).

SCC in situ, also referred to as Bowen's disease or intraepidermal carcinoma, usually presents as an asymptomatic well-defined erythematous scaly plaque. It has a predilection for sun-exposed areas, especially the face and legs, of fair-skinned older individuals.

Erythroplasia of Queyrat refers to SCC in situ of the penis [1,2]. It is found most commonly in the glans penis of uncircumcised men. It usually presents as a sharply demarcated asymptomatic, erythematous, shiny plaque. As in Bowen's disease, invasive carcinoma may arise in up to 10% of cases [2,4].

Keratoacanthomas (KAs) are fast-growing cutaneous neoplasms that usually show spontaneous regression. Clinically, they tend to be solitary neoplasms that are typically seen on sun-exposed areas of lighter skinned individuals. The most common locations include the face, forearms, and hands, and the peak incidence is usually in the sixth decade. They usually present as flesh-colored and dome-shaped papules with a central keratin plug. This tumor

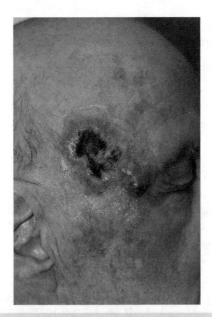

Fig. 1. Clinical presentation of cutaneous SCC. (*Courtesy of* M. MacCormack, MD; Burlington, MA, USA.)

usually grows rapidly to a size of 1 to 2 cm over a period of 2 months and involutes spontaneously after 3 to 6 months [1,4]. Controversy exists as to whether KAs are spontaneously regressing benign neoplasms or a true malignancy. Most practitioners, however, consider and treat KAs as a subtype of SCC [1,2,4].

Diagnosis of SCC and its variants is established histologically. Complete excision is curative in most cases. Occasionally, SCC invades along the perineural layer of peripheral nerves and extends well beyond the clinically apparent mass [3,4]. Local recurrence is more common in these instances, and when present on the head, direct intracranial extension may occur.

METASTATIC SQUAMOUS CELL CARCINOMA

Metastasis from cutaneous SCC usually presents 1 to 2 years after the initial diagnosis [4,53]. SCC typically spreads to local lymph node basins before distant metastases occur. The route of metastasis of SCC may occur through multiple mechanisms. In their analysis of the mechanism of metastasis, Brodland and Zitelli [58] suggested that this process follows six steps: detachment from a primary tumor, invasion into a vessel, circulation through hematogenous or lymphatic routes, stasis in a vessel, extravasation from vessels, and invasion into recipient bed.

To date, there have been a myriad of studies that have attempted to determine the overall metastatic rate for primary cutaneous SCC. The most comprehensive of these studies was performed in 1992 by Rowe and colleagues [53]. They analyzed data from more than 200 studies published from the 1930s into the 1990s, including all reports in which there was treatment of more than 20 patients who had SCC specified separately from BCC and wherein the results were separated by treatment modality. These studies did not have consistent follow-up intervals, and it is doubtful that the criteria for choosing among treatment modalities were similar; however, some features of SCC became clear. The metastatic rate for primary SCC of the sun-exposed areas was 5%, whereas the rates for SCC on the external ear, lip, and non–sun-exposed areas were 9%, 14%, and 38%, respectively. The survival rate associated with metastatic SCC of the skin was 44% with less than 5 years of follow-up and 34% with longer term follow-up. More recently, Weinberg and colleagues [59] reviewed the literature and found that even small tumors (less than 2 cm) and tumors with well-differentiated histology may metastasize.

Over the past decade, additional findings on the factors affecting metastatic potential have been published (Table 1). Presented here are those parameters that have been established to determine cutaneous SCCs that are at high risk for metastasis [59,60].

Tumor location

Tumor site influences prognosis. In their study of regional lymph node metastasis from cutaneous SCC, Kraus and colleagues [61] reported that the lip, ear, preauricular region, anterior scalp, and nose were the most common locations

Table 1
Risk factors for recurrence and metastasis of squamous cell carcinoma

Tumor location	Lip, ear
Size	Greater than 2 cm
Depth	Greater than 4 mm
	Clark's level IV
Histology	Poorly differentiated
	Perineural invasion
	Acantholytic type
	Desmoplastic type
	Spindle cell type
Host immune status	Immunosuppressed
Previous treatment	Site of prior radiation therapy

associated with regional lymph node spread. Others have cited tumors of ano-genital skin or SCC arising in areas of radiation or thermal injury and chronic inflammation as areas with increased potential for metastatic spread.

Tumor size and histologic depth of invasion

Despite the lack of randomized studies, many investigators agree that tumors greater than 2 cm in diameter are twice as likely to recur locally (15.2% versus 7.4%) and three times more likely to metastasize (30.3% versus 9.1%) than smaller tumors [9,61,62]. In addition, tumor thickness and depth of invasion may be important predictors of metastasis. Tumors greater than 4 mm in depth or extending down to the subcutis (Clark's level IV) are more likely to recur and metastasize (metastasis rate of 45.7%) compared with thinner tumors [9,62,63]. Recurrences and metastasis are less likely in tumors confined to the upper half of the dermis and less than 4 mm in depth (metastasis rate of 6.7%) [1,4,9,61–63].

Histologic subtypes

Some investigators have reported that perineural invasion (Fig. 2) and poorly differentiated tumors have a poorer prognosis with more than double the local recurrence and metastatic rate of well-differentiated SCC. Tumors with peri-neural invasion are more likely to recur and to metastasize [64–66].

Host immunosuppression

The incidence of metastatic SCC is significantly greater in individuals who have received allogenic organ transplants. These tumors behave more aggres-sively and patients who are immunosuppressed have a poorer prognosis. It is estimated that the metastatic rate of SCC is approximately 12.9% in the pres-ence of immunosuppression [45]. Dantal and colleagues [67] studied the effect of long-term immunosuppression on cancer incidence. In this study, they reported that those patients taking a lower dose of cyclosporine had an overall decreased incidence of skin cancer.

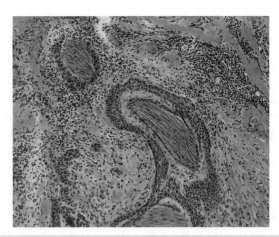

Fig. 2. SCC with perineural invasion (hematoxylin-eosin, original magnification ×40.)

Early detection of nodal disease may be beneficial in patients who have SCC in high-risk areas. The fact that distant spread in SCC is rarely seen in the absence of nodal involvement may indicate a possible role for early detection of subclinical nodal disease in SCC [4,5,45,49]. Recently, Ross and colleagues [68] reviewed the English literature for reports of sentinel lymph node biopsy (SLNB) in patients who have cutaneous SCC. This study collected data from 607 anogenital and 85 nonanogenital SCC cases. Their report identified positive lymph node biopsies in 24% of anogenital and 21% of nonanogenital SCC cases. Despite the lack of well-controlled clinical studies, this comprehensive review suggests that there may be a role in SLNB for cutaneous SCC to diagnose subclinical metastasis accurately [68].

TREATMENT MODALITIES

Most SCCs are low risk and amenable to many forms of treatment. The National Comprehensive Cancer Network (www.nccn.org) [69] and the American Academy of Dermatology (www.aad.org) [70] have published clinical practice guidelines for the treatment of SCC. In interpreting and applying these guidelines, one must keep in mind that there is a lack of multicenter randomized controlled trials (RCTs) comparing treatment approaches. Identification of those neoplasms that are at high risk is important. For these cases, the best approach is management by a multidisciplinary team with expertise in treating these tumors [4,5].

Aims of treatment and relevant outcomes

Treatment aims to remove or destroy the tumor completely and to reduce cosmetic and functional impairment. Success should therefore be measured by rates of recurrence or metastasis at fixed points in time. The morbidity of the procedure, as measured by acute or chronic pain, infection, scarring, and overall cosmesis, should be considered when choosing the appropriate treatment modality [4,71]. In addition, the cost and tolerance of the specific treatment modalities should be considered.

Treatment options may be divided into those that allow for histologic evaluation of margins (surgical excision and Mohs micrographic surgery [MMS]) and those that do not provide histologic margin control (chemotherapy, electrodesiccation and curettage [ED&C], cryotherapy, radiation, and photodynamic therapy [PDT]). This section summarizes the current treatment modalities of SCC (Table 2).

When choosing a treatment modality, it is important to be aware of the factors that may influence success. Destructive methods, such as ED&C, cryosurgery, and, to a lesser extent, radiotherapy, are all techniques in which outcome depends on appropriate tumor selection and the experience of the physician [70]. Although the same could be said for MMS and surgical excision, these latter two modalities provide tissue for complete histologic examination and margin evaluation, and thus are often the treatment of choice [4,71].

Imiquimod

Topical imiquimod may be effective in the treatment of SCC. The current literature on this modality in the treatment of SCC is scant, however, and this treatment is only validated by case reports and a few small open-label studies [72]. The mechanism of action of imiquimod is complex. This agent, considered to be an immune response modifier, binds to toll-like receptor (TLR)-7 and TLR-8 on dendritic cells, inducing and up-regulating the release of a variety of proinflammatory cytokines (eg, interferon-α, tumor necrosis factor) that, in turn, stimulate an antitumor immune response [72,73]. By modulating immune cytokines and IL-1, IL-6, IL-8, and IL-12, imiquimod activates T-lymphocyte helper type 1 cell-mediated immunity and promotes antitumor and antiviral behavior. In addition, tumor-selective apoptosis through bcl-2–dependent mitochondrial cytochrome c release and activation of caspase 3 and caspase 9 has been demonstrated in SCC cell lines with imiquimod [72].

In 2006, Peris and colleagues [73] designed a small open-label trial to evaluate the efficacy of imiquimod 5% cream in the treatment of invasive SCC and Bowen's disease. After daily application of imiquimod 5% cream five times a week for a maximum of 16 weeks, they examined tissue for histologic tumor clearance by means of a punch biopsy specimen with serial step sections. With

Table 2	
Treatment options for cutaneous squamous cell carcinoma	
Treatment	Options
Topical immune modulator	Imiquimod
Topical chemotherapy	5-Fluorouracil
Destruction (lack histologic margin control)	ED&C
	Cryotherapy
	Photodynamic therapy
	Radiation therapy
Surgery	Excisional surgery
	MMS

a small number of patients, they reported complete regression in four (80%) of five Bowen's disease lesions and in five (71.4%) of seven invasive SCCs after 12 weeks of treatment. Local adverse effects included local erythema, pruritus, irritation, and posttreatment hypopigmentation. They did not observe recurrence of invasive SCC lesions after a mean follow-up of 31 months. Other studies, mainly in the form of case reports and case series, have documented the efficacy of imiquimod in the treatment of Bowen's disease as a single agent and in combination with 5-fluorouracil (5-FU) [72–74]. Topical imiquimod may serve as an alternative beneficial approach to surgery in patients who have Bowen's disease and invasive SCC.

5-Fluorouracil

5-FU is the topical chemotherapeutic agent most widely used for nonmelanoma skin cancer [71,75]. This drug interferes with DNA synthesis and with the ability of abnormal cells to grow, causing cell death preferentially in malignant cell lines [75]. The standard dose of administration is usually once or twice daily for several weeks, resulting in increasing erythema and superficial erosions at affected sites. Although topical 5-FU has been used successfully to treat precancerous actinic keratosis lesions, its role in treating invasive SCC is challenged by its insufficient depth of penetration into the dermis. Topical 5-FU application has been limited to treating superficial BCC or SCC in situ because of the potential for persistent deeper invasive tumors to remain after treatment [75]. Advantages of this topical therapy include appealing to patient preference for a noninvasive approach and minimal scarring. Side effects include moderate to severe inflammation, pain, and pruritus. Close follow-up during the course of treatment to monitor response to the medication is recommended, in addition to long-term follow-up to identify recurrences early.

There are only a few studies providing details of the success rate for topical 5-FU as a first-line option for the treatment of SCC in situ. Most of these are open trials or small case series reporting recurrence rates ranging from 8% to 15%. The greatest success was reported by Sturm [76] in 1979. In this study, he used 1% to 3% preparations and additional keratolytics applied for an average of 9 weeks. Only three recurrences (8%) were reported in 41 lesions treated in 39 patients. There has not been a formal RCT comparing different treatment regimens of 5-FU.

The role of topical 5-FU in patients receiving a transplant who have rapid onset of multiple SCC has also been studied. In 2001, Smith and colleagues [77] reported a case series of five patients receiving a transplant who were treated with combined therapy using 5% 5-FU and 5% imiquimod for the treatment of SCC in situ. The treatment protocol was as follows: each patient used 5% imiquimod cream three times a week, alternating this with 5% 5-FU cream during the rest of the week. These investigators obtained histologic samples (by means of excision) of the treated areas at the 4-week follow-up after stopping both medications. They reported no residual epithelia dysplasia on sectioning through the blocks. The study reported no apparent systemic side effects.

Surgical excision

Surgical excision remains the major definitive treatment option for SCC less than 2 cm in diameter [69–71]. Caution is necessary when using this technique for larger SCCs or lesions in cosmetically complex areas, such as the face or hands. No large RCT has compared the effectiveness of surgical excision with any other treatment modality. Furthermore, no RCT has compared pre-determined margin widths for the surgical removal of SCC. Several case series demonstrate an excellent clearance of SCC lesions with surgical excision [71,78]. Freeman and colleagues [78] reported on 91 surgically excised SCCs, with a follow-up ranging from 1 to 5 years. Metastases developed in 3 of the 91 patients. These investigators did not note the size or location of the tumors. For SCC with clinically visible tumor less than 2 cm in diameter, surgical excision resulted in a 5-year disease-free survival rate of 96% (22 of 23 patients). For lesions clinically greater than 2 cm in diameter, 83% (10 of 12) of patients were free of disease 5 years later.

Although many researchers report low recurrence rates for excision with variable follow-up, the recommendations for the width of the margin of clinically normal skin excised has ranged from 4 mm to 1 cm. A pivotal study was done in 1992 by Brodland and Zitelli [79] to determine the appropriate margins for SCC. In this prospective study, 141 SCC lesions were excised with incremental 1-mm margins and subclinical extension of tumors was examined using MMS. With 4-mm surgical margins, low-risk tumors (less than 2 cm and well-differentiated histology) had a greater than 95% clearance, whereas high-risk tumors (clinically greater than 2 cm and invasive to fat, central face, or anogenital location) required at least 6-mm excision margins to achieve a greater than 95% clearance [79].

Mohs micrographic surgery

MMS seems to have lower recurrence rates than other treatment modalities [71,80,81]. Although MMS is frequently used in the treatment of SCC, there are no RCTs comparing MMS with other treatments for SCC. Because it uses sequential extirpation of tissue, it allows complete clearance of the tumor without taking large margins; thus, it is more sparing of adjacent normal tissue. This provides a cosmetic advantage for tumors located in functionally critical areas. The procedure is performed in an outpatient setting, and most patients tolerate it without difficulty.

Two large series document the safety of this procedure in an office setting [81,82]. In 3937 patients, Kimayai-Asadi and colleagues [81] found only one serious complication, which was gastrointestinal hemorrhage attributable to naproxen prescribed after surgery for auricular chondritis in 1 patient. In Cook and Perone's prospective study [82] of 1052 patients (1358 MMS cases), the overall complication incidence was 1.64%. Significantly, there were no serious complications that required involvement by another specialist or hospitalization of the patient. The technique avoids the delay associated with formalin-processed tissues and the need for multiple surgical procedures [80].

Mohs [83] reported a 5-year recurrence rate of 5% for primary SCC. In a case series analysis, Rowe and colleagues [53] found that MMS resulted in a lower rate of local recurrence compared with other treatment modalities. Holmkvist and Roenigk [84] report a recurrence rate for primary SCC of the lip of 5% after MMS for 50 patients in a 2- to 5-year average follow-up. Lawrence and Cottel [85] reported only three local recurrences of SCC in 44 patients with perineural invasion treated by MMS in a 1-year follow-up and further noted that predicted survival was higher than previously published survival rates for surgical excision.

MMS is expensive and is not accessible to all patients. Full extirpation of the tumor may require multiple stages over a period of many hours. Patients who cannot lie down because of a comorbid condition may not tolerate the potentially lengthy procedure. In addition, the processing of the frozen sections is labor-intensive. For low-risk small-diameter SCC (minimally invasive or in a low-risk site), other treatment modalities should be considered, because there is probably little to be gained in efficacy and much lost in terms of cost and time [80].

Electrodessication and curettage

ED&C is frequently used in the treatment of SCC, particularly for in situ or minimally invasive lesions on the trunk or limbs [4]. ED&C seems to be effective for minimally invasive SCC lesions less than 2 cm in diameter [86]. One clear advantage of ED&C over other modalities is that it is rapidly and easily performed by the experienced clinician. Although the healing time may be increased, ED&C is an affordable, effective, and rapid treatment option for SCC and should be considered for small or histologically less invasive tumors. Adequate follow-up is essential to recognize the rare recurrences.

ED&C is frequently used for SCC, but no RCTs have compared ED&C with other treatments. Several case series have examined the recurrence rate of ED&C for SCC lesions. Freeman and colleagues [78] treated 407 SCC lesions by ED&C over a 20-year period, with follow-up periods ranging from 1 to greater than 5 years. In patients with a greater than 5-year follow-up period, they found no recurrence in 96% (46 of 48) of SCCs less than 2 cm in diameter and in 100% (9 of 9) of SCCs greater than 2 cm in diameter. Of the 407 treated SCC lesions, 355 were less than 2 cm, suggesting the choice of this technique for smaller SCCs. Knox and colleagues [86] noted that only 4 SCC lesions recurred in 315 tumors treated with a follow-up of 4 months to 2 years. SCC lesions in this study were all less than 2 cm and without significant invasion. Honeycutt and Jansen [71] treated 281 invasive SCC lesions by ED&C and reported three recurrences in a follow-up period of up to 4 years. Of the patients who developed recurrences, two had had tumors greater than 2 cm. Whelan and Deckers [87] treated 26 SCC lesions on the trunk and extremities and reported no recurrence in 100% of lesions in a 2- to 9-year follow-up. In addition, they found that approximately 65% of lesions took 4 weeks to heal after ED&C.

Cosmetically, the scar from ED&C is usually a hypopigmented sclerotic disk, as compared with a thin line from excision. It is difficult to make comparisons of ED&C studies with studies of other treatments because this high success rate probably reflects, in part, a selection bias for smaller and less invasive lesions. Prolonged healing compared with surgical excision should be considered, particularly for lesions on the lower extremities [4,78]. Daily wound care is an essential part of ED&C, and diligence is required to prevent infection.

Finally, with the ED&C technique, there is no tissue obtained that can be examined microscopically to determine if the margins of the treatment are clear of tumor. If curettage develops a deep wound suggestive of deep tumor, it would be reasonable to consider excising the curettage wound with a 3- to 4-mm margin and sending that specimen for pathologic examination rather than completing the standard ED&C procedure [70,71].

Cryotherapy

Cryotherapy is effective for treating minimally invasive SCC on the trunk or limbs. Caution is warranted when treating SCC on the face, particularly near vital structures that are susceptible to cold injury or distortion from scarring [71]. This technique has been used for decades and is highly effective for treating small or minimally invasive SCC. The standard treatment protocol for cryotherapy consists of two cycles of freezing with liquid nitrogen lasting 1 to 5 minutes per cycle. The technique takes longer than ED&C but less time than surgical excision [4,71].

No RCTs have compared the effectiveness of cryotherapy with that of other treatments. Several case series have examined use of cryosurgery in SCC. Over an 18-year period, Zacarian [88] treated 4228 skin cancers with cryotherapy, which included 203 SCC lesions. He noted a 97% disease-free survival in a follow-up, ranging from less than 3 months to greater than 10 years. Most recurrences (87%) occurred in the first 3 years. Zacarian [88] further noted a healing time that ranged from 4 to 10 weeks. Kuflik and Gage [89] found a 96% 5-year disease-free survival rate for 52 SCC lesions.

With the cryotherapy procedure, no tissue is obtained for histologic examination. Because cryotherapy rarely destroys deep tissues, clinically suspected or biopsy-proved invasion into subcutaneous fat or deeper planes should be considered a relative contraindication [71]. Finally, in patients with abnormal cold tolerance, cryoglobulinemia, autoimmune deficiency, or platelet deficiency should not be treated with cryotherapy [68].

Photodynamic therapy

PDT is a procedure whereby a photosensitive topical compound is applied to the skin and the compound is activated by visible light. On activation, the compound releases reactive oxygen species, which causes tissue destruction [90]. This form of local treatment has been proved effective for actinic keratoses, and therefore is of interest in the treatment of SCC in situ. Although many photosensitizing compounds have been studied, amino levulinic acid and methyl aminolevulinate (MAL) [91], the ester of amino levulinic acid, are the two agents used currently. The light sources commonly used for activation include blue light, red light, and intense pulse light (IPL) devices.

Topical Aminolevulinic acid (ALA)-PDT has been shown to be effective in the treatment of SCC in situ and erythroplasia de Queyrat. Initial studies by Kennedy and colleagues [90] described a complete response in six patients who had SCC in situ. Patients used topical ALA applied for 3 to 6 hours, followed by red light irradiation. Morton and colleagues [92] compared ALA-PDT and cryotherapy for biopsy-proved SCC in situ of less than 2 cm in diameter. Forty tumors were randomized to a single treatment of cryotherapy or ALA-PDT. The protocol for this study used 20% topical ALA applied to tumors under occlusion for 4 hours, followed by irradiation with red light at 125 J/cm^2 (70 mW/cm^2). Results of this study were as follows: 50% of tumors treated with liquid nitrogen cryotherapy cleared versus 75% of SCC in situ lesions treated with ALA-PDT. All tumors cleared after a second course of ALA-PDT. Despite these positive results and overall good clearance rates, these results were not statistically significant.

Salim and colleagues [93] compared the effectiveness of ALA-PDT with 5-FU for treatment of SCC in situ. Forty patients who had biopsy-proved SCC in situ were selected for this study. Patients were treated with 5-FU once a day for 1 week and then twice a day for 3 weeks. The ALA-PDT group was treated with 20% ALA solution under occlusion for 4 hours followed by light at 100 J/cm^2 (50–90 mW/cm^2). At the end of the treatment time, 88% of patients in the ALA-PDT group had a complete response rate versus a 67% response rate in patients in the topical 5-FU group.

In 40 dermatology centers in 11 European countries, 225 patients who had biopsy-proved SCC in situ and no evidence of progression to invasive SCC were randomized to treatment with MAL-PDT (red light), placebo cream-PDT (red light), cryotherapy, or topical fluorouracil [92]. They were examined at 3 and 12 months after treatment for clinical response and cosmetic outcome. At the 12-month clinical follow-up, MAL-PDT had an 80% complete response compared with 67% for cryotherapy ($P = .047$) and 69% for fluorouracil ($P = .19$). In addition, MAL-PDT had a more acceptable cosmetic outcome that was maintained for 12 months. Based on these preliminary data, MAL-PDT seems to be adequate for treatment of SCC in situ, assuming that the patient is being seen regularly in follow-up to monitor for recurrence [91,92].

Overall, studies in the past decade show promising results for ALA-PDT treatment of in-situ keratinocyte neoplasia. ALA-PDT seems to be an effective treatment modality demonstrating fewer side effects and overall clearance response rate [90]. At this time, most investigators recommend that the primary treatment of SCC in situ with PDT should be considered in patients with large or multiple lesions and in those with patches involving poor healing sites. For more invasive tumors and for head and neck lesions, PDT should be considered as an adjuvant treatment modality but not as a first-line therapeutic modality [92].

Radiation therapy

Radiation therapy (RT) has been used as a primary treatment for SCC for the past century [71,75]. A wide variety of radioactive modalities and doses have been used, with irradiation techniques being adapted to tumor characteristics, such as location and size. RT for SCC generally involves superficial external irradiation of the lesion and its margins [9]. Uninvolved tissue is protected from radiation by the use of specially fitted lead masks or shields as necessary. Several fractionated doses of radiation are delivered over the course of a few weeks; administration of radiation in a single or few high-dose fractions is now less commonly used because of the increased risk for radionecrosis [94].

No standard protocols have been tested and generally adopted for RT for SCC, and no RCTs have examined the effectiveness of RT compared with other treatments for SCC. Several retrospective studies have examined the role of RT for SCC. Rowe and colleagues [53] analyzed the literature on SCC of the skin from 1940 to 1992 and found an average local recurrence rate of 10.0% after 5 or more years in 160 patients who had received RT for primary SCC. This was a higher recurrence rate than for ED&C (3.7% in 82 patients), surgical excision (8.1% in 124 patients), and MMS (3.1% in 2065 patients) 5 or more years after treatment. Several case studies in the radiation oncology literature have noted that increasing tumor size is associated with a progressively decreasing success rate in treating SCC with RT [94–97].

RT is the most expensive of all modalities to treat skin cancer and usually requires multiple treatment sessions, which may make it less convenient for patients. Unlike other standard treatments for SCC, ionizing radiation causes a small increased risk for cutaneous carcinoma within the treatment field [22,97–99]. Atrophy, hypopigmentation, alopecia, and telangiectases are also commonly seen late cutaneous sequelae of RT, yielding an eventual suboptimal cosmetic outcome in spite of excellent early cosmesis. These side effects make this modality of treatment for SCC less desirable for younger patients. Given the risk for radionecrosis, caution should also be exercised when considering RT for lesions overlying bone or cartilage.

The main advantages of RT include preservation of perilesional normal tissue and the tolerability of the treatment. RT does not require anesthesia, and patients who are medically unable to tolerate or who refuse a surgical procedure may be able to undergo RT [100]. RT seems to be an effective treatment for SCC, particularly for small lesions that have not been previously treated. Given that margin control is not assessed during treatment, treatment sites should be closely monitored at follow-up visits for possible recurrences.

FUTURE TREATMENT MODALITIES
Capecitabine
Oral capecitabine is an oral fluoropyrimidine converted into 5-FU preferentially by tumor cells and has been approved for the treatment of metastatic colorectal carcinoma and metastatic breast cancer [101]. Phase II and III trials have demonstrated that capecitabine is effective and offers a favorable safety profile compared with 5-FU, particularly with a low myelosuppression rate. In 2005, Wollina and colleagues [101] published a prospective case series using a combination of subcutaneous interferon-α with oral capecitabine in four

patients who had advanced SCC. Reported adverse effects include mucositis, mild nausea and vomiting, neutropenia, and inflammation of actinic keratosis. Early studies suggest that capecitabine offers an efficacy comparable to that of 5-FU and an improved safety profile [102,103].

SUMMARY

Cutaneous SCC is the second most common skin cancer among whites. Most cases of primary cutaneous SCC are induced by UV radiation. Chronic sun exposure is the major risk factor, and favored locations include the head and neck and other sun-exposed areas. Moreover, it is important for the clinician to recognize other risk factors associated with this malignancy, including HPV infection, occupational exposures, various genodermatoses, scarring dermatoses, chronic wounds, and burn scars. The allogenic transplant population is at most risk for developing cutaneous SCC. For these patients, aggressive patient education, control of immunosuppression, and clinical surveillance should be the standard of care.

Most patients who have primary SCC have an excellent prognosis, and treatment is usually straightforward. A substantial minority of these neoplasms, however, may recur or metastasize. Obtaining a complete history and performing a total-body skin examination can help to identify tumors at high risk for recurrence or metastasis in addition to those that may be more easily treated. For those individuals with metastatic disease, however, the long-term prognosis is guarded. Based on recent reports, in the future, there may be a role in SLNB for cutaneous SCC to diagnose subclinical metastasis accurately. Larger studies and better guidelines need to be developed before SLNB can be routinely used in the management of metastatic disease. Physicians should emphasize to their patients the benefits of sun avoidance and protection from sunlight, beginning in childhood, to minimize the risk for developing this potentially life-threatening neoplasm.

KEY POINTS

The following list has been modified from a table created by Liegeois and colleagues [104]:

Risk factors for recurrence of cutaneous SCC are treatment modality, size greater than 2 cm, depth greater than 4 mm, poor histologic differentiation, location on the ear or mucosal area, perineural involvement, location within scars or chronic inflammation, previously failed treatment, and immunosuppression.

Early detection of nodal disease may be beneficial in patients who have SCC in high-risk areas.

Cutaneous SCC occurs frequently and with great morbidity in recipients of solid organ transplants. Reducing immunosuppression in these patients is of prime therapeutic importance.

The evidence base for treatment of cutaneous SCC is poor.

None of the commonly used procedures have been tested in rigorous RCTs.

Case series that have followed up patients who had SCC treated by surgical excision, MMS, ED&C, cryotherapy, and RT all suggest 3- to 5-year recurrence rates of 10% or less.

Comparison of the recurrence rates among the major commonly used treatments is almost impossible because choice of treatment is probably based on likelihood of success (eg, only people with small uncomplicated SCCs are treated by destructive rather than excisional techniques).

Based on the available case series, there is no evidence to suggest that any of the commonly used treatments for SCC are ineffective.

Small thin tumors less than 2 cm in diameter in noncritical sites can probably be treated equally well by surgical excision with 4-mm margins, ED&C, or cryotherapy.

Larger tumors, especially in sites at which tissue sparing becomes vital, or tumors at high risk for recurrence are probably best treated by MMS.

RCTs with adequate long-term follow-up are needed to inform clinicians about the relative merits of the various treatments currently used for people who have SCC.

Such trials need to be large to exclude small but important differences, and they need to describe the sorts of people entered accurately in terms of risk factors for recurrences. Follow-up in such studies needs to be 5 years or longer.

References

[1] Kirkham N. Tumors and cysts of the epidermis. In: Elder D, Eleritas R, Jaworsky C, et al, editors. Lever's histopathology of the skin. Philadelphia: Lipincott-Raven; 1997. p. 685–746.
[2] Lohmann CM, Solomon AR. Clinicopathologic variants of cutaneous squamous cell carcinoma. Adv Anat Pathol 2001;8:27–36.
[3] Barksdale SK, O'Connor N, Barnhill R. Prognostic factors for cutaneous squamous cell and basal cell carcinoma. Determinants of risk of recurrence, metastasis, and development of subsequent skin cancers. Surg Oncol Clin N Am 1997;6:625–38.
[4] Preston DS, Stern RS. Nonmelanoma cancers of the skin. N Engl J Med 1992;327: 1649–62.
[5] Gray DT, Suman VJ, Siu WPD, et al. Trends in the population-based incidence of squamous cell carcinoma of the skin first diagnosed between 1984 and 1992. Arch Dermatol 1997;133:735–40.
[6] Christenson LJ, Barrowman TA, Vachon CM, et al. Incidence of basal cell and squamous cell carcinoma in a population younger than 40 years. JAMA 2005;294:681–90.
[7] Staples MP, Elwood M, Burton RC, et al. Non-melanoma skin cancer in Australia: the 2002 national survey and trends since 1985. Med J Aust 2006;184:6–10.
[8] Demers AA, Nugent Z, Mikhalcioiu C, et al. Trends of nonmelanoma skin cancer from 1960 through 2000 in a Canadian population. J Am Acad Dermatol 2005;53:320–8.
[9] Dinehart SM, Pollack SV. Metastases from squamous cell carcinoma of the skin and lip. An analysis of twenty-seven cases. J Am Acad Dermatol 1989;21:241–8.
[10] Stenbeck KD, Balanda KP, Williams MJ, et al. Patterns of treated non-melanoma skin cancer in Queensland—the region with the highest incidence rates in the world. Med J Aust 1990;153:511–5.
[11] Magnus K. The Nordic profile of skin cancer incidence. A comparative epidemiological study of the three main types of skin cancer. Int J Cancer 1991;47:12–9.
[12] Marks R, Staples M, Giles GG. The incidence of non-melanocytic skin cancers in an Australian population: results of a five-year prospective study. Med J Aust 1989;150:475–8.

[13] Giles GG, Marks P, Foley P. Incidence of non-melanocytic skin cancer treated in Australia. Br Med J (Clin Res Ed) 1988;296:13–7.

[14] Holt PJ. Cryotherapy for skin cancer: results over a 5-year period using liquid nitrogen spray cryosurgery. Br J Dermatol 1988;119:231–40.

[15] Scotto J, Kopf AW, Urbach F. Non-melanoma skin cancer among Caucasians in four areas of the United States. Cancer 1974;34:1333–8.

[16] Schreiber MM, Shapiro SI, Berry CZ, et al. The incidence of skin cancer in southern Arizona (Tucson). Arch Dermatol 1971;104:124–7.

[17] Serrano H, Scotto J, Shornick G, et al. Incidence of nonmelanoma skin cancer in New Hampshire and Vermont. J Am Acad Dermatol 1991;24:574–9.

[18] Hemminki K, Zhang H, Czene K. Time trends and familial risks in squamous cell carcinoma of the skin. Arch Dermatol 2003;139:885–9.

[19] Ramos J, Villa J, Ruiz A, et al. UV dose determines key characteristics of nonmelanoma skin cancer. Cancer Epidemiol Biomarkers Prev 2004;13(12):2006–11.

[20] Han J, Colditz GA, Samson LD, et al. Polymorphisms in DNA double-strand break repair genes and skin cancer risk. Cancer Res 2004;64(9):3009–13.

[21] Maier H, Schemper M, Ortel B, et al. In vitro sensitivity to ultraviolet B light and skin cancer risk: a case-control analysis. J Natl Cancer Inst 2005;97(24):1822–31.

[22] Karagas MR, McDonald JA, Greenberg ER, et al. Risk of basal cell and squamous cell skin cancers after ionizing radiation therapy. For the skin cancer prevention study group. J Natl Cancer Inst 1996;88(24):1848–53.

[23] Struijk L, Hall L, van der Meijden E, et al. Markers of cutaneous human papillomavirus infection in individuals with tumor-free skin, actinic keratoses, and squamous cell carcinoma. Cancer Epidemiol Biomarkers Prev 2006;15(3):529–35.

[24] Cassarino DS, Derienzo DP, Barr RJ. Cutaneous squamous cell carcinoma: a comprehensive clinicopathologic classification. Part one. J Cutan Pathol 2006;33(3):191–206 [review].

[25] Cassarino DS, Derienzo DP, Barr RJ. Cutaneous squamous cell carcinoma: a comprehensive clinicopathologic classification—part two. J Cutan Pathol 2006;33(4):261–79.

[26] Masini C, Fuchs PG, Gabrielli F, et al. Evidence for the association of human papillomavirus infection and cutaneous squamous cell carcinoma in immunocompetent individuals. Arch Dermatol 2003;139(7):890–4.

[27] Alam M, Caldwell JB, Eliezri YD. Human papillomavirus-associated digital squamous cell carcinoma: literature review and report of 21 new cases. J Am Acad Dermatol 2003;48(3):385–93.

[28] Harwood CA, Sasieni P, Proby CM, et al. Increased risk of skin cancer associated with the presence of epidermodysplasia verruciformis human papillomavirus types in normal skin. Br J Dermatolol 2004;15(5):949–57.

[29] Casabonne D, Michael KM, Waterboer T, et al. A prospective pilot study of antibodies against human papillomaviruses and cutaneous squamous cell carcinoma nested in the Oxford component of the European prospective investigation into cancer and nutrition. Int J Cancer 2007;121(8):1862–8.

[30] Karagas MR, Nelson HH, Sehr P, et al. Human papillomavirus infection and incidence of squamous cell and basal cell carcinomas of the skin. J Natl Cancer Inst 2006;98(6):389–95.

[31] Johnson TM, Rowe DE, Nelson BR, et al. Squamous cell carcinoma of the skin (excluding lip and oral mucosa). J Am Acad Dermatol 1992;26:467–84.

[32] Kwa RE, Campana K, Moy RL. Biology of cutaneous squamous cell carcinoma. J Am Acad Dermatol 1992;26:1–26.

[33] Euvrard S, Kanitakis J, Decullier E, et al. Subsequent skin cancers in kidney and heart transplant recipients after the first squamous cell carcinoma. Transplantation 2006;81(8):1093–100.

[34] Moloney FJ, Comber H, O'Lorcain P, et al. A population-based study of skin cancer incidence and prevalence in renal transplant recipients. Br J Dermatol 2006 Mar;154(3):498–504.

[35] Penn I. Tumors after renal and cardiac transplantation. Hematol Oncol Clin North Am 1993;7:431–45.

[36] Stasko T, Brown MD, Carucci JA, et al. International transplant-skin cancer collaborative; European skin care in organ transplant patients network. Guidelines for the management of squamous cell carcinoma in organ transplant recipients. Dermatol Surg 2004;30(4 Pt 2):642–50.

[37] Harvelt MM, Bavinck JN, Kootte AM, et al. Incidence of skin cancer after renal transplantation in the Netherlands. Transplantation 1990;49:506–9.

[38] Liddington M, Richardson AJ, Higgins RM, et al. Skin cancer in renal transplant recipients. Br J Surg 1989;76:1002–5.

[39] Hatton JL, Parent A, Tober KL, et al. Depletion of CD4+ cells exacerbates the cutaneous response to acute and chronic UVB exposure. J Invest Dermatol 2007;127(6):1507–15 [Epub 2007 Mar 15].

[40] Avaliable at: www.itscc.org. Accessed January 10, 2008.

[41] Martinez JC, Otley CC, Okuno SH, et al. Chemotherapy in the management of advanced cutaneous squamous cell carcinoma in organ transplant recipients: theoretical and practical considerations. Dermatol Surg 2004;30(4 Pt 2):679–86 [review].

[42] Moloney FJ, Kelly PO, Kay EW, et al. Maintenance versus reduction of immunosuppression in renal transplant recipients with aggressive squamous cell carcinoma. Dermatol Surg 2004;30(4 Pt 2):674–8.

[43] Otley CC, Maragh SL. Reduction of immunosuppression for transplant-associated skin cancer: rationale and evidence of efficacy. Dermatol Surg 2005;31(2):163–8.

[44] Harwood CA, Leedham-Green M, et al. Low-dose retinoids in the prevention of cutaneous squamous cell carcinomas in organ transplant recipients: a 16-year retrospective study. Arch Dermatol 2005;141(4):456–64.

[45] Dinehart SM, Chu DZ, Mahers AW, et al. Immunosuppression in patients with metastatic squamous cell carcinoma from the skin. J Dermatol Surg Oncol 1990;16:271–4.

[46] Boyle J, Mackie RM, Brigs JD, et al. Cancer, warts and sunshine in renal transplant patients. A case-control study. Lancet 1984;1(8379):702–5.

[47] George R, Weightman W, Russ GR, et al. Acitretin for chemoprevention of non-melanoma skin cancers in renal transplant recipients. Australas J Dermatol 2002;43(4):269–73.

[48] Vajdic CM, McDonald SP, McCredie MR, et al. Cancer incidence before and after kidney transplantation. JAMA 2006;296(23):2823–31.

[49] Laing ME, Dicker P, Moloney FJ, et al. Association of methylenetetrahydrofolate reductase polymorphism and the risk of squamous cell carcinoma in renal transplant patients. Transplantation 2007;84(1):113–6.

[50] Petter G, Haustein UF. Histologic subtyping and malignancy assessment of cutaneous squamous cell carcinoma. Dermatol Surg 2000;26:521–30.

[51] Suiqing C, Min Z, Lirong C. Overexpression of phosphorylated-STAT3 correlated with the invasion and metastasis of cutaneous squamous cell carcinoma. J Dermatol 2005;32:354–60.

[52] Koseki S, Aoki T, Ansai S, et al. An immunohistochemical study of E-cadherin expression in human squamous cell carcinoma of the skin: relationship between decreased expression of E-cadherin in the primary lesion and regional lymph node metastasis. J Dermatol 1999;26:416–22.

[53] Rowe DE, Carroll RJ, Day CL Jr. Prognostic factors for local recurrence, metastasis, and survival rates in squamous cell carcinoma of the skin, ear, and lip. Implications for treatment modality selection. J Am Acad Dermatol 1992;26:976–90.

[54] Keehn CA, Smoller BR, Morgan MB. Ets-1 immunohistochemical expression in non-melanoma skin carcinoma. J Cutan Pathol 2004;31:8–13.

[55] Kerkela E, Ala-aho R, Klemi P, et al. Metalloelastase (MMP-12) expression by tumour cells in squamous cell carcinoma of the vulva correlates with invasiveness, while that by macrophages predicts better outcome. J Pathol 2002;198:258–69.

[56] Niu Y, Liu F, Zhou Z, et al. Expression of CD44V6 and PCNA in squamous cell carcinomas. Med J 2002;115:1564–8.

[57] Rodriguez-Rodriguez L, Sancho-Torres I, Gibbon DG, et al. CD44–9v and CD44-10v are potential molecular markers for squamous cell carcinoma of the vulva. J Soc Gynecol Investig 2000;7:70–5.

[58] Brodland DG, Zitelli JA. Mechanism of metastasis. J Am Acad Dermatol 1992;27:1–8.

[59] Weinberg AS, Ogle CA, Shim EK. Metastatic cutaneous squamous cell carcinoma: an update. Dermatol Surg 2007;33:885–99.

[60] Breuniger H, Black B, Rassner G. Microstaging of squamous cell carcinomas. Am J Clin Pathol 1990;94:627–9.

[61] Kraus DH, Carew JF, Harrison LB. Regional lymph node metastasis from cutaneous squamous cell carcinoma. Arch Otolaryngol 1998;124:582–7.

[62] Clayman GL, Lee JJ, Holsinger FC, et al. Mortality risk from squamous cell skin cancer. J Clin Oncol 2005;23:759–65.

[63] Daniele E, Rodolico V, Leonardi V, et al. Prognosis in lower lip squamous cell carcinoma: assessment of tumor factors. Pathol Res Pract 1998;194:319–24.

[64] Breuninger H, Schaumburg-Lever G, Holzschuh J, et al. Desmoplastic squamous cell carcinoma of skin and vermilion ssurface. Cancer 1997;79:915–9.

[65] Friedman HI, Cooper PH, Wanebo HJ. Prognostic and therapeutic use of microstaging of cutaneous squamous cell carcinoma of the trunk and extremities. Cancer 1985;56:1099–1105.

[66] Kirkham N. Tumors and cysts of the epidermis. In: Elder D, editor. Lever's histopathology of the skin. 9th edition. Philadelphia: Lippincott Williams & Wilkins; 2005.

[67] Dantal J, Hourmant M, Cantarovich D, et al. Effect of long-term immunosuppression in kidney-graft recipients on cancer incidence: randomized comparison of two cyclosporin regimens. Lancet 1998;351:623–8.

[68] Ross AS, Delling A, Schmults C. Sentinel lymph node biopsy in cutaneous squamous cell carcinoma: a systematic review of the English literature. Dermatol Surg 2006;32:1309–21.

[69] National Cancer Network. Practice guidelines for oncology (squamous cell carcinoma). Ver. 1, January 2008. Available at: http://www.nccn.org/professionals/physician_gls/f_guidelines.asp. Accessed January 12, 2008.

[70] American Academy of Dermatology Website Clinical research and guidelines. Available at: http://www.aad.org/science/guidelines.htm Accessed January 12, 2008.

[71] Honeycutt WM, Jansen GT. Treatment of squamous cell carcinoma of the skin. Arch Dermatol 1973;108:670–2.

[72] Patel GK, Goodwin R, Chawla M, et al. Imiquimod 5% cream monotherapy for cutaneous squamous cell carcinoma in situ (Bowen's disease): a randomized, double-blind, placebo-controlled trial. J Am Acad Dermatol 2006;54(6):1025–32.

[73] Peris K, Micantonio T, Farnoli M. Imiquimod 5% cream in the treatment of Bowen's disease and invasive squamous cell carcinoma. J Am Acad Dermatol 2006;55(2):324–7.

[74] Rosen T, Harting M, Gibson M. Treatment of Bowen's disease with topical 5% imiquimod cream: retrospective study. Dermatol Surg 2007;33(4):427–31.

[75] Nguyen TH, Ho DQ. Nonmelanoma skin cancer. Curr Treat Options Oncol 2002;3(3):193–203.

[76] Sturm HM. Bowen's disease and 5-fluorouracil. J Am Acad Dermatol 1979;1:513–22.

[77] Smith KJ, Germain M, Skelton H. Squamous cell carcinoma in situ (Bowen's disease) in renal transplant patients treated with 5% imiquimod and 5% 5-fluorouracil therapy. Dermatol Surg 2000;27(6):561–4.

[78] Freeman RG, Knox JM, Heaton CL. The treatment of skin cancer: a statistical study of 1341 skin tumors comparing results obtained with irradiation, surgery, and curettage followed by electrodessication. Cancer 1964;17:535–8.

[79] Brodland DG, Zitelli JA. Surgical margins for excision of primary cutaneous squamous cell carcinoma. J Am Acad Dermatol 1992;27:241–8.

[80] Drake LA, Dinehart SM, Goltz RW, et al. Guidelines of care for Mohs micrographic surgery. J Am Acad Dermatol 1995;33:271–8.

[81] Kimayai-Asadi A, Goldberg LH, Peterson SR, et al. The incidence of major complications from Mohs micrographic surgery performed in office-based and hospital-based settings. J Am Acad Dermatol 2005;53:628–34.

[82] Cook JL, Perone JB. A prospective evaluation of the incidence of complications associated with Mohs micrographic surgery. Arch Dermatol 2003;139:143–52.

[83] Mohs FE. Chemosurgery: microscopically controlled surgery for skin cancer. Springfield (MA): Thomas CC; 1978.

[84] Holmkvist KA, Roenigk RK. Squamous cell carcinoma of the lip treated with Mohs micrographic surgery: outcome at 5 years. J Am Acad Dermatol 1998;38:960–6.

[85] Lawrence N, Cottel W. Squamous cell carcinoma of skin with perineural invasion. J Am Acad Dermatol 1994;31:30–3.

[86] Knox JM, Lyles TW, Shapiro EM, et al. Curettage and electrodessication in the treatment of skin cancer. Arch Dermatol 1960;82:197–204.

[87] Whelan CS, Deckers PJ. Electrocoagulation for skin cancer: an old oncologic tool revisited. Cancer 1981;47:2280–7.

[88] Zacarian SA. Cryosurgery of cutaneous carcinomas. An 18-year study of 3,022 patients with 4,228 carcinomas. J Am Acad Dermatol 1983;9:947–56.

[89] Kuflik EG, Gage AA. The five-year cure rate achieved by cryosurgery for skin cancer. J Am Acad Dermatol 1991;24:1002–4.

[90] Kennedy JC, Pottier RH, Pross DC. Photodynamic therapy with endogenous protoporphyrin IX: basic principles and present clinical experience. J Photochem Photobiol 1990;6: 143–8.

[91] Freeman M, Vinciullo C, Francis D, et al. A comparison of photodynamic therapy using topical methyl aminolevulinate (Metvix) with single cycle cryotherapy in patients with actinic keratosis: a prospective, randomized study. J Dermatolog Treat 2003;14:99–106.

[92] Morton C, Horn M, Leman J, et al. Comparison of topical methyl aminolevulinate photodynamic therapy with cryotherapy or fluorouracil for treatment of squamous cell carcinoma in situ: results of a multicenter randomized trial. Arch Dermatol 2006;142:729–35.

[93] Salim A, Leman JA, Chapman R. Randomized comparison of photodynamic therapy with topical 5-fluorouracil in Bowen's disease. Br J Dermatol 2003;148(3):539–43.

[94] Mazeron JJ, Chassagne D, Crook J, et al. Radiation therapy of carcinomas of the skin of nose and nasal vestibule: a report of 1676 cases by the Groupe Europeen de Curiethérapie. Radiother Oncol 1989;13:165–73.

[95] Petrovich Z, Parker RG, Luxton G, et al. Carcinoma of the lip and selected sites of head and neck skin. A clinical study of 896 patients. Radiother Oncol 1987;8:11–7.

[96] Lovett RD, Perez CA, Shapiro SJ, et al. External irradiation of epithelial skin cancer. Int J Radiat Oncol Biol Phys 1990;19:235–42.

[97] Silva JJ, Tsang RW, Panzarella T, et al. Results of radiotherapy for epithelial skin cancer of the pinna: the princess margaret hospital experience, 1982–1993. Int J Radiat Oncol Biol Phys 2000;47(2):451–9.

[98] Locke J, Karimpour S, Young G, et al. Radiotherapy for epithelial skin cancer. Int J Radiat Oncol Biol Phys 2001;51(3):748–55.

[99] Morrison WH, Garden AS, And KK. Radiation therapy for nonmelanoma skin carcinomas. Clin Plast Surg 1997;24:719–28.

[100] Goldman GD. Squamous cell cancer: a practical approach. Semin Cutan Med Surg 1998;17(2):80–95.

[101] Wollina U, Hansel G, Koch A, et al. Oral capecitabine plus subcutaneous interferon alpha in advanced squamous cell carcinoma of the skin. J Cancer Res Clin Oncol 2005;131(5): 300–8.

[102] Kaklamani VG, Gradishar WJ. Role of capecitabine (Xeloda) in breast cancer. Expert Rev Anticancer Ther 2003;3:137–44.

[103] Tewes M, Schleucher N, Achterrath W. Capecitabine and irinotecan as first line chemotherapy in patients with metastatic colorectal cancer: results of an extended phase I study. Ann Oncol 2003;14:1442–8.

[104] Liegeois NJ, Seo SJ, Olbricht SM. Squamous cell carcinoma. In: William H, Bigby M, Herxheimer A, editors. Evidence-based dermatology. London: BMJ Books; 2008. p. 248–55.

Epigenetics of Cutaneous Melanoma

Willmar D. Patino, MD[a], Joseph Susa, DO[b],*

[a]Department of Pathology, University of Texas Southwestern Medical Center in Dallas, 5323 Harry Hines Boulevard, Dallas, TX 75390, USA
[b]Department of Dermatology, Division of Dermatopathology, University of Texas Southwestern Medical Center in Dallas, 5323 Harry Hines Boulevard, Dallas, TX 75390, USA

EDITORIAL COMMENT

For many years genetic mutations have been known as important in the multistep theory of oncogenesis. What has become more evident in the last few years, however, is that alterations in the genome can be made without mutations and that these alterations can be important in the development of malignancy. This phenomenon is referred to as "epigenetics." In this article, the contribution of epigenetics to cutaneous malignancies is discussed in detail, especially with relation to melanoma. It is hoped that through better understanding of this process and how it relates to neoplasia, we will be better able to diagnose and treat conditions such as melanoma and other cutaneous malignancies.

Tumorigenesis is traditionally thought of as the result of the activation of oncogenes and the inactivation of tumor suppressor genes (TSGs). The development of these functional alterations in cancer cells is mainly caused by multiple genetic alterations, such as deletions, amplifications, translocations, and point mutations accumulating in the genome of neoplastic cells. In recent years, it has become evident that in addition to genetic abnormalities, epigenetic alterations are causally related to the development and progression of cancer [1]. Epigenetics refers to heritable DNA modifications that affect gene expression but do not involve changes in the underlying DNA sequence of the organism. These mechanisms include modification of DNA (hypo- and hypermethylation), changes in DNA packaging (histone modifications by acetylation, methylation, phosphorylation, and ubiquitination), and posttranslational modifications, such as RNA-associated silencing [2,3].

The best-studied epigenetic alteration in cancer is DNA methylation, a covalent modification of DNA in which a methyl group is transferred from S-adenosylmethionine to the C-5 position of cytosine by a family of DNA-methyltransferases [1]. This aberrant methylation, also known as hypermethylation,

*Corresponding author. E-mail address: jsusa@dermpathdiagnostics.com (J. Susa).

0882-0880/08/$ – see front matter
doi:10.1016/j.yadr.2008.09.003

occurs preferentially at the cytosine–phosphate–guanine dinucleotide-rich regions, known as CpG islands, which are located mainly in the promoter regions of most genes in the human genome. Under normal conditions, promoter regions are unmethylated. When abnormal methylation of the CpG islands occurs, there is no transcription; as a result, gene silencing occurs (Fig. 1). The transcriptional down-regulation that results from hypermethylation of TSG promoter regions can serve as a second hit for inactivation of TSG activity in tumorigenesis [2,4]. These epigenetic changes were first documented in colorectal cancer, but they have been reported in a large variety of cancers, including cutaneous neoplasms [2,5–7]. Different tumor types diverge with respect to the frequency and patterns of promoter hypermethylation [8,9].

Finally, epigenetic mechanisms are not only important for understanding the pathogenesis of cancer but also offer novel opportunities for cancer therapy. Hypermethylation of promoter regions can be reversed by DNA methyltransferase inhibitors or demethylating drugs, such as 5-aza-2′-deoxycytidine, which can lead to TSG reactivation. Different clinical trials have been completed using this approach, and many others are currently underway [10]. In this article we describe the different epigenetic mechanisms involved in the pathogenesis of cutaneous melanoma, particularly aberrant methylation of promoter regions and histone modifications. We also discuss some of the suggested interactions between environmental factors and epigenetic changes and the possible implications of these mechanisms in the treatment of melanoma.

EPIGENETIC ALTERATIONS IN MELANOMA
Aberrant methylation
Aberrant methylation, and in particular hypermethylation, is the most frequently documented epigenetic alteration in cutaneous melanoma. At least

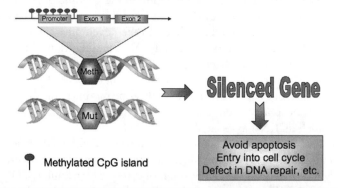

Fig. 1. Hypermethylation of TSGs serves as a second hit in tumorigenesis. An allele of a TSG is inactivated (Mut) by an inherited or acquired genetic alteration (mutation, deletion, translocation, etc). The second allele is inactivated by hypermethylation (Meth) of the CpG islands in the promoter region. The silenced gene can result in an abnormal phenotype, such as entry into cell cycle, avoidance of apoptosis, or a defect in DNA repair, which subsequently can result in the development of neoplasia.

50 different genes that exhibit hypermethylation of promoter regions have been reported in different studies using cultured melanoma cell lines and primary patient samples [2,3]. Table 1 summarizes the different genes that have been found to be hypermethylated in primary human cutaneous melanocytic lesions. The list of hypermethylated genes includes not only known TSGs but also genes involved in cell-cycle regulation, DNA repair, cell signaling, transcription, and apoptosis. Most of these studies used methylation-specific polymerase chain reaction in DNA samples isolated from primary or metastatic melanomas. Several studies also reported detection of hypermethylated genes using small amounts of circulating DNA from sera of patients with melanoma, however, which suggested that this strategy could potentially be used as a diagnostic tool [15,16].

One of the best characterized hypermethylated genes in melanoma is cyclin-dependent kinase inhibitor-2A (*CDKN2A*), which is considered one of the major genes involved in the pathogenesis of melanoma. Chromosomal deletions and inactivating mutations in the *CDKN2A* gene have been found in up to 25% of melanoma families [23–25]. *CDKN2A* is a TSG that encodes two separate gene products, p16 and p14ARF, which function as negative regulators of cell cycle progression [26]. Hypermethylation of this gene has been reported in up to 19% of primary cutaneous melanoma samples [13,14]. Straume and colleagues [14] reported loss of p16 protein expression because of hypermethylation in 11 of 59 melanoma samples. In that study, aberrant methylation *CDKN2A* was associated with increased tumor cell proliferation assessed by Ki-67 expression and a significant decrease in patient survival (31% versus 74%) after approximately 90 months of follow-up. Similarly, Hoon and colleagues [16] reported an association between disease progression and aberrant methylation of the promoter regions of the methylguanine-DNA methyltranferase (*MGMT*), RAS association domain family protein-1 (*RASSF1A*), and death-associated protein kinase (*DAPK*) genes. In their study, the frequency of hypermethylation of these genes was significantly higher in metastatic samples when compared with primary melanomas [16].

In addition to promoter hypermethylation, DNA hypomethylation has been reported in melanomas. The melanoma antigen (*MAGE*) gene family encodes for tumor-specific antigens that are recognized on melanoma cells by cytolytic T lymphocytes. These genes are only expressed by germ cells, and in somatic cells their expression is normally suppressed by promoter methylation. Abnormal expression of MAGE genes because of hypomethylation of the promoter regions has been reported in cutaneous melanoma cell lines. These reports suggested that hypomethylation of these genes is the result of a genome-wide demethylation process [27,28]. These observations also suggested that demethylating agents can be used to up-regulate the expression of different tumor antigens that can serve as targets for novel immunotherapy strategies [29].

Histone modification

DNA is packed into nucleosomes, which are composed of 146 base pairs of DNA coiled around a histone octomer composed of two molecules of each

Table 1
Hypermethylated genes in primary human melanocytic lesions

Gene	Function	Frequency	Reference
APC, adenomatous polyposis of the colon	Tumor suppression by antagonizing the WNT	9/54 (17%)	[11]
CDKN1B, p27 (Kip1), cyclin-dependent kinase inhibitor 1B	Negative regulation of cell cycle	4/45 (9%)	[12]
CDKN2a, cyclin-dependent kinase inhibitor-2a	Negative regulation of cell cycle	3/30 (10%) 11/59 (19%) 54% in metastatic and 75% in primary melanoma[a]	[13] [14] [15]
DAPK, death-associated protein kinase	Positive regulator of apoptosis	0% in primary and 19% of metastatic melanomas	[16]
MGMT, methylguanine-DNA methyltransferase	DNA repair	10% in primary and 34% of metastatic melanomas 15% in metastatic and 64% in primary melanoma[a]	[16] [15]
PRDX2, peroxiredoxin 2	Negative regulator of PDGF	3/36 (8%)	[17]
RASSF1a, RAS association domain family protein 1	Negative regulation of mitosis	24/44 (55%) 15% in primary and 57% of metastatic melanomas 62% in metastatic and 64% in primary melanoma[a]	[18] [16] [15]
RARB2, retinoic acid receptor-beta-2	Retinoic acid receptor signaling pathway	70% in both primary and metastatic melanomas 5/25 (20%)	[16] [19]
SOCS1, suppressor of cytokine signaling 1	Negatively regulate cytokine receptor signaling	31% in metastatic and 75% in primary melanoma[a]	[15]
SOCS2, suppressor of cytokine signaling 2	Negatively regulate cytokine receptor signaling	23% in metastatic and 43% in primary melanoma[a]	[15]
SOCS3, suppressor of cytokine signaling 3	Negatively regulate cytokine receptor signaling	3/5 melanomas (60%) and 1/2 nevi	[20]
THBD, thrombomodulin	Anticoagulant	12/20 (60%)	[21]
TMS1, target of methylation-induced silencing 1	Pro-apoptotic adaptor protein	5/10 (50%)	[22]
3-OST-2, 3-O-sulfotransferases 2	Heparan sulfate modification	14/25 (56%)	[19]

[a] Frequencies obtained using methylation-specific polymerase chain reaction from sera of patients with primary and metastatic melanomas.

of the four core histones (H2A, H2B, H3, and H4). The nucleosome forms a positively charged core around which the negatively charged DNA is wrapped. The H1 histone binds to the DNA between the nucleosomes at the DNA entry and exit sites. In turn, nucleosomes are fundamental in the organization of DNA in chromatin and chromosomes. Histone modification may affect chromatin remodeling and result in changes of accessibility of DNA for transcription or repair and can have global effects that result in DNA replication and chromosome segregation during mitosis.

The two main mechanisms of histone modification are chromatin remodeling by ATP-hydrolyzing enzymes and covalent modification of the histones at certain sites. Multisubunit ATP hydrolyzing enzymes may affect chromatin remodeling by altering the location of nucleosomes, removing or exchanging histones, or changing the relationship between DNA and histones to permit increased accessibility to regulating proteins. These complexes all share a common SNF-2–like subunit but are further classified into subfamilies of the imitation switch, chromodomain helicase-binding protein family, and SWItch/sucrose non-fermentable (SNF) [30]. Histone N-terminal tails protrude beyond the nucleosome, where at this exposed site they are subject to covalent modification by acetylation, methylation, phosphorylation, and ubiquitination [3].

Histone acetylation
In a simplified model, histone acetylation is generally associated with translationally active chromatin. Enzymes called histone acetyltransferases (HATs) transfer an acetyl group from acetyl-CoA to lysine residues on histone tails of all four histones of the nucleosome. Currently there are five known families of proteins, mostly transcriptional coactivators, with intrinsic HAT activity. The five classes are Gcn5-related acetyltransferases, histone acetyltransferases named for members MOZ, Ybf2/Sas3, Sas2, and Tip60 (MYST)-related HATS, p300/cyclic adenosine monophosphate response element binding proteins (p300/CBP HATS), general transcription factor HATS, and hormone-related HATs [31].

Researchers postulate that acetylation results in neutralization of the basic histone tails and leads to decompaction or relaxation of the chromatin, allowing access to transcription. Acetylation also may be important in forming recognitions sites for transcription co-factors. Conversely, histone deacetylation leads to chromatin condensation, diminished accessibility, and decreased transcription. This reversal is mediated by histone deacetylases (HDACs). Histone acetylation status is dynamically regulated by these two classes of enzymes. Currently there are 18 known histone deacetylases, which are subclassified into four classes (I–IV). Deacetylation of lysine residues is a prerequisite for methylation or ubiquitination, which also occurs at lysine residues in the histone tails. HDAC inhibitors recently have been used as a mechanism of action for a new class of chemotherapeutic drug.

Some histone acetylases function as tumor suppressors. Presumably one role of these enzymes is to acetylate chromatin at key target genes; however, acetylation and deacetylation are not restricted to histones. Transcription factors such as p53, signal transducer and activator of transcription 3 (STAT3), and nuclear factor–kappa beta are also targets of HATs and HDACs. Acetylation of the oncoprotein c-*myc* by the histone acetylase GCN-5 results in increased c-*myc* stability. C-*myc* has been implicated in tumorigenesis in several malignancies, including lung cancer and melanoma. Increased c-*myc* levels from increased expression or stability can drive unrestricted cellular proliferation, inhibit cellular differentiation, and promote vasculogenesis and metastasis [32]. Increased c-*myc* has been noted in advanced stages of melanoma, radial growth phase, and metastasis of melanoma [33,34]. Disregulation of the HDAC function has been associated with the ski oncogene, which has been linked to melanoma progression when overexpressed [35,36].

Histone methylation
Histone methylation occurs at lysine or arginine residues at several specific sites on histones H3 and H4. This modification may result in transcriptional activation or repression, depending on the sites affected. Histone methylation used to be regarded as a permanent epigenetic modification. The recent discovery of lysine-specific demethylase, an enzyme that can demethylate histone proteins, demonstrated that this is also a dynamic regulatory system [37]. Although the role of DNA methylation is well established, the role of histone methylation in melanoma is still an area to be well characterized.

Histone phosphorylation
Histone phosphorylation occurs at serine and threonine residues on certain histones, mostly H3. This change results in altered charge of the amino acids or facilitates binding of transcription or chromatin modeling factors, which leads to significant changes in chromatin structure [38]. Phosphorylation at certain histone serine residues is necessary for chromatin condensation and cell cycle progression. Histone phosphorylation of H3-serine 10 plays a role in transcriptional activation of immediate–early response genes c-*jun*, c-*fos*, and c-*myc* [39–41]. The role of histone phosphorylation in melanoma is not yet known.

Histone ubiquitination
Lysine residues on histone subunits, notably H2A and H2B, are targets for ubiquitination and modification by small ubiquitin-like modifier (SUMO). Ubiquitin and SUMO may directly compete for the same binding sites with directly opposing functions. Histone ubiquitination generally leads to increased gene expression, whereas SUMOylation generally leads to decreased gene expression. Ubiquitination, specifically nucleotide excision repair dependent mono-ubiquitination, occurs in the setting of ultraviolet damage in melanoma cells [42]. Still, the role of ubiquitination in melanoma in the setting of DNA damage and melanoma development has yet to be fully elucidated.

Implications of epigenetic alterations in treatment of melanoma
Epigenetic silencing of TSG is maintained during each cell cycle by continuous remethylation, which offers a potential target for treatment using DNA-methyltransferase inhibitors or demethylating agents. 5-Azacytidine and 5-aza-deoxycytidine (Decitabine) have been used in clinical trials for different solid tumors and are currently approved by the US Food and Drug Administration for the treatment of myelodysplastic syndrome [10]. Different

clinical trials involving melanoma have been completed with variable success. A phase II clinical trial using 5-aza-deoxycytidine in patients with melanoma showed stable disease in 22% of 18 patients and achieved a partial response in 1 of the patients [43]. A phase I trial of sequential low-dose Decitabine plus high-dose interleukin-2 demonstrated that Decitabine can be safely administered with high-dose interleukin-2 and may enhance the activity of interleukin-2 in melanoma patients [44]. Currently, an ongoing phase I study conducted by the National Cancer Institute and the University of California in San Diego is trying to elucidate the safety and efficacy of combining azacytidine and interferon in the treatment of patients with metastatic melanoma (http://clinicaltrials.gov).

Another way in which epigenetic mechanisms can be used for treatment of melanoma patients is by increasing susceptibility to chemotherapeutic agents. In contrast to basal cell carcinomas and squamous cell carcinomas, melanomas have a higher propensity to metastasize and are resistant to conventional chemotherapy. Soengas and colleagues [45] demonstrated that metastatic melanomas often lose expression of the apoptotic protease activating factor-1 gene (*Apaf-1*), a mediator of apoptosis that acts with cytochrome c and caspase-9 to mediate p53-dependent cell death. Loss of *Apaf-1* expression can be reversed by treatment with 5-aza-29-deoxycytidine and markedly enhances chemosensitivity in melanoma cell lines [45].

Histone deacetylases inhibitors
The first commercial chemotherapeutic HDAC inhibitor, vorinostat, became available in 2006. Trials of this drug and other substances in this class have demonstrated some promising results in vitro and in limited trials. Larger melanoma-specific clinical trials are currently being performed. Treatment with HDAC inhibitors in vitro alters levels of less than 10% of transcriptionally active genes, of which approximately half demonstrate increased expression and half demonstrate repression [46]. The affected genes include those involved with cell cycle regulation, apoptosis, and DNA replication [47]. Although HDAC inhibitors affect malignant and benign melanocytes, the normal melanocytes are resistant to HDAC inhibitor–mediated cell death [48]. The implication is that in addition to histone modification, there are also other effects, perhaps affected nonhistone proteins, or DNA repair mechanisms. HDAC inhibitors have several known effects, including cell cycle arrest, induction of apoptosis, induction of immune-mediated responses to tumor, and increasing susceptibility to complementary therapeutic modalities.

HDAC inhibitors are known to increase cyclin-dependent kinase inhibitor p21$^{WAF1/CiP1}$, which may lead to cell cycle arrest during the G1 phase [49]. Facchetti and colleagues [50] demonstrated inhibited melanoma proliferation with various HDAC inhibitors. HDAC inhibitors also have been shown to increase melanoma apoptosis independent of p53 levels [51]. A bacterial depsipeptide with HDAC inhibitor activity, FK228, decreased in vivo growth of subcutaneous melanoma xenografts in SCID mice [52]. The compound also nearly completely inhibited in vitro growth of melanoma cells while being significantly less toxic to normal human epidermal melanocytes.

HDAC inhibitors increase apoptosis of several malignancies, including melanoma [53]. Bandyopadhyay and colleagues [54] demonstrated that HDAC inhibition by sodium butyrate increases susceptibility to p53-mediated apoptosis. Researchers have postulated that HDAC inhibition leads to increased histone h3, h4, and p53 acetylation and later leads to upregulation of the proapoptotic protein BAX. HDAC inhibitors have been demonstrated to cause tumor cells to become capable of antigen presentation through the MHC II pathway [55]. In vitro treatment of a melanoma cell line by HDAC inhibitors demonstrated conversion to a cell capable of inducing interferon secretion by T lymphocytes by activation of the MHC-1 pathway [56]. HDAC inhibitors also increase susceptibility to other therapeutic treatments. Pretreatment of melanoma with sodium butyrate made it more sensitive to the effects of ionizing radiation but did not radiosensitize normal fibroblasts [57]. The mechanisms of action of HDAC are are still being elucidated. Although some promising results have been seen in the limited studied involving melanoma, the effects have not justified using HDAC inhibitors as primary treatment. HDAC inhibitors may play a role when used in combination with other agents to treat malignant melanoma. It is hoped that in the near future more clinical data will be available regarding the efficacy of epigenetic targets in the treatment of patients with melanoma.

Interactions between epigenetic alterations and environmental factors

Our understanding of the interactions between the environment and the different epigenetic mechanisms is still limited. Several lines of evidence suggest that environmental factors such as diet, chemicals, and radiation can affect the DNA methylation pattern [58,59]. The skin is a unique organ because it is continuously exposed to ultraviolet radiation, which is considered a major risk factor for development of skin cancer. Although still speculation, research suggests that ultraviolet radiation may directly or indirectly influence epigenetic changes in cells residing in the skin, thereby contributing to malignant transformation. Ultraviolet radiation induces cyclobutane pyrimidine dimers that give rise to C-T transitions. Research has suggested that DNA methylation can promote ultraviolet radiation–induced DNA damage because cyclobutane pyrimidine dimers form preferentially at dipyrimidine sequences with methylated cytosines [60,61]. Experimental data show that presence of a methyl group in a CpG dinucleotide increases the rate at which mutations are induced by ultraviolet radiation by shifting the absorption spectrum for cytosine [62]. Methylation of CpG sequences can create preferential targets for ultraviolet radiation. This interaction has been shown for CpG dinucleotides in the coding region of the p53 TSG during the development of skin cancer [63,64].

Experimental data from primary skin samples also suggest that abnormal methylation is directly related to sun exposure and begins before the development of cutaneous neoplasia. Sathyanarayana and colleagues [65] investigated the promoter methylation status of 12 different genes in benign and malignant skin lesions, including basal cell carcinomas, squamous cell carcinomas, and skin tags, and compared the results of lesions from sun-exposed and -protected regions. Among the 12 genes studied, E-cadherin, P-cadherin, Laminin A3, and Laminin C2 showed methylation frequencies more than 30% in one or more specimen types. The average age of the patients with skin tags was 10 to 20 years younger than persons with basal cell carcinomas or squamous cell carcinomas, which suggested that methylation begins in ultraviolet-exposed skin at a relatively early age before the onset of recognizable neoplasia. In their study, hypermethylation was significantly related to sun exposure, and samples from sun-protected skin had little or no methylation. Among the candidate genes, E-cadherin showed methylation that completely depended on sun exposure [65]. Similar studies have not been completed in melanoma samples. Downregulation of E-cadherin was reported in five of eight melanoma cell lines when compared with normal melanocytes, however. Methylation-specific polymerase chain reaction revealed CpG methylation of the promoter region of E-cadherin in two of the melanoma cell lines studied; treatment with 5-azacytidine led to re-expression of E-cadherin [66].

SUMMARY

Tumorigenesis is traditionally thought to be caused by the imbalance between oncogenes and tumor-suppressor genes. Epigenetics is a recently described phenomenon that uses an alternative mechanism to explain the transcriptional inactivation of tumor-suppressor genes predominantly by hypermethylation of the promoter regions. Hypermethylation of these regions has been described extensively in many neoplasms, including cutaneous melanoma. Histone modification, primarily by acetylation and deacetylation, is a current potential target for melanoma therapy, but more research is required to understand the mechanisms involved and the therapeutic effectiveness of regimens involving these agents. These mechanisms not only are important for understanding the origin and progression of neoplasms but also have important potential therapeutic implications. Understanding the epigenetic mechanisms involved in melanoma can provide valuable information with significant implications in diagnosis, treatment, and prevention.

References

[1] Feinberg AP. An epigenetic approach to cancer etiology. Cancer J 2007;13(1):70–4.

[2] Van Doorn R, Gruis NA, Willemze R, et al. Aberrant DNA methylation in cutaneous malignancies. Semin Oncol 2005;32(5):479–87.

[3] Rothhammer T, Bosserhoff AK. Epigenetic events in malignant melanoma. Pigment Cell Res 2007;20(2):92–111.

[4] Svensson Mansson S, Reis-Filho J, Landberg G. Transcriptional upregulation and unmethylation of the promoter region of p16 in invasive basal cell carcinoma cells and partial co-localization with the gamma 2 chain of laminin-332. J Pathol 2007;212(1):102–11.

[5] Goelz SE, Vogelstein B, Hamilton SR, et al. Hypomethylation of DNA from benign and malignant human colon neoplasms. Science 1985;228:187–90.

[6] Jones PA, Baylin SB. The epigenomics of cancer. Cell 2007;128(4):683–92.

[7] Esteller M. Cancer epigenomics: DNA methylomes and histone-modification maps. Nat Rev Genet 2007;8(4):286–98.

[8] Costello JF, Fruhwald MC, Smiraglia DJ, et al. Aberrant CpG-island methylation has non-random and tumour-type-specific patterns. Nat Genet 2000;24:132–8.

[9] Esteller M, Corn PG, Baylin SB, et al. A gene hypermethylation profile of human cancer. Cancer Res 2001;61:3225–9.

[10] Brueckner B, Kuck D, Lyko F. DNA methyltransferase inhibitors for cancer therapy. Cancer J 2007;13(1):17–22 [cells. Sb Lek 97:29–39, 1996].

[11] Worm J, Christensen C, Gronbaek K, et al. Genetic and epigenetic alterations of the APC gene in malignant melanoma. Oncogene 2004;23:5215–26.

[12] Worm J, Bartkova J, Kirkin AF, et al. Aberrant p27Kip1 promoter methylation in malignant melanoma. Oncogene 2000;19(44):5111–5.

[13] Gonzalgo ML, Bender CM, You EH, et al. Low frequency of p16/CDKN2A methylation in sporadic melanoma: comparative approaches for methylation analysis of primary tumors. Cancer Res 1997;57:5336–47.

[14] Straume O, Smeds J, Kumar R, et al. Significant impact of promoter hypermethylation and the 540 C>T polymorphism of CDKN2A in cutaneous melanoma of the vertical growth phase. Am J Pathol 2002;161:229–37.

[15] Marini A, Mirmohammadsadegh A, Nambiar S, et al. Epigenetic inactivation of tumor suppressor genes in serum of patients with cutaneous melanoma. J Invest Dermatol 2006;126(2):422–31.

[16] Hoon DS, Spugnardi M, Kuo C, et al. Profiling epigenetic inactivation of tumor suppressor genes in tumors and plasma from cutaneous melanoma patients. Oncogene 2004;23(22):4014–22.

[17] Furuta J, Nobeyama Y, Umebayashi Y, et al. Silencing of Peroxiredoxin 2 and aberrant methylation of 33 CpG islands in putative promoter regions in human malignant melanomas. Cancer Res 2006;66(12):6080–6.

[18] Spugnardi M, Tommasi S, Dammann R, et al. Epigenetic inactivation of RAS association domain family protein 1 (RASSF1A) in malignant cutaneous melanoma. Cancer Res 2003;63:1639–43.

[19] Furuta J, Umebayashi Y, Miyamoto K, et al. Promoter methylation profiling of 30 genes in human malignant melanoma. Cancer Sci 2004;95:962–8.

[20] Tokita T, Maesawa C, Kimura T, et al. Methylation status of the SOCS3 gene in human malignant melanomas. Int J Oncol 2007;30(3):689–94.

[21] Furuta J, Kaneda A, Umebayashi Y, et al. Silencing of the thrombomodulin gene in human malignant melanoma. Melanoma Res 2005;15:15–20.

[22] Guan X, Sagara J, Yokoyama T, et al. ASC/TMS1, a caspase-1 activating adaptor, is downregulated by aberrant methylation in human melanoma. Int J Cancer 2003;107:202–8.

[23] LeBoit PE, Burg G, Weedon D, et al, editors. Pathology and genetics of head and neck tumors: IARC WHO classification of tumors. World Health Organization; Lyon, France: IARC Press; 2005.

[24] Miller AJ, Mihm MC Jr. Melanoma. N Engl J Med 2006;355(1):51–65.

[25] Mittal A, Piyathilake C, Hara Y, et al. Exceptionally high protection of photocarcinogenesis by topical application of (-)-epigallocatechin-3-gallate in hydrophilic cream in SKH-1 hairless mouse model: relationship to inhibition of UVB-induced global DNA hypomethylation. Neoplasia 2003;5:555–65.

[26] Rocco JW, Sidransky D. p16(MTS-1/CDKN2/INK4a) in cancer progression. Exp Cell Res 2001;264(1):42–55.

[27] De Smet C, De Backer O, Faraoni I, et al. The activation of human gene MAGE-1 in tumor cells is correlated with genome-wide demethylation. Proc Natl Acad Sci U S A 1996;93(14):7149–53.

[28] Sigalotti L, Coral S, Nardi G, et al. Promoter methylation controls the expression of MAGE2, 3 and 4 genes in human cutaneous melanoma. J Immunother 2002;25(1):16–26.

[29] Coral S, Sigalotti L, Colizzi F, et al. Phenotypic and functional changes of human melanoma xenografts induced by DNA hypomethylation: immunotherapeutic implications. J Cell Physiol 2006;207(1):58–66.

[30] Van Grunsven LA, Verstappen G, Huylebroeck D, et al. Smads and chromatin modulation. Cytokine Growth Factor Rev 2005;16:495–512.

[31] Carrozza MJ, Utley RT, Workman JL, et al. The diverse functions of histone acetyltransferase complexes. Trends Genet 2003;19:321–9.

[32] Adhikary S, Eilers M. Transcriptional regulation and transformation by Myc proteins. Nat Rev Mol Cell Biol 2005;6:635–45.

[33] Bandyopadhyay D, Okan NA, Bales E, et al. Down-regulation of p300/CBP histone acetyltransferase activates a senescence checkpoint in human melanocytes. Cancer Res 2002;62:6231–9.

[34] Tulley PN, Neale M, Jackson D, et al. The relation between c-myc expression and interferon sensitivity in uveal melanoma. Br J Ophthalmol 2004;88:1563–7.

[35] Nomura T, Tanikawa J, Akimaru H, et al. Oncogenic activation of c-Myb correlates with a loss of negative regulation by TIF1beta and Ski. J Biol Chem 2004;279(16): 715–26.

[36] Reed JA, Lin Q, Chen D, et al. SKI pathways inducing progression of human melanoma. Cancer Metastasis Rev 2005;24:265–72.

[37] Shi Y, Lan F, Matson C, et al. Histone demethylation mediated by the nuclear amine oxidase homolog LSD1. Cell 2004;119:941–53.

[38] Dong Z, Bode AM. The role of histone H3 phosphorylation (Ser10 and Ser28) in cell growth and cell transformation. Mol Carcinog 2006;45:416–21.

[39] Dunn KL, Espino PS, Drobic B, et al. The Ras-MAPK signal transduction pathway, cancer and chromatin remodeling. Biochem Cell Biol 2005;83:1–14.

[40] Nowak SJ, Corces VG. Phosphorylation of histone H3: a balancing act between chromosome condensation and transcriptional activation. Trends Genet 2004;20:214–20.

[41] Santos-Rosa H, Caldas C. Chromatin modifier enzymes, the histone code and cancer. Eur J Cancer 2005;41:2381–402.

[42] Bergink S, Salomons FA, Hoogstraten D, et al. DNA damage triggers nucleotide excision repair-dependent monoubiquitylation of histone H2A. Genes Dev 2006;20: 1343–52.

[43] Abele R, Clavel M, Dodion P, et al. The EORTC early clinical trials cooperative group experience with 5-aza-2'-deoxycytidine (NSC 127716) in patients with colo-rectal, head and neck, renal carcinomas and malignant melanomas. Eur J Cancer Clin Oncol 1987;23(12):1921–4.

[44] Gollob JA, Sciambi CJ, Peterson BL, et al. Phase I trial of sequential low-dose 5-aza-2'-deoxycytidine plus high-dose intravenous bolus interleukin-2 in patients with melanoma or renal cell carcinoma. Clin Cancer Res 2006;12(15):4619–27.

[45] Soengas MS, Capodieci P, Polsky D, et al. Inactivation of the apoptosis effector Apaf-1 in malignant melanoma. Nature 2001;409(6817):141–4.

[46] Glaser KB, Staver MJ, Waring JF, et al. Gene expression profiling of multiple histone deacetylase (HDAC) inhibitors: defining a common gene set produced by HDAC inhibition in T24 and MDA carcinoma cell lines. Mol Cancer Ther 2003;2:151–63.

[47] Scwabe M, Lubbert M. Epigenetic lesions in malignant melanoma. Curr Pharm Biotechnol 2007;8:382–7.

[48] Boyle GM, Martyn AC, Parsons PG. Pigment Cell Res 2005;18(3):160–6.

[49] Saito A, Yamashita T, Mariko Y, et al. A synthetic inhibitor of histone deacetylase, MS-27-275, with marked in vivo antitumor activity against human tumors. Proc Natl Acad Sci U S A 1999;96:4592–7.

[50] Facchetti F, Previdi S, Ballarini M, et al. Modulation of pro- and anti-apoptotic factors in human melanoma cells exposed to histone deacetylase inhibitors. Apoptosis 2004;9: 573–82.

[51] Peltonen K, Kiviharju TM, Jarvinen PM, et al. Melanoma cell lines are susceptible to histone deacetylase inhibitor TSA provoked cell cycle arrest and apoptosis. Pigment Cell Res 2005;18:196–202.

[52] Kobayashi Y, Ohtsuki M, Murakami T, et al. Histone deacetylase inhibitor FK228 suppresses the Ras-MAP kinase signaling pathway by upregulating Rap1 and induces apoptosis in malignant melanoma. Oncogene 2006;25:512–24.

[53] Medina V, Edmonds B, Young GP, et al. Induction of caspase-3 protease activity and apoptosis by butyrate and trichostatin A (inhibitors of histone deacetylase): dependence on protein synthesis and synergy with a mitochondrial/cytochrome c-dependent pathway. Cancer Res 1997;57:3697–707.

[54] Bandyopadhyay D, Mishra A, Medrano EE. Overexpression of histone deacetylase 1 confers resistance to sodium butyrate-mediated apoptosis in melanoma cells through a p53-mediated pathway. Cancer Res 2004;64(21):7706–10.

[55] Chou S-D, Khan ANH, Magner WJ, et al. Histone acetylation regulates the cell type speciWc CIITA promoter, MHC class II expression and antigen presentation in tumor cells. Int Immunol 2005;17:1483–94.

[56] Kahn ANH, Gregorie CJ, Tomasi TB. Histone deacetylase inhibitors induce TAP, LMP, Tapasin genes and MHC class I antigen presentation by melanoma cells. Cancer Immunol Immunother 2008;57:647–54.

[57] Munshi A, Kurland JF, Nishikawa T, et al. Histone deacetylase inhibitors radiosensitize human melanoma cells by suppressing DNA repair activity. Clin Cancer Res 2005;11(13): 4912–22.

[58] Johanning GL, Heimburger DC, Piyathilake CJ. DNA methylation and diet in cancer. J Nutr 2002;132:3814S–8S.

[59] Weidman JR, Dolinoy DC, Murphy SK, et al. Cancer susceptibility: epigenetic manifestation of environmental exposures. Cancer J 2007;13(1):9–16.

[60] Pfeifer GP. p53 mutational spectra and the role of methylated CpG sequences. Mutat Res 2000;450:155–66.

[61] Tommasi S, Denissenko MF, Pfeifer GP. Sunlight induces pyrimidine dimers preferentially at 5-methylcytosine bases. Cancer Res 1997;57:4727–30.

[62] Sharonov A, Gustavsson T, Marguet S, et al. Photophysical properties of 5-methylcytidine. Photochem Photobiol Sci 2003;2:362–4.

[63] Denissenko MF, Chen JX, Tang MS, et al. Cytosine methylation determines hot spots of DNA damage in the human P53 gene. Proc Natl Acad Sci U S A 1997;94:3893–8.

[64] You YH, Pfeifer GP. Similarities in sunlight-induced mutational spectra of CpG-methylated transgenes and the p53 gene in skin cancer point to an important role of 5-methylcytosine residues in solar UV mutagenesis. J Mol Biol 2001;305:389–99.

[65] Sathyanarayana UG, Moore AY, Li L, et al. Sun exposure related methylation in malignant and non-malignant skin lesions. Cancer Lett 2007;245(1–2):112–22.

[66] Tsutsumida A, Hamada J, Tada M, et al. Epigenetic silencing of E- and P-cadherin gene expression in human melanoma cell lines. Int J Oncol 2004;25(5):1415–21.

Toll-Like Receptors in Skin

Lloyd S. Miller, MD, PhD

University of California Los Angeles, Division of Dermatology, Center for Health Sciences,
Room 52–121, 10833 Le Conte Avenue, Los Angeles, CA 90095, USA

EDITORIAL COMMENT

Dr. Miller and his colleagues at the University of California - Los Angeles have been national leaders in elucidating the roles of a family of proteins called Toll-like receptors (TLRs) in processes as diverse as *Staphylococcus aureus* skin infections, acne vulgaris, and leprosy infection. TLRs are a highly conserved family of pattern recognition receptors that have emerged as critical sensors of bacterial, fungal, and viral pathogens by recognizing conserved components of these microorganisms, such as bacterial lipopeptides and virally derived single-stranded and double-stranded RNA. The mechanism of action of current FDA-approved drugs, such as imiquimod, are based on the ability of these agents to activate TLRs. Agents that activate TLRs may also be very helpful in cancer therapy as vaccine adjuvants; conversely, inhibition of TLR-mediated signaling may help to down-regulate unwanted inflammation. Interestingly, TLRs have been implicated in cutaneous immune responses against a wide range of skin infections, including infections caused by *Staphylococcus aureus*, *Mycobacterium leprae*, *Candida albicans*, and viruses such as herpes simplex and varicella-zoster, and may contribute to the pathophysiology of common skin diseases such as atopic dermatitis, psoriasis, and acne vulgaris. Therefore, understanding the biology of the TLRs may give us new insights and, potentially, treatments for a variety of skin conditions.

Sam Hwang

I n addition to its role as a physical barrier between the host and the environment, the skin also has an important immunologic role in detecting invading pathogens [1–3]. The skin immune system can be divided into early innate immune responses, which promote cutaneous inflammation, and adaptive immune responses, which promote memory responses against foreign antigens [4,5]. Toll-like receptors (TLRs) are a recently identified group of pattern recognition receptors (PRRs) that are involved in mechanisms of host defense against a wide range of pathogenic microorganisms [6–8]. TLRs are thought to function by detecting the presence of components of microorganisms and subsequently activating different gene programs, which promote various innate

E-mail address: llmiller@mednet.ucla.edu.

0882-0880/08/$ – see front matter
doi:10.1016/j.yadr.2008.09.004

and adaptive immune responses [6–8]. There are many different types of cells in the skin that express TLRs, including keratinocytes and Langerhans cells (LCs) in the epidermis; resident and trafficking immune system cells such as monocytes/macrophages, dendritic cells (DCs), T and B lymphocytes, and mast cells in the dermis; endothelial cells of the skin microvasculature; and stromal cells such as fibroblasts and adipocytes [3]. All of the cells through their distinct expression of TLRs can recognize different components of microorganisms and initiate host defense mechanisms [3]. Thus, TLRs expressed by cells in skin enable these cells to play an integral role in cutaneous immune responses against microbial pathogens. In addition, TLRs have been implicated in the pathogenesis of certain skin diseases [1–3].

INNATE AND ADAPTIVE IMMUNITY

Innate immunity was once considered to be an early nonspecific proinflammatory response whose primary function was to recruit and activate phagocytes such as neutrophils and monocytes/macrophages to phagocytize microorganisms [9,10]. It is now known that the innate immune response has considerable specificity that is directed against conserved molecular patterns of components of microorganisms, which are called pathogen-associated molecular patterns (PAMPs) [9,10]. The receptors on immune system cells that recognize PAMPs are called pattern recognition receptors (PRRs) [9,10]. TLRs are a major class of PRRs and each TLR recognizes a different PAMP (see later in this article) [6–10]. In contrast, adaptive immunity is mediated by T and B lymphocytes, which have somatically generated receptors on their cell surface [4,6]. The receptors of the adaptive immune system cells are not PRRs and do not recognize PAMPs, but instead recognize a diverse array of foreign antigenic components [4,6]. These adaptive immunity receptors are generated by somatic hypermutation and genomic DNA recombination of antigen receptor gene segments [4,6]. This process allows for a small number of genes to produce a vast array of different antigen receptors on each T and B lymphocyte with each receptor having a unique affinity for a given antigen [4,6]. In addition, since the gene rearrangement is permanent, all of the progeny of a given T or B lymphocyte will express the same antigen receptor [4,6]. This results in the production of "memory" T and B lymphocytes, which are responsible for mediating long-lived immunologic memory responses [4,6]. Interestingly, T and B cells, in addition to expressing these adaptive immune receptors, also express TLRs, which can modify the immune responses generated by these cells [3]. The early immune response to an invading pathogen is largely mediated by innate immunity, whereas the subsequent cell-mediated and humoral immune responses and ensuing memory responses are mediated by T and B lymphocytes of the of the adaptive immune response [4,6].

TOLL-LIKE RECEPTORS

TLRs are transmembrane glycoproteins that contain an ectodomain of leucine-rich motifs, which is involved in recognition of components of microbes [6–8].

TLRs also contain a transmembrane domain and a cytoplasmic tail domain that is homologous to the interleukin-1 receptor and is responsible for initiating various intracellular signaling cascades (Fig. 1) [6–8]. These signaling cascades include activation of nuclear factor-κB (NF-κB), which is a key transcription factor that promotes expression of genes involved in immune responses such as cytokines, chemokines, and co-stimulatory and adhesion molecules [6–8]. Thus far, 10 TLRs have been identified in humans (Fig. 2) [6–8]. Interestingly, each TLR recognizes a distinct PAMP [6–8]. TLR2 can form a heterodimer with either TLR1 or TLR6 to recognize tri- or di-acyl lipopeptides of bacteria, respectively [6–8]. TLR2/6, along with CD36, has also been shown to recognize lipoteichoic acid (which is diacylated) of gram-positive bacteria [6–8]. In addition, TLR2 recognizes peptidoglycan of most bacterial species and can also recognize components of fungi [6–8]. TLR3 recognizes double-stranded RNA (dsRNA), which is found during the replication cycle of most viruses [6–8]. TLR4 along with CD14 recognizes lipopolysaccharide (LPS) of gram-negative bacteria [6–8]. TLR5 recognizes bacterial flagellin [6–8]. TLR7 and TLR8 recognize single-stranded RNA (ssRNA) found in certain viruses and also recognize the imidazoquinoline compounds, imiquimod and resiquimod (R-848) [6–8,11]. Imiquimod (Aldara) is the first TLR ligand that has been

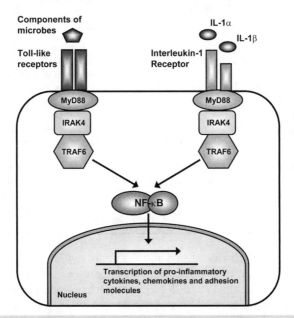

Fig. 1. TLRs and IL-1R share a similar signaling cascade to initiate immune responses. TLRs and IL-1R share a similar signaling cascade, which involves activation of the adapter molecule MyD88. MyD88 forms an initial signaling complex with IRAK4 and TRAF6. Formation of this complex results in activation of a signaling cascade that eventually leads to activation of NF-κB (and other pathways) to promote transcription of proinflammatory cytokines, chemokines, and co-stimulatory and adhesion molecules involved in innate and adaptive immune responses.

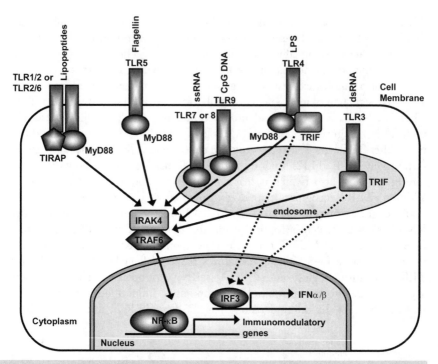

Fig. 2. PAMPs recognized by TLRs, the cellular location of TLRs and the different MyD88 adapters used by TLRs that promote distinct immune responses. Each TLR recognizes a different microbial component. TLR2 forms a heterodimer with TLR1 or TLR6 to recognize tri- and di-acyl lipopeptides, respectively. TLR4 recognizes LPS and TLR5 recognizes flagellin. These TLRs are located on the cell membrane and become internalized into phagosomes after interaction with their ligands. In contrast, TLR3 recognizes viral dsRNA, TLR7 and TLR8 recognize viral ssRNA, and TLR9 recognizes hypomethylated DNA (CpG motifs) of both bacteria and viruses and are located in intracellular membranes of endosomes and lysosomes. TLRs use MyD88 and TRIF adapters to initiate signaling. All TLRs except TLR3 can signal via MyD88. TLR2 and TLR4 also require the presence of TIRAP. MyD88 initiates a signaling cascade that eventually results in activation of NF-κB (and other pathways) to promote transcription of immunomodulatory genes. In contrast, TLR3 and TLR4 can also signal via TRIF in a MyD88-independent pathway. The TRIF pathway is critical in activating IRF3 (and IRF7), which promotes production of type I interferon (ie, IFNα and IFNβ) and antiviral immune responses.

used to treat human disease. Imiquimod is approved by the Food and Drug Administration (FDA) to treat genital warts, actinic keratoses, and superficial basal cell carcinomas [11,12]. TLR9 recognizes hypomethylated CpG motifs of bacterial double-stranded DNA (dsDNA) and DNA generated during the replication process of dsDNA viruses such as herpes simplex virus [6–8]. The PAMP recognized by TLR10 is unknown.

TLRs can also be classified into two groups based on cellular location (Fig. 2) [6–8]. TLRs 1, 2, 4, 5, and 6 are found on the cell membrane and can be activated by extracellular PAMPs. In contrast, TLRs 3, 7, 8, and 9 are found in membranes of intracellular compartments, such as endosomes and lysosomes

[6–8]. The intracellular location of TLRs 3, 7, 8, and 9 enable them to detect nucleic acids (ie, DNA or RNA) that have been released from viruses or bacteria that are degraded within endosomes and lysosomes inside the cell [6–8].

TOLL-LIKE RECEPTOR SIGNALING AND IMMUNE RESPONSES

Activation of TLRs by their ligands results in initiation of several signaling cascades, which eventually result in expression of cytokines (eg, tumor necrosis factor [TNF]α, interleukin [IL]-1β, IL-6, IL-12), chemokines (IL-8, growth-regulated oncogene [GRO]-α, monocyte chemoattractant protein [MCP]-1, -2, -3, -4, macrophage inflammatory protein [MIP]1α/β, and Regulated upon Activation, Normal T-cell Expressed, and Secreted [RANTES]), antimicrobial peptides, (beta-defensins and cathelicidin), co-stimulatory molecules (CD40, CD80, and CD86), and adhesion molecules (ICAM-1) that are involved in innate and adaptive immune responses (Fig. 3) [6–8,13,14]. In certain

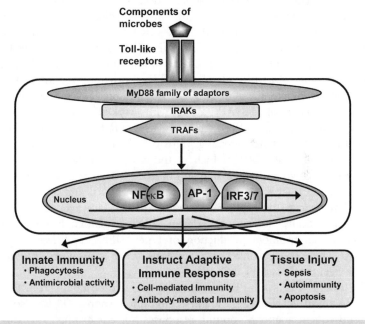

Fig. 3. Immune responses generated by activation of TLRs. TLRs recognize various microbial components and transduce signals via the family of MyD88 adapter molecules. MyD88 adapters recruit IL-1R-associated kinases (IRAKs) and tumor necrosis factor receptor-associated factors (TRAFs) to form the initial signaling complexes that lead to activation of downstream signaling pathways, including activation of transcription factors such as NF-κB, AP-1 (activator protein-1), and IRF3/7 (interferon regulatory factors 3 and 7). These signaling pathways are responsible for distinct gene programs involved in different innate and acquired immune responses. TLRs have also been implicated in tissue injury in conditions such as sepsis, autoimmunity, and apoptosis.

instances, TLRs can cause tissue injury in conditions such as sepsis, autoimmunity, and apoptosis of cells [7,13,14]. The early signaling events initiated by TLR activation is mediated by members of the myeloid differentiation factor 88 (MyD88) family of adapter proteins [7,13,14]. Activation of MyD88 adapters results in recruitment of IL-1 receptor-associated kinases (IRAKs) and TNF receptor-associated factors (TRAFs) (especially IRAK4 and TRAF6), which form the initial signaling complex [7,13,14]. Formation of this complex eventually leads to activation of downstream signaling pathways, including activation of members of the MAP kinases (mitogen-activated protein kinases) such as ERK (extracellular-signal-regulated kinase), JNK (c-Jun-NH$_2$-terminal kinase), and p38, and also activates transcription factors such as NF-κB and AP-1 (activator protein-1) [7,13,14]. Activation of these pathways leads to expression of inflammatory cytokine genes and subsequent immune responses [6–8,13].

Interestingly, despite the common use of several signaling molecules, the different MyD88 adapter proteins are only used by certain TLRs [7,13,14]. This difference in adapters leads to activation of distinct signaling pathways and gene programs that contribute to different cellular responses (Fig. 2). These different adapters include MyD88, TIRAP (Toll-interleukin 1 receptor domain-containing adapter protein), TRIF (Toll-interleukin 1 receptor domain-containing adapter-inducing interferon-β), and TRAM (TRIF-related adapter molecule) [7,13,14]. All of the TLRs, with the exception of TLR3, use MyD88 to initiate signaling (Fig. 2). In addition, TLRs 2 and 4 also require the presence of TIRAP (along with MyD88) to initiate signaling [7,13,14]. Interestingly, TLR3 exclusively uses TRIF in a MyD88-independent pathway to initiate signaling [7,13,14]. TLR4, in addition to using MyD88, can also use TRIF (which in the case of TLR4 also requires the presence of TRAM) to initiate signaling [7,13,14]. Use of the TRIF pathway by TLR3 or TLR4 results in the activation both NFκB and MAP kinases in a similar manner as the MyD88 pathway [7,13,14]. However, TRIF, but not MyD88, specifically activates interferon (IFN)-regulatory factors 3 and 7 (IRF3/7), which promote production of type I IFN (ie, IFNα and IFNβ) [7,13,14]. These type I interferon responses are critical in the immune response against viruses [6–8,13,14].

Even though TLRs are PRRs and are thought to be involved in the early sensing of an infection during the innate immune response, TLRs also can instruct subsequent adaptive immune responses [6]. For example, activation of TLRs on dendritic cells (DCs) can promote up-regulation of co-stimulatory molecules such as CD40, CD80, and CD86 and production of IL-12 [6]. CD80 and CD86 are important co-stimulatory molecules that help promote interaction and stimulation of antigen-specific T cells of the adaptive immune response [6]. In addition, IL-12 produced by TLR-stimulated DCs specifically promotes the induction of T helper 1 (Th-1) cell-mediated immune responses [6]. Thus, in certain instances, TLR activation can instruct adaptive immune responses by inducing a Th-1–type immune response [6].

TOLL-LIKE RECEPTORS CAN INDUCE A VITAMIN D-DEPENDENT ANTIMICROBIAL PATHWAY

Recently, Liu and colleagues [15,16] demonstrated that activation of TLR2/1 on human monocytes/macrophages up-regulated a vitamin D-1-hydroxylase (CYP27B1) and the vitamin D receptor (VDR) (Fig. 4). This activity of TLR2/1 resulted in the conversion of the inactive form of vitamin D (25D3) to its active form (1,25D3), which subsequently activated the VDR and led to the production of the antimicrobial peptide cathelicidin [15,16]. Since cathelicidin has microbicidal activity against a variety of pathogenic microorganisms, TLR2 induction of a vitamin D–dependent antimicrobial pathway may be an important mechanism for host defense. Similarly, Schauber and colleagues [17] demonstrated that wounding of skin or stimulation of keratinocytes with transforming growth factor (TGF)-β resulted in increased expression of TLR2 and CYP27B1 expression by keratinocytes (Fig. 4). This resulted in increased cathelicidin expression via a vitamin D–dependent pathway [17]. Taken together, these studies demonstrate that TLRs can increase cellular antimicrobial

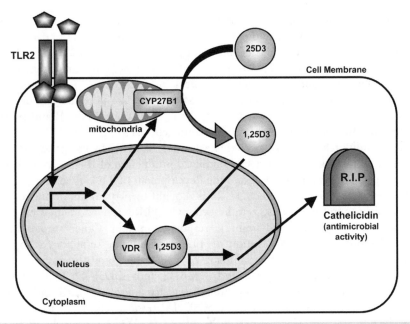

Fig. 4. TLR2 activates a vitamin D–dependent antimicrobial pathway. Activation of TLR2 on human monocytes/macrophages or keratinocytes from healing wounds (or keratinocytes stimulated with TGF-β) results in increased expression of the vitamin D-1-hydroxylase CYP27B1 and the vitamin D receptor (VDR). CYP27B1 converts the inactive form of vitamin D (25D3) to its active form (1,25D3). 1,25D3 binds to and activates the VDR, which induces production of the antimicrobial peptide cathelicidin. Since cathelicidin has microbicidal activity against a variety of pathogenic microorganisms, TLR2 induction of a vitamin D-dependent antimicrobial pathway may be an important mechanism for cutaneous host defense.

responses via a vitamin D–dependant pathway and represent another way that TLRs can protect the skin against infection.

TOLL-LIKE RECEPTOR EXPRESSION AND FUNCTION OF SKIN-SPECIFIC CELLS

There are many different cell types in human skin that express TLRs [1–3]. In the epidermis, keratinocytes have been shown to express functional TLRs. In addition, there are resident and trafficking immune system cells in the skin that express TLRs, including Langerhans cells (LCs), monocytes/macrophages, dendritic cells (DCs), T and B lymphocytes, and mast cells [1–3]. Last, endothelial cells of the microvasculature and stromal cells such as fibroblasts and adipocytes also express TLRs [1–3]. Each of these cell types has distinct TLR expression patterns and likely contributes to cutaneous immune responses [1–3]. This section will discuss TLR expression and function on keratinocytes and Langerhans cells.

Keratinocytes

Keratinocytes of the epidermis not only play an important role in maintaining the physical barrier between the host and the environment, but also participate in cutaneous immune responses [5,18]. In particular, keratinocytes have been shown to express TLRs 1 to 6 and 9, which can help keratinocytes act as first-responders against pathogenic microorganisms [17,19–31]. For example, activation of TLR2 on keratinocytes by *Staphylococcus aureus* or its components, peptidoglycan and lipoteichoic acid, results in activation of NF-κB and subsequent production of the neutrophil chemotactic factor IL-8 and iNOS [26]. Other studies have demonstrated that activation of TLR3 by its ligand, dsRNA (poly I:C), on human keratinocytes induced production of IL-8, TNFα, IL-18, and type I interferon (IFNα/β) and the development of Th-1–type immune responses [20,24,25,30,32]. Since TLR3 is thought to play an important role in recognizing viral infections, keratinocytes via TLR3 activation may play an important role in antiviral immune responses in skin. Other studies have also demonstrated that activation of TLR5 on human keratinocytes by its ligand, flagellin, resulted in production of TNFα, IL-8, and the antimicrobial peptides, human β-defensins 2 and 3 (hBD2 and hBD3) [25,32,33]. Lebre and colleagues [25]. have demonstrated that activation of TLR3 and TLR9 on keratinocytes (by poly I:C and CpG DNA, respectively) leads to selective production of the chemokines, CXCL9 and CXCL10, which promote memory T-cell responses and production of type I interferon. Another study by Miller and colleagues [27] found that the keratinocyte growth and differentiation factor, TGFα, which is found at high levels in healing wounds, upregulated expression and function of TLR5 and TLR9. Thus, TGFα may not only stimulate keratinocytes to repair the barrier after wounding, but may also increase the ability of keratinocytes to sense an infection via increasing their functional responsiveness to TLR ligands [27].

Langerhans cells

Langerhans cells (LCs) are a subset of dendritic cells (DCs) that are found in the epidermis. LCs express the protein, langerin, which is found in birbeck granules, the intracellular organelle of LCs. Several studies have demonstrated that LCs express TLRs and may participate in mediating TLR responses [34–39]. A previous study by Renn and colleagues [40] demonstrated that LC-like DCs that were derived from human cord blood express mRNA for TLRs 1 to 10. LC-like DCs were most responsive to TLR2 ligands and TLR7/8 ligands [40]. Furthermore, activation of LC-like DCs by TLR3 stimulation resulted in production of type I interferon (IFNα/β), suggesting a role for LC-like DCs in antiviral immunity [34,40]. However, recently, a study by Flacher and colleagues [41]. demonstrated that freshly isolated LCs that were purified from human skin express only TLRs 1, 2, 3, 5, 6, and 10. These skin LCs responded to ligands to TLR2 and TLR3 and produced IL-6, IL-8, and TNFα, but not IL-12 or IFNα/β [41]. Interestingly, in response to peptidoglycan stimulation, the skin-derived LCs produced the Th2 cytokine, IL-10, suggesting that LCs may play a role in tolerance against commensal grampositive bacteria [41]. Taken together, there are significant differences among TLR expression and function of LC-like DCs and LCs purified from human skin. The LCs purified from human skin appear to play an important role in immunologic tolerance.

TOLL-LIKE RECEPTORS IN THE PATHOPHYSIOLOGY OF SKIN DISEASE

Atopic dermatitis

Atopic dermatitis or eczema is an inflammatory skin disease that is associated with a hereditary predisposition to atopic conditions, which include allergic rhinitis, allergic keratoconjuntivitis, asthma, and eczema [5]. Clinically, atopic dermatitis is characterized by the presence of inflammatory skin lesions that are extremely pruritic [5]. Like other allergic diseases, the pathophysiology of atopic dermatitis involves a Th-2 type immune response in the skin. The role of TLRs in the pathophysiology of atopic dermatitis is not entirely understood. However, the skin lesions of atopic dermatitis are highly susceptible to superinfection by bacterial and viral pathogens such as *S aureus* and herpes simplex virus [42–45]. Several studies have demonstrated that the skin lesions of atopic dermatitis have decreased levels of various antimicrobial peptides (beta-defensins, cathelicidin, and dermcidin) as compared with normal skin or psoriatic skin lesions and these lower levels of antimicrobial peptides may contribute to the increased susceptibility to infection [42–45]. Recent studies have identified the presence of certain polymorphisms in TLRs or TLR signaling molecules in patients with atopic dermatitis. One study found that a specific polymorphism in TLR2 (R753Q), which was previously associated with a subset of patients with severe *S aureus* infections [46], defined a group of atopic dermatitis patients with a severe phenotype [47]. However, another study did not show an association with TLR2 polymorphisms among patients with atopic dermatitis [48]. Other studies have demonstrated that polymorphism in the TLR9 promoter or in TOLLIP, an inhibitory adapter protein within the TLR pathway, were also associated with atopic dermatitis [49,50]. Last, monocytes from patients with atopic dermatitis have been shown to have a significant impairment in TLR2-mediated production of proinflammatory cytokines [51]. Taken together, polymorphisms in TLRs or TLR signaling molecules may impair the functional responsiveness of TLRs (especially TLR2 and TLR9) in patients with atopic dermatitis. This impairment in TLR function may contribute the increased susceptibility of lesions of atopic dermatitis to bacterial and viral superinfection and may also contribute to the pathophysiology of the disease.

Psoriasis

Psoriasis is an inflammatory skin disease that is characterized clinically by cutaneous erythematous plaques with thick slivery scale [5]. Histologic examination of psoriasis lesions reveals epidermal hyperplasia (acanthosis), dilation of papillary dermal blood vessels, and a dermal inflammatory infiltrate composed of predominantly of T cells and histiocytes [5,52]. In contrast to atopic dermatitis, psoriasis has been associated with a Th-1 cytokine profile and more recently a Th-17 cytokine profile [5,52]. Also, it is well known that psoriatic plaques are highly resistant to superinfection by pathogenic bacteria such as *S aureus* [53]. This increased resistance to infection may be partly explained by the high levels of antimicrobial peptides found in psoriatic scales [42,43,54,55]. In addition, several studies have found that keratinocytes in psoriatic lesions have increased levels of TLRs 1, 2, 4, 5, and 9 compared with normal skin [19–21,27,56]. As mentioned above, Miller and colleagues [27] demonstrated that the keratinocyte growth factor TGFα, which is found at high levels in healing wounds and in psoriatic lesions, increased expression of TLRs 5 and 9 and increased TLR-dependent production of proinflammatory cytokines (eg, IL-8) and beta-defensins. Therefore, TLRs may contribute to the increased levels of antimicrobial peptides and cutaneous immune responses in psoriatic lesions. Interestingly, a previous report demonstrated that topical application of the TLR7 agonist imiquimod induced the spreading of a psoriatic plaque [57]. Thus, TLR activation may also play a role in the pathophysiology of psoriasis by exacerbating the disease process [57]. Last, a recent study demonstrated that the antimicrobial peptide cathelicidin (LL-37), which is found at high levels in psoriatic skin, can convert otherwise nonstimulatory self-DNA into a potent activator of TLR9 on plasmacytoid DCs resulting in production of IFNα [58]. This may be one important mechanism of how TLRs can promote autoimmunity in psoriasis [58].

Acne vulgaris

Acne vulgaris is an inflammatory skin disease that occurs mostly during adolescence and involves inflammation of the pilosebaceous unit. The anaerobic bacterium *Propionibacterium acnes* has been associated with the inflammation in acne lesions. Kim and colleagues [59] demonstrated that TLR2 on human monocytes can be activated by *P acnes* in vitro, resulting in increased production of IL-12 and IL-8. Furthermore, macrophages expressing TLR2 were found surrounding pilosebaceous units of histologic sections of acne lesions from patients [59]. Interestingly, topical retinoids such as all-trans retinoic acid and adapalene, which are used clinically to treat acne, have been shown to decrease TLR2 expression [60,61]. Liu and colleagues [60] demonstrated that all-trans retinoic acid can decrease TLR2 expression and function on cultured human monocytes. Tenaud and colleagues [61] demonstrated that adapalene can decrease TLR2 expression on epidermal keratinocytes of explants of normal human skin and explants of acne lesions. Thus, TLR2 has been implicated in the inflammatory process in acne vulgaris and topical retinoids may help decrease the inflammation in acne lesions by decreasing expression and function of TLR2.

TOLL-LIKE RECEPTORS IN SKIN INFECTIONS
Staphylococcus aureus
S aureus is a gram-positive bacterium that is the most common cause of bacterial skin infections in humans such as impetigo, folliculitis/furunculosis, and cellulitis. TLR2 has been shown to recognize various components of *S aureus*, including peptidoglycan and lipopeptides [62–64]. In addition, the TLR2/6 heterodimer along with CD36 has been shown to recognize *S aureus* lipoteichoic acid [65]. A recent study demonstrated that TLR2 on primary human keratinocytes contributed to up-regulation of human beta-defensin 3 (hBD3), which has potent microbicidal activity against *S aureus* [66]. Other studies in mice have shown that mice deficient in TLR2 developed larger skin lesions in response to *S aureus* skin infection [65,67]. However, mice deficient in MyD88-developed much larger lesions than TLR2-deficient mice, suggesting that other receptors that signal via MyD88 may be important in cutaneous host defense against *S aureus* [67]. Miller and colleagues [67] determined that mice deficient in IL-1 receptor (IL-1R), which also signals via MyD88, developed large lesions that closely resembled those of MyD88-deficient mice, suggesting that IL-1R may play a more prominent role in cutaneous host defense against *S aureus* than TLR2.

Mycobacterium leprae
Mycobacterium leprae is an intracellular bacterium that causes the clinical disease leprosy [68]. Clinically, leprosy has a broad clinical spectrum. The tuberculoid form has few skin lesions, rare bacteria seen by histology, and is associated with a Th-1–type cell-mediated immune response [68]. In contrast, the lepromatous form has numerous skin lesions, readily detectable bacteria by histology and is associated with a Th-2 type antibody-mediated immune response [68]. There is considerable evidence that TLRs are involved in the immune response against leprosy. In vitro studies by Krutzik and colleagues [69] have found that lipoproteins from *M leprae* mediate cellular activation via TLR2/1. Furthermore, another study demonstrated that TLR2 induced apoptosis of Schwann cells, which may contribute to the nerve damage seen in leprosy patients [70].

In addition, individuals with polymorphisms in TLR2, which impair TLR2 function, have been shown to have an increased susceptibility to leprosy and the development of the lepromatous form [71–73]. In particular, peripheral blood leukocytes isolated from patients with these polymorphisms produced less TNFα and Th-1 cytokines (eg, IL-2, IL-12, and IFNγ) and increased IL-10 levels compared with individuals without the polymorphism [71,72]. Thus, TLR2 has shown to be important in host defense against *M leprae*, but may also increase nerve damage seen in leprosy lesions by increasing apoptosis of Schwann cells.

Candida albicans

Candida albicans is a fungal pathogen that causes mucocutaneous infections and even life-threatening infections, especially in immunocompromised individuals [74]. TLR2 recognizes *C albicans* phospholipomannan [75]. In contrast, TLR4 recognizes *C albicans* O-bound mannan [76]. In human keratinocyte cultures, Pivarcsi and colleagues [28] demonstrated that keratinocyte-induced killing of *C albicans* was dependent upon TLR2 and TLR4 activation. These studies suggest that TLR2 and TLR4 not only can recognize components of *C albicans*, but also play a role in keratinocyte antimicrobial activity against *C albicans*.

Herpes Simplex and Varicella-Zoster Virus

Herpes simplex virus (HSV) and varicella-zoster virus (VZV) are viral pathogens of the Herpesviridae family of dsDNA viruses that commonly infect human skin and mucosa [77,78]. Infections by HSV and VZV typically result in grouped vesicles that ulcerate and then heal [77,78]. VZV is responsible for the clinical manifestations of varicella (chicken pox) during the first exposure and zoster (shingles) during reactivation of latent viral infection [78]. Several TLRs have been implicated in the immune response to HSV. Individuals with genital HSV infections who had polymorphisms in TLR2, which caused impairment of TLR2 activity, had increased viral shedding and more recurrent infections than patients without TLR2 polymorphisms [79]. Furthermore, individuals deficient in TLR3 had increased spreading of HSV infection from keratinocytes to cranial nerves, resulting in an increased susceptibility to HSV encephalitis [80]. In cultures systems, TLR2 and TLR9 have been shown to recognize HSV glycoproteins and HSV dsDNA, respectively, and promote production of inflammatory cytokines [81–84]. Similarly, TLR2 can be activated by VZV to induce production of proinflammatory cytokines [78]. Taken together, there is evidence that TLRs 2, 3, and 9 are involved in the cutaneous innate immune response against HSV and VZV infections.

Toll-like receptor–based treatments of skin disease

Since activation of TLRs promotes immune responses, there has been a growing interest in pharmacologic targeting of TLRs in the treatment of various medical conditions, including certain skin diseases and skin cancer. In fact, imiquimod 5% topical cream (Aldara), which is a nucleoside analog and a TLR7 agonist, has already been FDA approved to treat genital warts, actinic keratoses, and superficial basal cell carcinomas [85,86]. Through activation of TLR7, imiquimod induces expression of proinflammatory cytokines such as IFNα, TNFα, IL-6, IL-8, and IL-12 that promote a Th-1–type immune response [85,86]. Furthermore, imiquimod has been shown to have pro-apoptotic activity against tumors, which may explain its activity against skin cancers such as basal cell carcinomas [86]. In addition, other studies have demonstrated that TLR9 agonists (ie, CpG oligodeoxynucleotides) can be used as adjuvants in anticancer vaccines, which may be important in promoting specific anticancer immune responses against malignant melanoma and perhaps other cancers [87–89]. Thus, pharmacologic targeting of the immunomodulatory effects of TLRs may provide a basis for future therapies or vaccine development against certain skin diseases, skin cancer, and infections.

SUMMARY
TLRs have emerged as a major class of PRRs that are involved in detecting invading pathogens in the skin and initiating cutaneous immune responses. TLRs are expressed on many different cell types in the skin, including keratinocytes and Langerhans cells in the epidermis. Each TLR can recognize a different microbial component and there are differences among the TLR signaling pathways, which lead to distinct immune responses against a given pathogen. Certain TLRs have been implicated in the pathogenesis of skin diseases, such as atopic dermatitis, psoriasis, and acne vulgaris. In addition, TLRs have been shown to be important in cutaneous host defense mechanisms against common bacterial, fungal, and viral pathogens in the skin, such as *S aureus*, *C albicans*, and HSV. Since the discovery that topical TLR agonists promote antiviral and antitumor immune responses, there has been considerable interest in the development of TLR-based therapies for skin diseases, skin cancer, and infections. Future research involving TLRs in skin will hopefully provide new insights into host defense against skin pathogens and novel therapeutic targets aimed at treating skin disease and skin cancer.

References
[1] Kang SS, Kauls LS, Gaspari AA. Toll-like receptors: applications to dermatologic disease. J Am Acad Dermatol 2006;54(6):951–83.
[2] McInturff JE, Modlin RL, Kim J. The role of toll-like receptors in the pathogenesis and treatment of dermatological disease. J Invest Dermatol 2005;125(1):1–8.
[3] Miller LS, Modlin RL. Toll-like receptors in the skin. Semin Immunopathol 2007;29(1): 15–26.
[4] Clark R, Kupper T. Old meets new: the interaction between innate and adaptive immunity. J Invest Dermatol 2005;125(4):629–37.
[5] Kupper TS, Fuhlbrigge RC. Immune surveillance in the skin: mechanisms and clinical consequences. Nat Rev Immunol 2004;4(3):211–22.
[6] Iwasaki A, Medzhitov R. Toll-like receptor control of the adaptive immune responses. Nat Immunol 2004;5(10):987–95.
[7] Kawai T, Akira S. TLR signaling. Semin Immunol 2007;19(1):24–32.
[8] Trinchieri G, Sher A. Cooperation of Toll-like receptor signals in innate immune defence. Nat Rev Immunol 2007;7(3):179–90.

[9] Medzhitov R. Toll-like receptors and innate immunity. Nat Rev Immunol 2001;1:135–45.

[10] Medzhitov R, Janeway C Jr. Innate immunity. N Engl J Med 2000;343:338–44.

[11] Schiller M, Metze D, Luger TA, et al. Immune response modifiers—mode of action. Exp Dermatol 2006;15(5):331–41.

[12] Gupta AK, Cherman AM, Tyring SK. Viral and nonviral uses of imiquimod: a review. J Cutan Med Surg 2004;8(5):338–52.

[13] Modlin RL, Cheng G. From plankton to pathogen recognition. Nat Med 2004;10(11): 1173–4.

[14] O'Neill LA, Bowie AG. The family of five: TIR-domain-containing adaptors in Toll-like receptor signalling. Nat Rev Immunol 2007;7(5):353–64.

[15] Liu PT, Stenger S, Tang DH, et al. Cutting edge: vitamin D-mediated human antimicrobial activity against Mycobacterium tuberculosis is dependent on the induction of cathelicidin. J Immunol 2007;179(4):2060–3.

[16] Liu PT, Stenger S, Li H, et al. Toll-like receptor triggering of a vitamin D-mediated human antimicrobial response. Science 2006;311(5768):1770–3.

[17] Schauber J, Dorschner RA, Coda AB, et al. Injury enhances TLR2 function and antimicrobial peptide expression through a vitamin D-dependent mechanism. J Clin Invest 2007;117(3): 803–11.

[18] Robert C, Kupper TS. Inflammatory skin diseases, T cells, and immune surveillance. N Engl J Med 1999;341:1817–28.

[19] Baker BS, Ovigne JM, Powles AV, et al. Normal keratinocytes express toll-like receptors (TLRs) 1, 2 and 5: modulation of TLR expression in chronic plaque psoriasis. Br J Dermatol 2003;148:670–9.

[20] Begon E, Michel L, Flageul B, et al. Expression, subcellular localization and cytokinic modulation of Toll-like receptors (TLRs) in normal human keratinocytes: TLR2 up-regulation in psoriatic skin. Eur J Dermatol 2007;17(6):497–506.

[21] Curry JL, Qin JZ, Bonish B, et al. Innate immune-related receptors in normal and psoriatic skin. Arch Pathol Lab Med 2003;127:178–86.

[22] Kawai K, Shimura H, Minagawa M, et al. Expression of functional toll-like receptor 2 on human epidermal keratinocytes. J Dermatol Sci 2002;30(3):185–94.

[23] Kawai K. Expression of functional toll-like receptors on cultured human epidermal keratinocytes. J Invest Dermatol 2003;121:217–8.

[24] Lebre MC, Antons JC, Kalinski P, et al. Double-stranded RNA-exposed human keratinocytes promote Th1 responses by inducing a Type-1 polarized phenotype in dendritic cells: role of keratinocyte-derived tumor necrosis factor alpha, type I interferons, and interleukin-18. J Invest Dermatol 2003;120(6):990–7.

[25] Lebre MC, van der Aar AM, van BL, et al. Human keratinocytes express functional toll-like receptor 3, 4, 5, and 9. J Invest Dermatol 2006;127(2):331–41.

[26] Mempel M, Voelcker V, Kollisch G, et al. Toll-like receptor expression in human keratinocytes: nuclear factor kappaB controlled gene activation by Staphylococcus aureus is toll-like receptor 2 but not toll-like receptor 4 or platelet activating factor receptor dependent. J Invest Dermatol 2003;121(6):1389–96.

[27] Miller LS, Sorensen OE, Liu PT, et al. TGF-alpha regulates TLR expression and function on epidermal keratinocytes. J Immunol 2005;174(10):6137–43.

[28] Pivarcsi A, Bodai L, Rethi B, et al. Expression and function of toll-like receptors 2 and 4 in human keratinocytes. Int Immunol 2003;15(6):721–30.

[29] Pivarcsi A, Koreck A, Bodai L, et al. Differentiation-regulated expression of toll-like receptors 2 and 4 in HaCaT keratinocytes. Arch Dermatol Res 2004;296:120–4.

[30] Prens EP, Kant M, van DG, et al. IFN-alpha enhances poly-IC responses in human keratinocytes by inducing expression of cytosolic innate RNA receptors: relevance for psoriasis. J Invest Dermatol 2007;128(4):932–8.

[31] Song PI, Park YM, Abraham T, et al. Human keratinocytes express functional CD14 and toll-like receptor 4. J Invest Dermatol 2002;119(2):424–32.

[32] Kollisch G, Kalali BN, Voelcker V, et al. Various members of the toll-like receptor family contribute to the innate immune response of human epidermal keratinocytes. Immunology 2005;114(4):531–41.

[33] Miller LS, Modlin RL. Human keratinocyte toll-like receptors promote distinct immune responses. J Invest Dermatol 2007;127(2):262–3.

[34] Fujita H, Asahina A, Mitsui H, et al. Langerhans cells exhibit low responsiveness to double-stranded RNA. Biochem Biophys Res Commun 2004;319(3):832–9.

[35] Takeuchi J, Watari E, Shinya E, et al. Down-regulation of toll-like receptor expression in monocyte-derived Langerhans cell-like cells: implications of low-responsiveness to bacterial components in the epidermal Langerhans cells. Biochem Biophys Res Commun 2003;306(3):674–9.

[36] Burns RP Jr, Ferbel B, Tomai M, et al. The imidazoquinolines, imiquimod and R-848, induce functional, but not phenotypic, maturation of human epidermal Langerhans cells. Clin Immunol 2000;94(1):13–23.

[37] Gatti E, Velleca MA, Biedermann BC, et al. Large-scale culture and selective maturation of human Langerhans cells from granulocyte colony-stimulating factor-mobilized CD34+ progenitors. J Immunol 2000;164(7):3600–7.

[38] van der Aar AM, Sylva-Steenland RM, Bos JD, et al. Loss of TLR2, TLR4, and TLR5 on Langerhans cells abolishes bacterial recognition. J Immunol 2007;178(4):1986–90.

[39] Sugita K, Kabashima K, Atarashi K, et al. Innate immunity mediated by epidermal keratinocytes promotes acquired immunity involving Langerhans cells and T cells in the skin. Clin Exp Immunol 2007;147(1):176–83.

[40] Renn CN, Sanchez DJ, Ochoa MT, et al. TLR activation of Langerhans cell-like dendritic cells triggers an antiviral immune response. J Immunol 2006;177(1):298–305.

[41] Flacher V, Bouschbacher M, Verronese E, et al. Human Langerhans cells express a specific TLR profile and differentially respond to viruses and gram-positive bacteria. J Immunol 2006;177(11):7959–67.

[42] Nomura I, Goleva E, Howell MD, et al. Cytokine milieu of atopic dermatitis, as compared to psoriasis, skin prevents induction of innate immune response genes. J Immunol 2003;171: 3262–9.

[43] Ong PY, Ohtake T, Brandt C, et al. Endogenous antimicrobial peptides and skin infections in atopic dermatitis. N Engl J Med 2002;347:1151–60.

[44] Howell MD, Gallo RL, Boguniewicz M, et al. Cytokine milieu of atopic dermatitis skin subverts the innate immune response to vaccinia virus. Immunity 2006;24(3):341–8.

[45] Rieg S, Steffen H, Seeber S, et al. Deficiency of dermcidin-derived antimicrobial peptides in sweat of patients with atopic dermatitis correlates with an impaired innate defense of human skin in vivo. J Immunol 2005;174(12):8003–10.

[46] Lorenz E, Mira JP, Cornish KL, et al. A novel polymorphism in the toll-like receptor 2 gene and its potential association with staphylococcal infection. Infect Immun 2000;68(11): 6398–401.

[47] Ahmad-Nejad P, Mrabet-Dahbi S, Breuer K, et al. The toll-like receptor 2 R753Q polymorphism defines a subgroup of patients with atopic dermatitis having severe phenotype. J Allergy Clin Immunol 2004;113(3):565–7.

[48] Weidinger S, Novak N, Klopp N, et al. Lack of association between toll-like receptor 2 and toll-like receptor 4 polymorphisms and atopic eczema. J Allergy Clin Immunol 2006;118(1):277–9.

[49] Novak N, Yu CF, Bussmann C, et al. Putative association of a TLR9 promoter polymorphism with atopic eczema. Allergy 2007;62(7):766–72.

[50] Schimming TT, Parwez Q, Petrasch-Parwez E, et al. Association of toll-interacting protein gene polymorphisms with atopic dermatitis. BMC Dermatol 2007;7:3.

[51] Hasannejad H, Takahashi R, Kimishima M, et al. Selective impairment of toll-like receptor 2-mediated proinflammatory cytokine production by monocytes from patients with atopic dermatitis. J Allergy Clin Immunol 2007;120(1):69–75.

[52] van Beelen AJ, Teunissen MB, Kapsenberg ML, et al. Interleukin-17 in inflammatory skin disorders. Curr Opin Allergy Clin Immunol 2007;7(5):374–81.

[53] Henseler T, Christophers E. Disease concomitance in psoriasis. J Am Acad Dermatol 1995;32:982–6.

[54] Harder J, Bartels J, Christophers E, et al. Isolation and characterization of human beta-defensin-3, a novel human inducible peptide antibiotic. J Biol Chem 2001;276:5707–13.

[55] Harder J, Bartels J, Christophers E, et al. A peptide antibiotic from human skin. Nature 1997;387:861.

[56] Seung NR, Park EJ, Kim CW, et al. Comparison of expression of heat-shock protein 60, Toll-like receptors 2 and 4, and T-cell receptor gammadelta in plaque and guttate psoriasis. J Cutan Pathol 2007;34(12):903–11.

[57] Fitzgerald KA, O'Neill LA. The role of the interleukin-1/toll-like receptor superfamily in inflammation and host defence. Microbes Infect 2000;2(8):933–43.

[58] Lande R, Gregorio J, Facchinetti V, et al. Plasmacytoid dendritic cells sense self-DNA coupled with antimicrobial peptide. Nature 2007;449(7162):564–9.

[59] Kim J, Ochoa MT, Krutzik SR, et al. Activation of toll-like receptor 2 in acne triggers inflammatory cytokine responses. J Immunol 2002;169(3):1535–41.

[60] Liu PT, Krutzik SR, Kim J, et al. Cutting edge: all-trans retinoic acid down-regulates TLR2 expression and function. J Immunol 2005;174(5):2467–70.

[61] Tenaud I, Khammari A, Dreno B. In vitro modulation of TLR-2, CD1d and IL-10 by adapalene on normal human skin and acne inflammatory lesions. Exp Dermatol 2007;16(6): 500–6.

[62] Takeuchi O, Hoshino K, Kawai T, et al. Differential roles of TLR2 and TLR4 in recognition of gram-negative and gram-positive bacterial cell wall components. Immunity 1999;11(4): 443–51.

[63] Schroder NW, Morath S, Alexander C, et al. Lipoteichoic acid (LTA) of *Streptococcus pneumoniae* and *Staphylococcus aureus* activates immune cells via Toll-like receptor (TLR)-2, lipopolysaccharide-binding protein (LBP), and CD14, whereas TLR-4 and MD-2 are not involved. J Biol Chem 2003;278(18):15587–94.

[64] Hashimoto M, Tawaratsumida K, Kariya H, et al. Not lipoteichoic acid but lipoproteins appear to be the dominant immunobiologically active compounds in *Staphylococcus aureus*. J Immunol 2006;177(5):3162–9.

[65] Hoebe K, Georgel P, Rutschmann S, et al. CD36 is a sensor of diacylglycerides. Nature 2005;433(7025):523–7.

[66] Menzies BE, Kenoyer A. Signal transduction and nuclear responses in *Staphylococcus aureus*-induced expression of human beta-defensin 3 in skin keratinocytes. Infect Immun 2006;74(12):6847–54.

[67] Miller LS, O'Connell RM, Gutierrez MA, et al. MyD88 mediates neutrophil recruitment initiated by IL-1R but not TLR2 activation in immunity against *Staphylococcus aureus*. Immunity 2006;24(1):79–91.

[68] Walker SL, Lockwood DN. Leprosy. Clin Dermatol 2007;25(2):165–72.

[69] Krutzik SR, Ochoa MT, Sieling PA, et al. Activation and regulation of toll-like receptors 2 and 1 in human leprosy. Nat Med 2003;9:525–32.

[70] Oliveira RB, Ochoa MT, Sieling PA, et al. Expression of Toll-like receptor 2 on human Schwann cells: a mechanism of nerve damage in leprosy. Infect Immun 2003;71(3): 1427–33.

[71] Bochud PY, Hawn TR, Aderem A. Cutting edge: a toll-like receptor 2 polymorphism that is associated with lepromatous leprosy is unable to mediate mycobacterial signaling. J Immunol 2003;170(7):3451–4.

[72] Kang TJ, Lee SB, Chae GT. A polymorphism in the toll-like receptor 2 is associated with IL-12 production from monocyte in lepromatous leprosy. Cytokine 2002;20(2):56–62.

[73] Kang TJ, Chae GT. Detection of Toll-like receptor 2 (TLR2) mutation in the lepromatous leprosy patients. FEMS Immunol Med Microbiol 2001;31(1):53–8.

[74] Netea MG, Brown GD, Kullberg BJ, et al. An integrated model of the recognition of *Candida albicans* by the innate immune system. Nat Rev Microbiol 2008;6(1):67–78.

[75] Jouault T, Ibata-Ombetta S, Takeuchi O, et al. *Candida albicans* phospholipomannan is sensed through Toll-like receptors. J Infect Dis 2003;188(1):165–72.

[76] Netea MG, Gow NA, Munro CA, et al. Immune sensing of *Candida albicans* requires cooperative recognition of mannans and glucans by lectin and Toll-like receptors. J Clin Invest 2006;116(6):1642–50.

[77] Barton GM. Viral recognition by Toll-like receptors. Semin Immunol 2007;19(1):33–40.

[78] Wang JP, Kurt-Jones EA, Shin OS, et al. Varicella-zoster virus activates inflammatory cytokines in human monocytes and macrophages via Toll-like receptor 2. J Virol 2005;79(20):12658–66.

[79] Bochud PY, Magaret AS, Koelle DM, et al. Polymorphisms in TLR2 are associated with increased viral shedding and lesional rate in patients with genital herpes simplex virus Type 2 infection. J Infect Dis 2007;196(4):505–9.

[80] Zhang SY, Jouanguy E, Ugolini S, et al. TLR3 deficiency in patients with herpes simplex encephalitis. Science 2007;317(5844):1522–7.

[81] Sato A, Linehan MM, Iwasaki A. Dual recognition of herpes simplex viruses by TLR2 and TLR9 in dendritic cells. Proc Natl Acad Sci U S A 2006;103(46):17343–8.

[82] Aravalli RN, Hu S, Rowen TN, et al. Cutting edge: TLR2-mediated proinflammatory cytokine and chemokine production by microglial cells in response to herpes simplex virus. J Immunol 2005;175(7):4189–93.

[83] Lund JM, Linehan MM, Iijima N, et al. Cutting edge: plasmacytoid dendritic cells provide innate immune protection against mucosal viral infection in situ. J Immunol 2006;177(11):7510–4.

[84] Kurt-Jones EA, Chan M, Zhou S, et al. Herpes simplex virus 1 interaction with Toll-like receptor 2 contributes to lethal encephalitis. Proc Natl Acad Sci U S A 2004;101(5):1315–20.

[85] Hemmi H, Kaisho T, Takeuchi O, et al. Small anti-viral compounds activate immune cells via the TLR7 MyD88-dependent signaling pathway. Nat Immunol 2002;3(2):196–200.

[86] Schon MP, Schon M. Imiquimod: mode of action. Br J Dermatol 2007;157(Suppl 2):8–13.

[87] Krieg AM. Development of TLR9 agonists for cancer therapy. J Clin Invest 2007;117(5):1184–94.

[88] Pashenkov M, Goess G, Wagner C, et al. Phase II trial of a Toll-like receptor 9-activating oligonucleotide in patients with metastatic melanoma. J Clin Oncol 2006;24(36):5716–24.

[89] Speiser DE, Lienard D, Rufer N, et al. Rapid and strong human CD8+ T cell responses to vaccination with peptide, IFA, and CpG oligodeoxynucleotide 7909. J Clin Invest 2005;115(3):739–46.

Advances in Dermatology 24 (2008) 89–103

ADVANCES IN DERMATOLOGY

Application of Angiogenesis to Clinical Dermatology

Levi E. Fried, BA, Jack L. Arbiser, MD, PhD*

Department of Dermatology, Emory University School of Medicine, WMB 5309,
101 Woodruff Circle Atlanta, GA 30322, USA

EDITORIAL COMMENT

As defined in this article by Drs. Fried and Arbiser, angiogenesis is "the process by which normal and pathologic tissue derives a blood supply." Increasingly, angiogenesis has been shown to play critical roles in inflammatory as well as neoplastic processes. Understanding the molecular basis of angiogenesis, including the homing of bone marrow endothelial cell precursors to newly established sites of angiogenesis, has given us many potential therapeutic targets related to formation or maintenance of blood vessels. The recent approval of an anti-VEGF antibody, bevacizumab, for cancer therapy is one such example and many more appear to be on their way. Dr. Jack Arbiser, the senior author of this review, has been a leader in elucidating the molecular basis of angiogenesis (eg, the role of reactive oxygen species) as well as a pioneer in using new and established drugs (eg, gentian violet) to block angiogenesis in a variety of settings, including the treatment of hemangiomas, that have relevance in dermatology.

Sam Hwang

A ngiogenesis is the process through which normal and pathologic tissue derives a blood supply, which is necessary for the perfusion of these tissues with oxygen and removal of waste. Impairment of angiogenesis to normal tissues or abnormal tissues has immediate consequences, including central necrosis and apoptosis. When this occurs in normal tissue, this is called infarction, which can have life-ending consequences (myocardial infarction, stroke). When this occurs in pathologic tissues, ie, tumors or inflammatory processes, central necrosis and apoptosis may occur, and this may be therapeutically beneficial. Excess angiogenesis underlies many disease processes in dermatology, from those that seem obvious (neoplastic disease), but

J.L.A. was supported by the grant RO1 AR47901 and P30 AR42687 Emory Skin Disease Research Core Center Grant from the National Institutes of Health, and a Veterans Administration Hospital Merit Award.

*Corresponding author. E-mail address: jarbise@emory.edu (J.L. Arbiser).

0882-0880/08/$ – see front matter
doi:10.1016/j.yadr.2008.09.010

also in ulceration, in which excess angiogenesis prevents reepithelialization, to inflammatory processes (psoriasis, atopic dermatitis, lupus), and even chronic infections like leprosy. In this article, we discuss common disorders that are angiogenic and discuss how novel and existing treatments may be used to treat these disorders.

Angiogenesis is the process in which tissue recruits blood vessels to form a neovasculature to vascularize the tissue. In most cases, the tissue experiences physiologic hypoxia, in which the tissue generates angiogenic growth factors such as vascular endothelial growth factors (VEGF A, B, C, D), basic fibroblast growth factor (bFGF, FGF-2), placenta growth factor (PLGF), stromal-derived factor (SDF-1), corticotrophin-releasing hormone (CRH), angiopoietins 1 and 2, leptin, monocyte chemotactic factor (MCP-1), and others [1–8]. These factors encourage both local angiogenesis, through mobilizing small vessel endothelial cells from preexisting capillaries, as well as recruitment of bone marrow endothelial precursors. The ability of processes to recruit endothelial cells from these processes differs between processes and in different individuals, and may be different between males and females because of estrogenic stimuli. Tumors injected into mice are highly dependent on recruitment of bone marrow precursors, while tumors that are induced in mice through chemical carcinogenesis are dependent on local recruitment. Evidence of this is provided by the Id-1/Id-3 knockout mice, which are highly resistant to implanted tumors but are not resistant to carcinogen-induced tumors [9,10].

Once endothelial cells are attracted to the source of blood vessels, they must form a functional lumen, allowing for the transport of red blood cells and metabolic wastes. Initial lumen formation is a state in which blood vessels are not invested with pericytes, and is thus unstable. This vasculature, called a neovasculature, is leaky and unstable, and is prone to constant remodeling. Interestingly, tumors that have a high degree of vascular remodeling have a poor prognosis [11–13]. If the neovasculature is not actively remodeling, it becomes invested with pericytes and becomes stabilized and has a decreased ability to remodel. Pericytes are cells with smooth muscle characteristics that invest small blood vessels. It is harder to regress blood vessels that have been stabilized with pericytes, but these vessels may have less capability to vascularize a rapidly proliferating tumor [14,15]. There is thus a tradeoff between vessel growth and stability.

Targeting the neovasculature has been a focus of pharmacologic efforts to inhibit angiogenesis. Most neovasculatures are characterized by high levels of VEGF, but also angiopoeitin-2 (ang-2), which has the dual effect of destabilizing vessels and attracting endothelial precursor cells. Tumors with high levels of ang-2 have a poor prognosis compared with tumors with low levels of ang-2. Both ang-2 and ang-1 bind to the same receptor, and stimulate similar signaling cascades, but ang-2 causes leaky vessels and vascular leak, while ang-1 decreases vascular leak and promotes vessel stabilization [16,17]. These findings have been thought to be counterintuitive, but more recent studies show that ang-1 and ang-2 are both survival factors for endothelial cells under different combinations of growth factors, and that ang-2 promotes endothelial cell survival under conditions of severe stress, such as the acidotic and hypoxic environment of a solid tumor. For the clinician, the important thing to remember is that redness is often a sign not just of angiogenesis, but vascular leak, and that these conditions are often accompanied by high-level expression of ang-2.

VASCULAR LEAK AS A TARGET FOR THERAPY

Vascular leak is a common component of multiple pathologic processes, which may be systemic or local. Dramatic evidence of systemic vascular leak is seen in sepsis, which is often accompanied by peptides that enhance vascular leak, such as tumor necrosis factor alpha (TNF-α). The edema of a glioblastoma multiforme or toxoplasmosis causing the enhancing ring phenomenon on radiography is an example of vascular leak in an area that is compressed. In areas that are not compressed, such as the peritoneum or pleura, vascular leak manifests itself as ascites. In the skin, vascular leak, if rapid, manifests itself as bullae, which may account for the blisters seen in pemphigus or pemphigoid. Lower-level vascular leak manifests as microvesicles, such as seen in allergic contact dermatitis, dermatitis herpetiformis, psoriasis, and atopic dermatitis [18–22]. Vascular leak is associated in most cases with a limited genetic repertoire, consisting of an inflammatory cytokine (often TNF-α), nuclear factor kappa beta (NFkB) activation, endothelial expression of surface intercellular adhesion molecule (ICAM)-1, vascular cell adhesion molecule (VCAM)-1, and E-selectin, which promotes lymphocytic, neutrophil, and platelet adherence to endothelial cells, and high levels of VEGF and ang-2 [23,24]. These processes can be seen in a variety of infection processes as well, ranging from soft tissue cellulitis to meningococcal meningitis to cerebral malaria [25]. Currently the major treatment of vascular leak is systemic glucocorticoids, which decrease vascular leak and have lytic effects on neutrophils and lymphocytes, which perpetuate the inflammatory effects. Unfortunately, steroids are highly immunosuppressive and have other effects, such as promotion of insulin resistance. This may be because of increased production of reactive oxygen as a downstream effect of glucocorticoid action [26], and may explain the flare of psoriasis seen when systemic steroids are used to treat psoriasis and tapered off.

TARGETING REACTIVE OXYGEN TO TREAT SKIN DISEASES

Oxygen is the major component of cellular respiration. When fully metabolized, oxygen is converted to water. However, oxygen has additional metabolic fates, such as conversion to superoxide by enzymes such as the NADPH oxidase complex (Nox) [27]. This is a family of enzymes that converts molecular oxygen to superoxide, a highly reactive and potentially destructive molecule. Superoxide has many physiologic functions, such as the destruction of pathogens by neutrophils, as neutrophils can use superoxide directly or metabolites of superoxide, such as hypochloric acid (bleach) to kill organisms. Deficiency of the ability to produce superoxide is manifested in chronic granulomatous disorder (CGD), the most common form is X-linked CGD, in which Nox2 is deficient [28,29].

The Nox enzyme family in humans consists of five Nox genes and two dual oxygenase (Duox genes). Nox2, which is the primary gene of CGD, resides at the cell membrane in a complex with other genes, such as gp22phox, gp47phox, p67phox, and the small GTPases rac1 and rac2. Deficiency in any of these genes can result in a CGD-like phenotype, in which neutrophils can engulf bacteria but not destroy them, leading to granulomas that are inflammatory. Rac is required for the activity of Nox 1, 2, and 3, while gp22phox is required for the activity of Nox4 [30].

Generation of superoxide has several important physiologic consequences for cells, whether or not the cells are specialized to kill pathogens. Superoxide oxidizes IkB, resulting in activation of NFkB and downstream target genes, such as ICAM-1, VCAM-1, E-selectin, ang-2, and VEGF [31–33]. Superoxide can also promote tumors through epigenetic phenomena including hypermethylation of tumor suppressor genes and oxidation of other tumor suppressor genes, such as phosphatase and tensin homolog (PTEN) [34]. Hyperproliferative activity of reactive oxygen may be halted by activation of the tumor suppressor gene p53 [35].

Reactive oxygen has been shown to control angiogenesis in many tumors, especially those deficient in the tumor suppressor gene p16ink4a [36]. Prominent among them are melanomas, the third most common form of skin cancer and the cancer responsible for most death attributable to a skin condition. Most melanomas exhibit a phenomenon called the "reactive-oxygen driven tumor" in which angiogenesis and resistance to apoptosis are mediated by a reactive oxygen (superoxide)-NFkB mechanism [37,38]. Blockade of reactive oxygen may sensitize these tumors to chemotherapy and radiation, in part by reducing NFkB-mediated angiogenesis. Recently, we have found that triphenylmethane dyes, such as gentian violet, block the activity of Nox2 and Nox4 and eliminate the growth of experimental hemangiomas in mice [39]. Gentian violet has been shown to be clinically effective against oral hairy leukoplakia, a condition caused by epithelial infection with Epstein Barr virus (EBV), which causes reactive oxygen generation [40,41]. Currently, novel derivatives of gentian violet are being synthesized for systemic use against solid and hematopoietic tumors that use reactive oxygen for signaling.

ANGIOGENESIS AND PSORIASIS

Psoriasis is a common papulosquamous disorder that is present in 1% to 2% of the US population, and can range in severity from a few asymptomatic plaques to total body involvement [3,42]. Psoriasis can overlap with other rheumatologic disorders, including arthritis and inflammatory bowel disease. Psoriasis is seen exclusively in humans, and results from a complex interaction between lymphocytes and keratinocytes. The earliest evidence of increased angiogenesis in psoriasis was elucidated by Braverman and colleagues, who demonstrated increased vascularity in the psoriatic lesion and determined that the epidermis was the major source of the angiogenic activity (Fig. 1) [43–45]. A major component of that activity was found to be VEGF, and transgenic overexpression

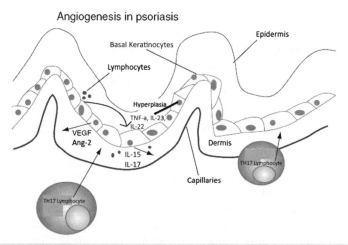

Fig. 1. Angiogenesis in psoriasis. Lymphocytes act to release TNF-α, IL-23, and IL-22, which induced hyperplasia in basal keratinocytes. This causes the release of VEGF, Ang2, IL-15, and IL-17 into the dermis, which causes inflammation.

of VEGF-A in the epidermis gives rise to some features of the psoriatic pheno-type [46,47]. The dependence of the psoriatic process on lymphocytes was el-egantly demonstrated by Wrone-Smith and Nickoloff [48], who transplanted uninvolved psoriatic skin onto SCID mice, infused stimulated lymphocytes into the mice, and demonstrated regeneration of the psoriatic lesion along with a vigorous neovasculature.

Psoriasis was once thought to be attributable to a Th1 lymphocytic process, but more recently has been demonstrated to be mediated by a Th17 lympho-cytic process, mediated by T cells that have some similarity to NK cells [49–55]. This finding might explain why psoriasis often worsens in patients with ad-vanced HIV infection, in which Th1 function is severely dysfunctional. Infil-trating T lymphocytes in psoriasis produce IL-17, which stimulates NFkB targets in keratinocytes, including ICAM-1 [53,56,57]. Synergistic activity is seen with interferon gamma, and other cytokines potentiate the inflammatory and angiogenic response, including interleukins 15, 22, and 23, as well as TNF-α. Interleukin (IL)-23 shares the p40 subunit of its receptor with the IL-12 receptor, and a recent clinical trial has shown efficacy of targeted therapy in patients with psoriasis. IL-22 has shown to cause epidermal hyperplasia, and possibly increased epidermal angiogenesis. These cytokines are controlled by TNF-α, and blockade of TNF-α has been shown to be efficacious in reduc-ing levels of IL-22 and IL-23. Inhibitors of TNF-α, including traps and blocking antibodies, are in widespread use in psoriasis, although complicated by expense and side effects [58–60]. The side effects include reactivation of chronic infections, ie, tuberculosis, worsening of autoimmune diseases that may be con-trolled by TNF-α (lupus, multiple sclerosis), or worsening of congestive heart failure. In virtually all cases, psoriasis returns after cessation of TNF inhibitor therapy, necessitating long-term therapy for efficacy.

Other drugs used in psoriasis may have antiangiogenic properties. Methotrexate was once the most popular systemic drug against psoriasis, and has been demonstrated to have antiangiogenic properties. Other compounds used against psoriasis, including cyclosporine, retinoids, and vitamin D analogs, have also been shown to have antiangiogenic properties. Coal tar, one of the oldest remedies for psoriasis, has been shown to induce long-term remissions in psoriasis. Recently, we fractionated coal tar and found an angiogenesis inhibitor, carbazole, which blocks rac-stat3 function and may account for the therapeutic activity of coal tar in psoriasis, as well as block production of IL-15 [61]. Antimicrobial peptides that are overexpressed in psoriasis stimulate generation of reactive oxygen. Thus, it is likely that psoriasis represents a reactive oxygen–driven process, and that inhibitors of this process may be beneficial in the treatment of angiogenesis associated with psoriasis [62,63].

ANGIOGENESIS AND VASCULAR LESIONS

Vascular lesions comprise a large and heterogeneous population of lesions that are not fully understood. While the molecular events of only a few of these lesions are understood, the clinical course of these lesions fits into one of three possibilities: rapid growth and regression (hemangioma), growth proportional to growth of patient without regression, and growth with local invasion and metastasis without regression (malignant endothelial tumor). Of these categories, hemangioma is the most common, found in 1% of all births and up to 10% of premature infants. Risk factors for hemangioma include female sex (fourfold increase), premature birth, and chorionic villus biopsy [64]. The endothelial cells that comprise hemangiomas express placental markers, so it was proposed that hemangiomas arise from placental rests. Clonality has been assigned to hemangiomas, but their true neoplastic nature has not been elucidated. Currently, the most likely hypothesis is that hemangiomas represent populations of embryonic bone marrow endothelium that homes to skin (or other organs). Factors that may play a role in this phenomenon are ang-2, which is highly expressed in hemangiomas of infancy, as well as a mouse model, bend3 cells, derived from polyoma middle T transformation of embryonic endothelial cells. Bend3 cells form tumors exclusively by recruiting host endothelial cells, and of interest, polyoma middle T only transforms embryonic or neonatal endothelial cells, and not cells from older mice, suggesting that like in humans [65]. Intriguingly, verruga peruana, caused by infection of endothelial cells by *Bartonella bacilliformis*, is associated with rac elevation and increased production of ang-2, and is histologically indistinguishable from hemangiomas [66,67].

Hemangiomas exhibit a distinct "life cycle," which has been divided into three phases [64]. The proliferative state is characterized by rapid growth of the lesion. The second state is spontaneous involution, in which endothelial apoptosis is noted. The final stage is the involuted state, in which the hemangiomas are replaced by a connective tissue scar. Unlike other angiogenic lesions, hemangiomas do not use VEGF as their major angiogenic factor, but use ang-2, which recruits endothelial precursor cells [68]. Finally, we demonstrated that polyoma-transformed endothelial cells produce high levels of ang-2 compared to VEGF, and the growth of these cells in vivo could be inhibited by a trap against ang-2. Therefore, strategies that block the production of ang-2 might be potentially useful in the treatment of hemangiomas [39]. To this end, we demonstrated that triphenylmethane dyes, which block the production of ang-2 in endothelial cells, block the growth of polyoma-transformed murine hemangiomas in vivo. To determine whether these findings could be translated into human disease, we treated ulcerated hemangiomas in infants with the triphenylmethane eosin (manuscript submitted), and showed significant efficacy.

Vascular malformations are the second-most common class of endothelial lesions (Fig. 2) [69]. Unlike hemangiomas, vascular malformations do not regress with time, and often have large lumens with diminished smooth muscle investment. This is commonly seen in Sturge-Weber syndrome. Recently, we demonstrated that overexpression of Akt in endothelial cells could reproduce the large vessel phenotype. Interestingly, while there is evidence that hemangiomas also have high levels of Akt, they also express reactive oxygen markers such as ICAM-1 and Wilms tumor 1 (WT-1), whereas hemangiomas do not [70–72]. Thus, large vessel vascular malformations use Akt, while hemangiomas use both Akt and reactive oxygen. Another class of small vessel vascular hemangiomas includes the acquired vascular disorder, rosacea. We hypothesize that while large vessel malformations use Akt alone, and hemangiomas use Akt/reactive oxygen, rosacea may use reactive oxygen alone. Rosacea can be treated with tetracycline class antibiotics, which inhibit matrix metalloproteinases, or by drugs such as metronidazole, which inhibits reactive oxygen. Finally, sulfacetamide is also a reducing agent that may inhibit reactive oxygen.

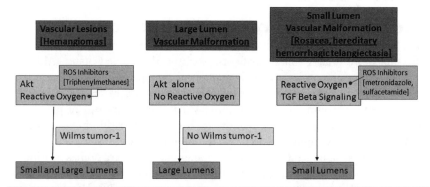

Fig. 2. Pathways of different vascular diseases. Vascular diseases such as malformations and lesions have differing pathways that lead to the creation of lumens of varying size.

ANGIOGENESIS AND MELANOMA

Melanoma is the third most common skin cancer, but is the leading cause of death attributable to a dermatologic condition. The factors that make melanoma such a lethal cancer are its propensity to metastasize and the resistance of metastatic tumors to chemotherapy and radiation. Both of these adverse prognostic factors are directly related to angiogenesis. Most melanomas arise as a result of mutations in B-raf or N-ras in the setting of loss of the tumor suppressor p16ink4a, and this combination of oncogenes and tumor suppressor genes may account for up to 90% of cutaneous melanomas [36]. We have previously demonstrated an association between loss of p16ink4a and activation of p42/44 MAP kinase and reactive oxygen/akt activation. This association holds true in cutaneous melanoma. Over 90% of early melanomas are positive for MAP kinase activation and expression of VEGF [73,74]. Introduction of MAP kinase into immortalized melanocytes results in induction of VEGF. In deeper melanomas, VEGF is similarly highly expressed, but MAP kinase activation is replaced by activation of Akt/reactive oxygen. These discoveries lead to potential therapies for melanoma [38].

Sorafenib is a small molecule inhibitor of B-raf and VEGFR2 tyrosine kinases. The impetus for the development of sorafenib is the high rate of B-raf mutations in melanoma. However, sorafenib did not have appreciable activity in melanoma as monotherapy [75,76]. The likeliest reason for this result is that in deeper melanomas, additional signaling pathways can substitute for MAP kinase activation. Blockade of additional signaling pathways will be required to treat melanoma. Interferon alpha is currently the treatment of choice in high-risk melanoma, but yields only a 10% survival advantage. Resistance to interferon may be because of induction of Akt by both endothelial and tumor cells. Avastin (bevacizumab), an anti-VEGF antibody, has been tried in combination with interferon alpha [77]. Avastin alone had modest effects, and the addition of interferon did not increase efficacy. It is becoming clear that treatment of melanoma will require multiple drug cocktails, similar to our treatment of HIV infection.

ANGIOGENESIS AND NONMELANOMA SKIN CANCER

Basal and squamous cell carcinomas represent the most common skin cancers, affecting more than 1 million patients yearly in the United States. Although most of these tumors are curable through local excision and destructive modalities, a minority of these tumors exhibit aggressive and metastatic properties. These are most commonly seen in tumors that arise in transplant patients or in the setting of chronic inflammation, ie, carcinomas arising in scars, ulcers, and recessive dystrophic epidermolysis bullosa (RDEB). We have demonstrated that a significant number of squamous cell carcinomas arising in RDEB exhibit loss of p16ink4a, in contrast to the mutations in p53 most commonly seen in cutaneous nonmelanoma skin cancers [5,78]. We have previously demonstrated that p16ink4a-deficient tumors signal differently than mutant p53 tumors, with trends toward increased aggressiveness.

The major angiogenic factor in basal cell carcinoma is bFGF; in squamous cell carcinoma the major angiogenic factor is VEGF [79]. The reason for this difference remains unclear, but may explain why basal cell carcinoma is usually less aggressive than squamous cell carcinoma. Both tumors require an angiogenic switch between local inhibitors of angiogenesis (interferon alpha, IL-12) and local stimulators of angiogenesis (bFGF, VEGF) [80,81]. Angiogenesis inhibitors are already in use for the treatment of nonmelanoma skin cancers. These include imiquimod, which is approved by the Food and Drug Administration (FDA) for nonmelanoma skin cancers, as well as warts, which are also angiogenic. Imiquimod is a TLR7 agonist that induces local production of interferon. Other topical antiangiogenic agents include topical vitamin D, whereas systemic agents that have antiangiogenic activity include retinoids and tyrosine kinase inhibitors that inhibit VEGF, EGFR, and her2/neu (geftinib, herceptin, erlotinib, sunitinib, and so forth). However, these agents are probably likely to be ineffective as monotherapy because activation of oncogenic ras genes leads to resistance to these targeted therapies (Table 1) [82].

Kaposi's sarcoma (KS) has been a prime focus for angiogenesis inhibition. KS is thought to originate from HHV8 infection of lymphatic endothelial cells. Drugs that have demonstrated efficacy against KS include thalidomide, rapamycin, liposomal doxorubicin, and docetaxol, all of which have antiangiogenic activities [83–88]. Additive therapies that induce lytic replication of HHV8 in KS cells in combination with antiangiogenic agents, such as valproic acid and other HDAC inhibitors, may provide additional benefit in KS [89,90].

ANGIOGENESIS AND INFECTION

The host response to both acute and chronic infection requires angiogenesis. While it is important not to inhibit the host response to acute infection, chronic infection may require angiogenesis for maintenance. Most chronic infections result from intracellular colonization of bacteria, or adherence of bacteria to a foreign object, impairing bacterial clearance.

Bacterial infections associated with intracellular colonization include mycobacterial infections (leprosy, tuberculosis), syphilis (endothelial colonization), and bartonella (endothelial colonization). Each of these colonizations activates signaling abnormalities in the host cell to allow both persistence and maintenance. For example, bartonella infection induces rac activation and ang-2 production to mimic a hemangioma [66,67]. Increased angiogenesis is seen in lepromatous leprosy, in which an ineffective immune response, due in part to loss of interleukin-12 and other angiogenesis inhibitors, allows engorgement of cells into tumorlike masses [91]. We have recently shown that lepromatous leprosy is highly angiogenic, and that administration of angiogenesis inhibitors may shorten the duration of therapy needed to treat mycobacterial infections, such as leprosy and tuberculosis.

Chronic viral infections often induce angiogenesis through oncogenes. Human papillomavirus (HPV) contains two oncogenes that can impact angiogenesis. E6 binds p53 and E7 binds Rb. The action of either or both of these

Table 1
The most common angiogenesis stimulators

Angiogenesis stimulators	Description
Vascular endothelial growth factor (VEGF)	VEGF is a primary contributor to the growth of capillaries in a given network. In the presence of VEGF, endothelial cells will undergo angiogenesis. VEGF causes a large tyrosine kinase signaling cascade in endothelial cells. This cascade causes other factors to be produced and these factors stimulate proliferation (survival) via bFGF, migration via MMP and differentiation into mature blood vessels. The up-regulation of VEGF is the main operator in the physiological response during exercise. Muscle contraction increases the blood flow to the affected areas. This increased flow causes an increase in the mRNA production of VEGF receptors 1 and 2. This increase in receptors increases the signaling cascades related to angiogenesis.
Basic fibroblast growth factor (bFGF)	Basic fibroblast growth factor is a member of the fibroblast growth factor family. In normal tissue, basic fibroblast growth factor is present in basement membranes and in the subendothelial extracellular matrix of blood vessels. bFGF stays membrane-bound as long as there is no signal peptide. During both wound healing of normal tissues and tumor development, the action of heparan sulphate–degrading enzymes activates bFGF, thus mediating the formation of new blood vessels (angiogenesis).
Matrix metalloproteinase (MMP)	MMPs help degrade the proteins that keep the vessel walls solid. This proteolysis allows the endothelial cells to escape into the interstitial matrix as seen in sprouting angiogenesis. These enzymes are highly regulated during the vessel formation process because this destruction of the extracellular matrix would destroy the integrity of the microvasculature. MMP2 and MMP9 are the two proteinases linked to angiogenesis.
Cyclooxygenase-2–prostaglandin E$_2$ (COX2-PGE2)	COX-2 inhibitors are a class of nonsteroidal anti-inflammatory drugs (NSAIDs) that selectively block the COX-2 enzyme. This action impedes the production of the chemical messengers (prostaglandins) that cause the pain and swelling of arthritis inflammation. Being that COX-2 inhibitors selectively block the COX-2 enzyme and not the COX-1 enzyme, these drugs are uniquely different from traditional NSAIDs.
Platelet-derived growth factor (PDGF)	PDGF is a dimer that activates its signaling pathway by a ligand-induced receptor dimerization and autophosphorylation. PDGF has provided a market for protein receptor antagonists to treat disease. These antagonists include specific antibodies that target the molecule of interest.

genes is sufficient to increase angiogenesis. Epstein-Barr virus, which causes Burkitt's lymphoma, oral hairy leukoplakia, and leiomyosarcoma, expresses oncogenes such as LMP-1, which activate angiogenesis [40]. HHV8 also expresses an oncogenic G protein that induces angiogenesis.

Chronic infections resist immune clearance by several mechanisms. These include VEGF, which impairs dendritic cell maturation, secretion of immunosuppressive cytokines, such as IL-10, and decreased expression of antigen-presenting molecules. These may be controlled by similar pathways, such as phosphoinositol-3 kinase/Akt and reactive oxygen signaling. Blockade of these pathways may enhance clearance of chronic infection through angiogenesis inhibition and enhanced immune response.

ANGIOGENESIS INHIBITION—AN OVERVIEW
Most conditions in dermatology are characterized by excess angiogenesis. These include inflammatory processes such as psoriasis; atopic dermatitis; rosacea; acne; venous ulcers; neoplastic conditions, such as melanoma, nonmelanoma skin cancer, and benign neoplasia; and chronic infections. As part of routine dermatologic practice, we use angiogenesis inhibition often without recognizing it. Drugs already in use are tetracycline antibiotics, which inhibit the activity of matrix metalloproteinases; retinoids, which inhibit the synthesis of matrix metalloproteinases; interferon and interferon inducers (imiquimod); gentian violet, which inhibits NADPH oxidases; topical glucocorticoids; and TNF-α inhibitors/blockers. Drugs that are used in other specialties also affect cutaneous angiogenesis. These include statins, tyrosine kinase inhibitors, Avastin, and PPAR agonists. Finally, dietary supplements such as curcumin and tea polyphenols may systemically affect the angiogenic state of the patient. Knowledge of these basic mechanisms will enhance dermatologic therapy.

References
[1] Folkman J, Merler E, Abernathy C, et al. Isolation of a tumor factor responsible for angiogenesis. J Exp Med 1971;133:275–88.
[2] Fischer C, Jonckx B, Mazzone M, et al. Anti-PlGF inhibits growth of VEGF(R)-inhibitor-resistant tumors without affecting healthy vessels. Cell 2007;131:463–75.
[3] Arbiser JL. Angiogenesis and the skin: a primer. J Am Acad Dermatol 1996;34:486–97.
[4] Arbiser JL, Karalis K, Viswanathan A, et al. Corticotropin-releasing hormone stimulates angiogenesis and epithelial tumor growth in the skin. J Invest Dermatol 1999;113:838–42.
[5] Arbiser JL, Fine JD, Murrell D, et al. Basic fibroblast growth factor: a missing link between collagen VII, increased collagenase, and squamous cell carcinoma in recessive dystrophic epidermolysis bullosa. Mol Med 1998;4:191–5.
[6] Jin DK, Shido K, Kopp HG, et al. Cytokine-mediated deployment of SDF-1 induces revascularization through recruitment of CXCR4+ hemangiocytes. Nat Med 2006;12:557–67.
[7] Petit I, Jin D, Rafii S. The SDF-1-CXCR4 signaling pathway: a molecular hub modulating neo-angiogenesis. Trends Immunol 2007;28:299–307.
[8] Li S, Takeuchi F, Wang JA, et al. MCP-1 overexpressed in tuberous sclerosis lesions acts as a paracrine factor for tumor development. J Exp Med 2005;202:617–24.
[9] Lyden D, Young AZ, Zagzag D, et al. Id1 and Id3 are required for neurogenesis, angiogenesis and vascularization of tumour xenografts. Nature 1999;401:670–7.

[10] Sikder H, Huso DL, Zhang H, et al. Disruption of Id1 reveals major differences in angiogenesis between transplanted and autochthonous tumors. Cancer Cell 2003;4:291–9.

[11] Tanaka S, Mori M, Sakamoto Y, et al. Biologic significance of angiopoietin-2 expression in human hepatocellular carcinoma. J Clin Invest 1999;103:341–5.

[12] Kalomenidis I, Kollintza A, Sigala I, et al. Angiopoietin-2 levels are elevated in exudative pleural effusions. Chest 2006;129:1259–66.

[13] Hu B, Jarzynka MJ, Guo P, et al. Angiopoietin 2 induces glioma cell invasion by stimulating matrix metalloprotease 2 expression through the alphavbeta1 integrin and focal adhesion kinase signaling pathway. Cancer Res 2006;66:775–83.

[14] Berger M, Bergers G, Arnold B, et al. Regulator of G-protein signaling-5 induction in pericytes coincides with active vessel remodeling during neovascularization. Blood 2005;105:1094–101.

[15] Hirschi KK, Rohovsky SA, D'Amore PA. PDGF, TGF-beta, and heterotypic cell-cell interactions mediate endothelial cell-induced recruitment of 10T1/2 cells and their differentiation to a smooth muscle fate. J Cell Biol 1998;141:805–14.

[16] Daly C, Pasnikowski E, Burova E, et al. Angiopoietin-2 functions as an autocrine protective factor in stressed endothelial cells. Proc Natl Acad Sci U S A 2006;103:15491–6.

[17] Fiedler U, Reiss Y, Scharpfenecker M, et al. Angiopoietin-2 sensitizes endothelial cells to TNF-alpha and has a crucial role in the induction of inflammation. Nat Med 2006;12:235–9.

[18] Voskas D, Jones N, Van SP, et al. A cyclosporine-sensitive psoriasis-like disease produced in Tie2 transgenic mice. Am J Pathol 2005;166:843–55.

[19] Lind AJ, Wikstrom P, Granfors T, et al. Angiopoietin 2 expression is related to histological grade, vascular density, metastases, and outcome in prostate cancer. Prostate 2005;62:394–9.

[20] Thurston G, Wang Q, Baffert F, et al. Angiopoietin 1 causes vessel enlargement, without angiogenic sprouting, during a critical developmental period. Development 2005;132:3317–26.

[21] Kim I, Kim JH, Moon SO, et al. Angiopoietin-2 at high concentration can enhance endothelial cell survival through the phosphatidylinositol 3'-kinase/Akt signal transduction pathway. Oncogene 2000;19:4549–52.

[22] Hammes HP, Lin J, Wagner P, et al. Angiopoietin-2 causes pericyte dropout in the normal retina: evidence for involvement in diabetic retinopathy. Diabetes 2004;53:1104–10.

[23] Lee KH, Lawley TJ, Xu YL, et al. VCAM-1-, ELAM-1-, and ICAM-1-independent adhesion of melanoma cells to cultured human dermal microvascular endothelial cells. J Invest Dermatol 1992;98:79–85.

[24] Mattila P, Majuri ML, Mattila PS, et al. TNF alpha-induced expression of endothelial adhesion molecules, ICAM-1 and VCAM-1, is linked to protein kinase C activation. Scand J Immunol 1992;36:159–65.

[25] Ockenhouse CF, Tegoshi T, Maeno Y, et al. Human vascular endothelial cell adhesion receptors for Plasmodium falciparum-infected erythrocytes: roles for endothelial leukocyte adhesion molecule 1 and vascular cell adhesion molecule 1. J Exp Med 1992;176:1183–9.

[26] Houstis N, Rosen ED, Lander ES. Reactive oxygen species have a causal role in multiple forms of insulin resistance. Nature 2006;440:944–8.

[27] Lambeth JD. NOX enzymes and the biology of reactive oxygen. Nat Rev Immunol 2004;4:181–9.

[28] Babior BM, Curnutte JT. Chronic granulomatous disease—pieces of a cellular and molecular puzzle. Blood Rev 1987;1:215–8.

[29] Dinauer MC, Orkin SH, Brown R, et al. The glycoprotein encoded by the X-linked chronic granulomatous disease locus is a component of the neutrophil cytochrome b complex. Nature 1987;327:717–20.

[30] Bokoch GM, Zhao T. Regulation of the phagocyte NADPH oxidase by Rac GTPase. Antioxid Redox Signal 2006;8:1533–48.

[31] Lopes NH, Vasudevan SS, Gregg D, et al. Rac-dependent monocyte chemoattractant protein-1 production is induced by nutrient deprivation. Circ Res 2002;91:798–805.

[32] Chen XL, Zhang Q, Zhao R, et al. Superoxide, H2O2, and iron are required for TNF-alpha-induced MCP-1 gene expression in endothelial cells: role of Rac1 and NADPH oxidase. Am J Physiol Heart Circ Physiol 2004;286:H1001–7.

[33] Yu L, Zhen L, Dinauer MC. Biosynthesis of the phagocyte NADPH oxidase cytochrome b558. Role of heme incorporation and heterodimer formation in maturation and stability of gp91phox and p22phox subunits. J Biol Chem 1997;272:27288–94.

[34] Kwon J, Lee SR, Yang KS, et al. Reversible oxidation and inactivation of the tumor suppressor PTEN in cells stimulated with peptide growth factors. Proc Natl Acad Sci U S A 2004;101: 16419–24.

[35] Govindarajan B, Klafter R, Miller MS, et al. Reactive oxygen-induced carcinogenesis causes hypermethylation of p16(Ink4a) and activation of MAP kinase. Mol Med 2002;8:1–8.

[36] Shields JM, Thomas NE, Cregger M, et al. Lack of extracellular signal-regulated kinase mitogen-activated protein kinase signaling shows a new type of melanoma. Cancer Res 2007;67:1502–12.

[37] Fried L, Arbiser JL. The reactive oxygen-driven tumor: relevance to melanoma. Pigment Cell Melanoma Res 2008;21:117–22.

[38] Govindarajan B, Sligh JE, Vincent BJ, et al. Overexpression of Akt converts radial growth melanoma to vertical growth melanoma. J Clin Invest 2007;117:719–29.

[39] Perry BN, Govindarajan B, Bhandarkar SS, et al. Pharmacologic blockade of angiopoietin-2 is efficacious against model hemangiomas in mice. J Invest Dermatol 2006;126(10): 2316–22.

[40] Cerimele F, Battle T, Lynch R, et al. Reactive oxygen signaling and MAPK activation distinguish Epstein-Barr Virus (EBV)-positive versus EBV-negative Burkitt's lymphoma. Proc Natl Acad Sci U S A 2005;102:175–9.

[41] Bhandarkar SS, Mackelfresh J, Fried L, et al. Targeted therapy of oral hairy leukoplakia with gentian violet. J Am Acad Dermatol 2008;58:711–2.

[42] Arbiser JL, Grossman K, Kaye E, et al. Use of short-course class 1 topical glucocorticoid under occlusion for the rapid control of erythrodermic psoriasis. Arch Dermatol 1994;130:704–6.

[43] Braverman IM, Sibley J. Role of the microcirculation in the treatment and pathogenesis of psoriasis. J Invest Dermatol 1982;78:12–7.

[44] Malhotra R, Stenn KS, Fernandez LA, et al. Angiogenic properties of normal and psoriatic skin associate with epidermis, not dermis. Lab Invest 1989;61:162–5.

[45] Braverman IM, Sibley J. The response of psoriatic epidermis and microvessels to treatment with topical steroids and oral methotrexate. J Invest Dermatol 1985;85:584–6.

[46] Detmar M, Brown LF, Claffey KP, et al. Overexpression of vascular permeability factor/vascular endothelial growth factor and its receptors in psoriasis. J Exp Med 1994;180:1141–6.

[47] Kunstfeld R, Hirakawa S, Hong YK, et al. Induction of cutaneous delayed-type hypersensitivity reactions in VEGF-A transgenic mice results in chronic skin inflammation associated with persistent lymphatic hyperplasia. Blood 2004;104:1048–57.

[48] Wrone-Smith T, Nickoloff BJ. Dermal injection of immunocytes induces psoriasis. J Clin Invest 1996;98:1878–87.

[49] Nickoloff BJ, Xin H, Nestle FO, et al. The cytokine and chemokine network in psoriasis. Clin Dermatol 2007;25:568–73.

[50] Nickoloff BJ, Bonish BK, Marble DJ, et al. Lessons learned from psoriatic plaques concerning mechanisms of tissue repair, remodeling, and inflammation. J Investig Dermatol Symp Proc 2006;11:16–29.

[51] Zenz R, Eferl R, Kenner L, et al. Psoriasis-like skin disease and arthritis caused by inducible epidermal deletion of Jun proteins. Nature 2005;437:369–75.

[52] Ma HL, Liang S, Li J, et al. IL-22 is required for Th17 cell-mediated pathology in a mouse model of psoriasis-like skin inflammation. J Clin Invest 2008;118:597–607.

[53] Fitch E, Harper E, Skorcheva I, et al. Pathophysiology of psoriasis: recent advances on IL-23 and Th17 cytokines. Curr Rheumatol Rep 2007;9:461–7.

[54] Elder JT. IL-15 and psoriasis: another genetic link to Th17? J Invest Dermatol 2007;127: 2495–7.

[55] Li J, Chen X, Liu Z, et al. Expression of Th17 cytokines in skin lesions of patients with psoriasis. J Huazhong Univ Sci Technolog Med Sci 2007;27:330–2.

[56] Zheng Y, Danilenko DM, Valdez P, et al. Interleukin-22, a T(H)17 cytokine, mediates IL-23-induced dermal inflammation and acanthosis. Nature 2007;445:648–51.

[57] Zaba LC, Cardinale I, Gilleaudeau P, et al. Amelioration of epidermal hyperplasia by TNF inhibition is associated with reduced Th17 responses. J Exp Med 2007;204: 3183–94.

[58] Kimball AB, Gordon KB, Langley RG, et al. Safety and efficacy of ABT-874, a fully human interleukin 12/23 monoclonal antibody, in the treatment of moderate to severe chronic plaque psoriasis: results of a randomized, placebo-controlled, phase 2 trial. Arch Dermatol 2008;144:200–7.

[59] Gottlieb AB, Matheson RT, Lowe N, et al. A randomized trial of etanercept as monotherapy for psoriasis. Arch Dermatol 2003;139:1627–32.

[60] Tyring S, Gordon KB, Poulin Y, et al. Long-term safety and efficacy of 50 mg of etanercept twice weekly in patients with psoriasis. Arch Dermatol 2007;143:719–26.

[61] Arbiser JL, Govindarajan B, Battle TE, et al. Carbazole is a naturally occurring inhibitor of angiogenesis and inflammation isolated from antipsoriatic coal tar. J Invest Dermatol 2006;126:1396–402.

[62] Zheng Y, Niyonsaba F, Ushio H, et al. Cathelicidin LL-37 induces the generation of reactive oxygen species and release of human alpha-defensins from neutrophils. Br J Dermatol 2007;157:1124–31.

[63] Buchau AS, Gallo RL. Innate immunity and antimicrobial defense systems in psoriasis. Clin Dermatol 2007;25:616–24.

[64] Takahashi K, Mulliken JB, Kozakewich HP, et al. Cellular markers that distinguish the phases of hemangioma during infancy and childhood. J Clin Invest 1994;93:2357–64.

[65] Williams RL, Risau W, Zerwes HG, et al. Endothelioma cells expressing the polyoma middle T oncogene induce hemangiomas by host cell recruitment. Cell 1989;57:1053–63.

[66] Cerimele F, Brown LF, Bravo F, et al. Infectious angiogenesis: Bartonella bacilliformis infection results in endothelial production of angiopoetin-2 and epidermal production of vascular endothelial growth factor. Am J Pathol 2003;163:1321–7.

[67] Verma A, Ihler GM. Activation of Rac, Cdc42 and other downstream signalling molecules by Bartonella bacilliformis during entry into human endothelial cells. Cell Microbiol 2002;4:557–69.

[68] Yu Y, Varughese J, Brown LF, et al. Increased Tie2 expression, enhanced response to angiopoietin-1, and dysregulated angiopoietin-2 expression in hemangioma-derived endothelial cells. Am J Pathol 2001;159:2271–80.

[69] Chiller KG, Frieden IJ, Arbiser JL. Molecular pathogenesis of vascular anomalies: classification into three categories based upon clinical and biochemical characteristics. Lymphat Res Biol 2003;1:267–81.

[70] Perry B, Banyard J, McLaughlin ER, et al. AKT1 overexpression in endothelial cells leads to the development of cutaneous vascular malformations in vivo. Arch Dermatol 2007;143: 504–6.

[71] Shirazi F, Cohen C, Fried L, et al. Mammalian target of rapamycin (mTOR) is activated in cutaneous vascular malformations in vivo. Lymphat Res Biol 2007;5:233–6.

[72] Lawley LP, Cerimele F, Weiss SW, et al. Expression of Wilms tumor 1 gene distinguishes vascular malformations from proliferative endothelial lesions. Arch Dermatol 2005;141: 1297–300.

[73] Cohen C, Zavala-Pompa A, Sequeira JH, et al. Mitogen-actived protein kinase activation is an early event in melanoma progression. Clin Cancer Res 2002;8:3728–33.

[74] Govindarajan B, Bai X, Cohen C, et al. Malignant transformation of melanocytes to melanoma by constitutive activation of mitogen-activated protein kinase kinase (MAPKK) signaling. J Biol Chem 2003;278:9790–5.

[75] Eisen T, Ahmad T, Flaherty KT, et al. Sorafenib in advanced melanoma: a Phase II randomised discontinuation trial analysis. Br J Cancer 2006;95(5):581–6.

[76] Ratain MJ, Eisen T, Stadler WM, et al. Phase II placebo-controlled randomized discontinuation trial of sorafenib in patients with metastatic renal cell carcinoma. J Clin Oncol 2006;24:2505–12.

[77] Varker KA, Biber JE, Kefauver C, et al. A randomized phase 2 trial of bevacizumab with or without daily low-dose interferon alfa-2b in metastatic malignant melanoma. Ann Surg Oncol 2007;14:2367–76.

[78] Arbiser JL, Fan CY, Su X, et al. Involvement of p53 and p16 tumor suppressor genes in recessive dystrophic epidermolysis bullosa-associated squamous cell carcinoma. J Invest Dermatol 2004;123:788–90.

[79] Arbiser JL, Byers HR, Cohen C, et al. Altered basic fibroblast growth factor expression in common epidermal neoplasms: examination with in situ hybridization and immunohistochemistry. J Am Acad Dermatol 2000;42:973–7.

[80] Meeran SM, Katiyar S, Elmets CA, et al. Interleukin-12 deficiency is permissive for angiogenesis in UV radiation-induced skin tumors. Cancer Res 2007;67:3785–93.

[81] Yusuf N, Nasti TH, Long JA, et al. Protective role of Toll-like receptor 4 during the initiation stage of cutaneous chemical carcinogenesis. Cancer Res 2008;68:615–22.

[82] Arbiser JL. Why targeted therapy hasn't worked in advanced cancer. J Clin Invest 2007;117:2762–5.

[83] Kolhe N, Mamode N, Van der WJ, et al. Regression of post-transplant Kaposi's sarcoma using sirolimus. Int J Clin Pract 2006;60:1509–12.

[84] Campistol JM, Gutierrez-Dalmau A, Torregrosa JV. Conversion to sirolimus: a successful treatment for posttransplantation Kaposi's sarcoma. Transplantation 2004;77:760–2.

[85] Campistol JM, Schena FP. Kaposi's sarcoma in renal transplant recipients—the impact of proliferation signal inhibitors. Nephrol Dial Transplant 2007;22(Suppl 1):i17–22.

[86] Fife K, Howard MR, Gracie F, et al. Activity of thalidomide in AIDS-related Kaposi's sarcoma and correlation with HHV8 titre. Int J STD AIDS 1998;9:751–5.

[87] Cooley T, Henry D, Tonda M, et al. A randomized, double-blind study of pegylated liposomal doxorubicin for the treatment of AIDS-related Kaposi's sarcoma. Oncologist 2007;12: 114–23.

[88] Krown SE. Therapy of AIDS-associated Kaposi's sarcoma: targeting pathogenetic mechanisms. Hematol Oncol Clin North Am 2003;17:763–83.

[89] Shaw RN, Arbiser JL, Offermann MK. Valproic acid induces human herpesvirus 8 lytic gene expression in BCBL-1 cells. AIDS 2000;14:899–902.

[90] Klass CM, Krug LT, Pozharskaya VP, et al. The targeting of primary effusion lymphoma cells for apoptosis by inducing lytic replication of human herpesvirus 8 while blocking virus production. Blood 2005;105:4028–34.

[91] Bhandarkar SS, Cohen C, Kuruvila M, et al. Angiogenesis in cutaneous lesions of leprosy: implications for treatment. Arch Dermatol 2007;143:1527–9.

Uncommon Benign Infantile Vascular Tumors

Odile Enjolras, MD[a,*], Véronique Soupre, MD[a], Arnaud Picard, MD[a,b,c]

[a]Centre de Référence des Pathologies Neurovasculaires Malformatives, Site Trousseau, Pr MP Vazquez, Consultation des Angiomes, Service de Chirurgie Maxillo-Faciale et Chirurgie Plastique, AP-HP, Hôpital d'Enfants Armand Trousseau, Avenue du Dr Arnold Netter, Paris F-75012, France
[b]Université Pierre et Marie Curie-Paris 6, UFR de Médecine Pierre et Marie Curie, Paris F-75005, France
[c]Centre de Recherche des Cordeliers, UMRS 872 INSERM, équipe 5, Laboratoire de Biologie Oro-faciale et Pathologies, Paris F-75005, France

EDITORIAL COMMENT

There have been significant advances in the understanding of congenital vascular tumors during the past 2 decades. In this article, Dr. Odile Enjolras, an expert in the discipline of vascular anomalies, highlights this progress and shares her clinical experience. She updates the reader on the latest literature pertaining to congenital vascular tumors. She compares and contrasts the clinical, histologic, and radiologic characteristics of infantile hemangiomas and less common vascular tumors such as congenital hematomas, kaposiform hemangioendotheliomas, and tufted angiomas. She reviews the potentially life-threatening condition Kasabach-Merritt phenomenon and the multimodal approach to its management. Dr. Enjolras enhances this useful clinical information with photographs that clearly illustrate the heterogenous clinical presentations of these challenging tumors.

Amy Nopper, MD

Over the centuries, one single benign vascular tumor was recognized in infants: the hemangioma, also known as a "capillary," "lobular," or "cellular" hemangioma. It often was referred to as "cavernous" hemangioma, a somewhat misleading adjective because this term also was used for venous malformations. This lesion now is referred to as "infantile hemangioma." This common vascular tumor has a female:male predilection that ranges from 2.5 to 3:1 for minor lesions (about 80% of cases) to 9:1 for the most serious cases (such as posterior fossa anomalies, facial hemangioma, arterial anomalies [intra- and extracranial], aortic arch coarctation and cardiac congenital defects, eye abnormalities, and sternal malformations [PHACES]

Corresponding author. E-mail address: secretariat.enjolras@trs.aphp.fr (O. Enjolras).

0882-0880/08/$ – see front matter
doi:10.1016/j.yadr.2008.09.008

syndrome) [1]. Although hemangiomas are histologically benign tumors, infantile hemangiomas can have significant associated morbidity. Some infantile vascular tumors, including infantile hemangioma, may be locally extensive and aggressive, creating cosmetic and functional problems, and other, high-risk lesions may develop life-threatening complications. During the last 20 years, the complexity of the "hemangioma group" has been established, and the existence of other vascular tumors has been documented.

Congenital vascular tumors, fully grown in utero, had been reported occasionally and were included in the spectrum of hemangioma, but their clinical and pathologic differences and their distinctive postnatal course led to their being categorized separately as congenital hemangiomas. These lesions have a prenatal growth phase, as opposed to the postnatal proliferating phase of infantile hemangioma [2]. Then, because there are two divergent postnatal courses, congenital hemangiomas were divided into two subtypes: rapidly involuting congenital hemangioma (RICH) and noninvoluting congenital hemangioma (NICH) [2–4]. NICH also have been called "congenital nonprogressive hemangioma" [5].

With the HIV epidemic came the emergence of numerous, often atypical, cases of Kaposi sarcoma. Pathologists focused their attention on the recognition of other vascular tumors composed of spindled cells. These tumors had some pathologic resemblance to Kaposi sarcoma, but they were not linked to HIV contamination or to human herpesvirus 8 (HHV8) infection. In 1993, Zukerberg [6] described kaposiform hemangioendothelioma (KHE). This tumor also was identified in infants who had rare lethal visceral growths described as "hemangioma with Kaposi's sarcoma features" [7] and as "Kaposi-like infantile hemangioendothelioma" [8]. The label "KHE" has prevailed. KHE usually is a congenital or a neonatal neoplasm that often is complicated by a thrombocytopenic coagulopathy, the Kasabach-Merritt syndrome (KMS) or phenomenon (KMP). The primary tumor in KMS is either superficial or visceral. Working independently, two groups (the authors' group in Paris and the Vascular Anomalies Program in Boston) reached the same conclusion: two types of vascular tumors are able to develop into KMS/KHE and tufted angioma (TA). Infantile hemangioma is not implicated in this thrombocytopenic coagulopathy [9,10]. TA was described in 1989 in the English literature based on the distinctive pathologic distribution of the vascular lesions in skin [11], but TA has long been reported in the Japanese literature as "angioblastoma of Nakagawa." KHE should not be confused with another rare vascular tumor which is composed of spindle cells but is not linked to KMS and TA: the spindle cell hemangioendothelioma. Spindle cell hemangioendothelioma may be present at birth or develop in childhood or later; in some patients, spindle cell hemangioendothelioma is a component of the soft tissue lesions of Maffucci syndrome. Two other red vascular tumors, the hemangiopericytoma and infantile myofibromatosis, sometimes are mistaken for infantile hemangioma.

In the literature KMS, the transient hematologic and coagulopathic disorder occurring in infancy and childhood, which first was documented clearly by Kasabach and Merritt in the 1940s, sometimes is confused with the lifelong localized intravascular coagulopathy associated with venous malformations [12] or lymphatic–venous malformations or with the coagulopathy occurring with some malignancies such as angiosarcoma or fibrosarcoma. This inaccurate identification still persists in recent papers [13,14].

In summary, based on the classification of the International Society for the Study of Vascular Anomalies (ISSVA) [1], in addition to the common infantile hemangioma, the main group of benign vascular tumors includes a number of uncommon tumors: congenital hemangiomas of the RICH or NICH subtypes, KHE, and TA (Fig. 1). Other very rare vascular tumors are also differentiated with a name joining a descriptive feature to the label "hemangioma" or "hemangioendothelioma" (Box 1). This article reviews these less common infantile vascular tumors and discusses the distinguishing features that should differentiate these entities from the common infantile hemangioma. It also highlights clinical features that may help distinguish benign vascular tumors from the less common malignant congenital tumors, namely congenital fibrosarcoma and rhabdomyosarcoma, because these tumors can present a significant diagnostic challenge at birth or (in the case of a tumor with prominent vascularization) when detected prenatally.

UNCOMMON INFANTILE VASCULAR TUMORS
Congenital hemangiomas
Congenital hemangiomas are unusual tumors that, unlike infantile hemangiomas, have no female predominance. Congenital hemangiomas are fully grown in utero and do not have a postnatal growth phase. Infantile hemangioma, on the other hand, has a three-phase course with rapid postnatal growth over months, very slow involution over years, and an involuted stage, often with some sequelae. When a large infantile hemangioma is both superficial and deep, its superficial crimson islands usually are distributed irregularly over its deep component, and the surface is papillomatous or folded (Fig. 2). Congenital hemangiomas lack these characteristic clinical features.

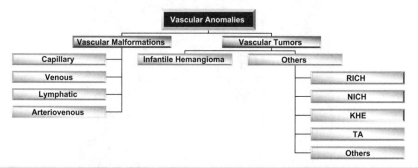

Fig. 1. The ISSVA classification. KHE, kaposiform hemangioendothelioma; NICH, noninvoluting congenital hemangioma; RICH, rapidly involuting congenital hemangioma; TA, tufted angioma.

Box 1: Other (often uncommon) vascular tumors

Hemangioendotheliomas

Spindle cell hemangioendothelioma (and Maffucci syndrome)

Retiform hemangioendothelioma

Epithelioid (or histiocytoid) hemangioendothelioma (or angiolymphoid hyperplasia with eosinophilia)—not a rare lesion

Composite hemangioendothelioma

Polymorphous hemangioendothelioma

Malignant endovascular papillary angioendothelioma (Dabska tumor)

Benign lymphangioendothelioma (acquired progressive lymphangioma)

Hemangiomas

Acquired elastotic hemangioma

Glomeruloid hemangioma

Targetoid hemosiderotic hemangioma (or hobnail hemangioma)

Microvenular hemangioma

Sinusoidal hemangioma

Lobular capillary hemangioma (pyogenic granuloma)—a common lesion

Sudoriparous angioma (eccrine angiomatous hamartoma)

Furthermore, complex developmental anomalies are associated with infantile hemangiomas and are known by acronymic descriptions. These anomalies include PHACES syndrome; the spinal dysraphism, anogenital, cutaneous, renal, and urologic anomalies, and angioma of lumbosacral localization (SACRAL)

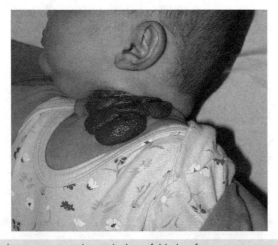

Fig. 2. Infantile hemangioma with a red, shiny, folded surface.

syndrome; and the perineal hemangioma, external genitalia malformations, lipomyelomeningocele, vesicorenal abnormalities, imperforate anus, and skin tag (PELVIS) syndrome. These complex developmental anomalies never have been reported in conjunction with congenital hemangiomas. Finally, unequivocal differences in the pathologic features of infantile hemangiomas and congenital hemangiomas solidified the distinction of the two tumor types as separate entities: on glucose transporter 1 (GLUT-1) staining, 100% of infantile hemangiomas are positive, and congenital hemangiomas are all negative (Box 2) [1].

Thus congenital hemangiomas clearly differ from the common infantile hemangioma based on clinical features, pathology, and immunophenotype [15]. Congenital hematomas are categorized further by two different outcomes observed after birth as either RICH, which regress within about 1 year after birth, or NICH, which persist indefinitely [4] Current evaluation of the tumor immunophenotype tries to explain potential clinical and pathologic links between RICH and NICH and between both these entities and infantile hemangioma [16]

Rapidly involuting congenital hemangiomas
RICH most often are located on a limb close to a joint (mainly knee, ankle, hip, or elbow), on the forehead, cheek, scalp, or around the ear. They also can develop on the occipital scalp or nape of the neck. They do not seem to occur in the centrofacial area as do focal infantile hemangioma. RICH appears as a large, round or oval, bulging tumor, usually with a smooth surface but

---

Box 2: The main characteristics of infantile hemangiomas

Initial presentation: at birth (possibly a pink or white macule or patch as a premonitory precursor) or shortly thereafter within first month of life

Sex predilection (F:M): 3:1 to 9:1 (depending on seriousness)

Skin involvement: superficial (strawberry mark), deep (subcutaneous), or both (mixed)

Distinctive configuration on the facial area: focal or segmental

Course: three-phase: proliferation, involution, sequelae (or restoration of normal skin)

Pathology:

Proliferating: dense lobules of capillaries with virtual lumen

Involuting: larger vessels

Sequelae, if any: fibrofatty residuum

Immunophenotype: "placental" immunophenotype of infantile hemangioma endothelial cells: GLUT-1+, Lewis Y Ag+, Fcγ RII (CD 32)+, merosin+

Complications: rapid extension/expansion, ulceration, visceral locations, cardiac failure, associated structural malformations (PHACES, PELVIS syndrome)

occasionally with an unevenly bossed presentation. Slight variants are noted (Fig. 3). The color of the surface ranges from pale pink to purple. Prominent telangiectasias often are seen on the surface of the RICH, and long telangiectasias sometimes are distributed in a radial arrangement. The center of the mass may be nodular or a have a linear central scar or necrotic area with or without crust. A subtle white ring or halo commonly encircles the mass. Spontaneous regression usually occurs in 6 to 14 months.

Because of the volume and vascularity of these tumors, RICH now are increasingly detected during prenatal ultrasound (US) investigations, usually during the third trimester but sometimes as early as the sixteenth week of gestation. A RICH appears as an exophytic, hypoechoic mass traversed by multiple compressible channels with a predominantly venous flow [17]. RICH have a solid homogeneous or heterogeneous aspect, close to placental echogenicity, with some venous lakes mimicking a cystic component, hemosiderin deposits, and small calcifications. Most of the heterogeneous aspect is related to vessels. If a RICH is noted on prenatal US, an antenatal MRI is recommended to define better the characteristics of the vascular tumor. Depending on the size, site, and vascularization of the tumor, a cesarean section may be indicated. Lesions may have a very fast flow during the prenatal period and appear less vascularized on postnatal US or MRI investigations. It is worth repeating an US and MRI at birth, particularly if there is a central necrotic area, to appraise further the risk of bleeding in case of large, fast-flow vessels located

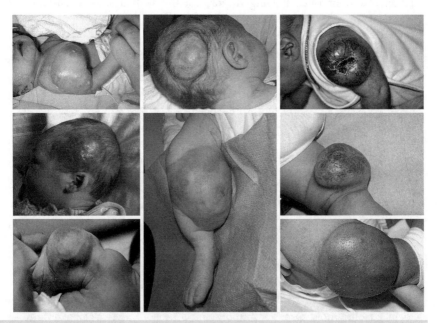

Fig. 3. Various presentations of rapidly involuting congenital hemangioma.

just underneath the damaged surface. On MRI, the tumor has intermediate signal intensity on T1 sequences and is hyperintense on T2 sequences. It enhances intensely after intravenous gadolinium administration; large vessels with rapid flow show linear tubular flow voids, principally in the periphery of the tumor and less frequently inside the mass. Angiographic findings are those of a fast-flow vascular anomaly with inhomogeneous parenchymal staining, direct arteriovenous shunts, arterial aneurysms, and also thrombi [18]. In the scalp area, bone flattening and even bone erosion, lytic changes, and intracranial invasion may occur (Fig. 4A, B). The pathologic features of a RICH include large and small lobules of vessels embedded in fibrosis, as well as extralobular vessels. Some vessels have a moderately plump endothelium; endothelial cells are negative for GLUT-1.

Occasionally, in some large RICH, a moderate thrombocytopenia with elevated D-dimer level and low fibrinogen is documented soon after birth. These alterations are transient and generally do not require treatment. By definition, a RICH is an auto-involuting tumor. After regression, however, some of these tumors leave cosmetically disturbing sequelae such as areas of lipoatrophy, excess wrinkled skin, or a slightly telangiectasic or pale bluish macule. At birth, when a wound exposes large vessels to erosion, the feasibility of early surgical excision is considered to avoid life-threatening hemorrhage [19].

Noninvoluting congenital hemangiomas
A NICH is less impressive at birth than a RICH. The tumor usually is flat, rarely bossed, and is round or oval in shape. The outer area is white (Fig. 5). The center varies from pinkish, with minor telangiectasia, to deep purple. The locations for NICH are similar to those of RICH: 43% occur in the head and neck, 38% in the limbs, and 19% in the trunk [3]. Prenatal US detects NICH less commonly than RICH. After birth, a NICH is fast-flow by

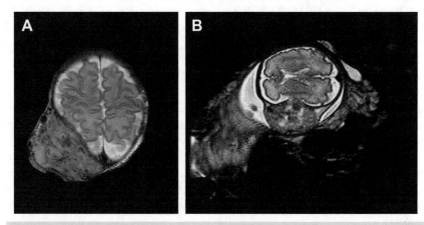

Fig. 4. (A) Postnatal MRI of a RICH on the scalp (axial spin-echoT2 image): heterogeneous tumor with bone flattening and erosion. (B) Prenatal MRI of a RICH of the scalp showing a large vault defect with the tumor coming in contact with the meninges.

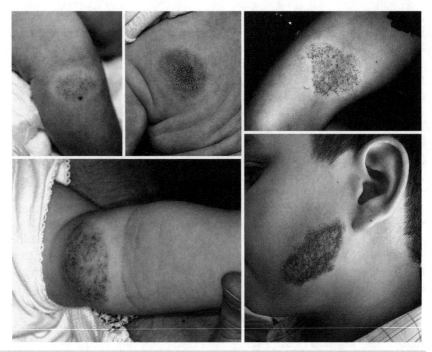

Fig. 5. Various presentations of noninvoluting congenital hemangioma.

US-Doppler evaluation, and it may reveal minor arteriovenous fistulas. On MRI, it appears isointense on T1 sequences, hyperintense on T2 sequences, and intensely enhanced after intravenous gadolinium administration.

The pathology of a NICH includes rather large lobules made of small capillaries lined by endothelial cells with hobnailed nuclei. Lobules are separated by an often dense fibrous tissue. In the center of the lobules, elongated thin-walled vessels and often a prominent stellate vessel are separated by fibrosis. Extralobular vessels are large, and this intralobular vascular component may be so prominent that, were it not for an occasional lobule, the pathologist might make the diagnosis of a vascular malformation (usually capillary-venous malformation) [3,4]. Calcifications may be seen also. Histologically, numerous alpha-actin positive cells are observed in the lobules. Endothelial cells lack immunoreactivity for GLUT-1 [4,5]. Pathologic features of NICH have been found in atypical large congenital vascular anomalies of the neck and shoulder area [1]. They create ill-defined, telangiectasic, large plaquelike lesions extending from the chin to the shoulders along the neck, with bluish, pale, irregular borders.

Unlike a RICH, a NICH never involutes. In contrast, some NICH show a moderate vascular increase during childhood, with equatorial draining veins developing in and around the lesion. The only therapeutic option is surgical excision. The authors have found arterial embolization alone to be of no help. When performed 24 hours before excision, arterial embolization helps prevent excess intraoperative bleeding in some large NICH with arteriovenous fistulas detected by Doppler US.

Missing links?
RICH and NICH may be part of a same spectrum [20]. The authors base this hypothesis on a number of clinical and histopathologic observations. In the authors' experience, large RICH shrink only partially in about 30% of affected infants (unpublished data). These RICH leave a residual tumor, the pattern of which suggests a NICH. Some commonalities are found on radiologic imaging and on pathology samples. With the improvement in prenatal US and Doppler evaluations, the onset of prenatal regression of large intrauterine tumors of the RICH type has been documented in some fetuses during the third trimester of gestation. The current hypothesis is that NICH could be the end point of the in utero involution of a RICH.

Some infants who have a RICH or a NICH at birth develop a typical GLUT-1–positive infantile hemangioma on another cutaneous area in the postnatal period. This finding suggests that RICH, NICH, and infantile hemangioma might be part of a common spectrum of vascular tumors, despite their different clinical courses and distinct cellular immunophenotypes. The authors emphasize again, however, that no structural malformations (PHACES or other such syndromes) have been reported in association with RICH and NICH. Interestingly, although it was long thought that congenital hemangiomas were exclusively cutaneous tumors, an infantile auto-involuting solitary liver tumor with negative GLUT-1 expression has been categorized as a considered a liver RICH [20,21].

Some cellular phenotypic markers indicate molecular evidence for a relationship between congenital hemangiomas and infantile hemangiomas. Insulin-like growth factor-2 (IGF-2) was expressed strongly in infantile hemangioma and correlated with the level of expression of vascular epithelial growth factor receptor 2 (VEGF-R2) [22]. IGF-2 also was detected in RICH and NICH, although IGF-2 mRNA transcript levels were low, similar to levels observed in the late stage of involuting infantile hemangioma [16]. On the other hand, increased expression of membrane-associated fms-like tyrosine kinase-1 receptor (FLT-1)/VEGF-R1 mRNA was found in RICH and NICH; levels were higher in congenital hemangiomas than in proliferating, involuting, or involuted infantile hemangioma and were comparable with those observed in full-term human placenta [16]. These findings provide molecular evidence for a close biologic relationship between the two fetal vascular tumors RICH and NICH. Hence, the low levels of membrane-associated FLT-1 in infantile hemangioma prompt the speculation that the regulation and function of this VEGF receptor are altered in common infantile hemangioma.

Kaposiform hemangioendothelioma
KHE is a rare and locally aggressive vascular tumor involving superficial or deep soft tissues and, rarely, bones. This tumor was long referred to as an

"hemangioma." It can occur at any age but generally is congenital or acquired during infancy or childhood; cases first manifesting in adults seem to be uncommon [23]. There is no female predominance, as seen in true infantile hemangioma. The clinical course often is protracted as the tumor expands slowly and covers large areas of skin. Cases developing over decades, from infancy into adulthood, have been observed [24]. In infants, when KHE is complicated by the thrombocytopenic coagulopathy KMS, the clinical aspect of the tumor changes suddenly [10]. The term "hemangioendothelioma" is somewhat confusing, because it suggests a borderline malignancy. Although KHE has been found in regional lymph nodes [9,25], distant metastases have not been reported. The tumor becomes life threatening only if KMS engrafts on it, because of potentially fatal hemorrhagic, infectious, or cardiac complications and iatrogenic adverse effects. Nevertheless, even without KMS, KHE can cause significant local morbidity [23].

In most patients, KHE is a single or regional tumor [24]. Infrequently, a multifocal onset has been described [26,27]. Cutaneous patterns vary (Fig. 6). Color ranges from scarlet to purple. The lesion is infiltrative and plaquelike or nodular. The surface often is smooth and shiny but may be thick like an orange rind. Rarely, a full-limb massive and diffuse infiltration occurs. One reported congenital case was especially puzzling: an infant had multifocal, red-bluish nodules scattered over the head, extremities, and trunk [27].

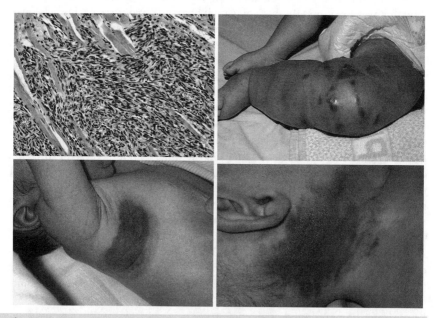

Fig. 6. Various presentations of kaposiform hemangioendothelioma (*top right, bottom left and right*). H&S original magnification × 10 (*top left*).

MRI demonstrates an ill-defined dense lesion crossing tissue planes with stranding of subcutaneous fat. The tumor is hyperintense on T2 sequences with flow voids representing rapid-flowing feeding and draining vessels [28]. Deep retroperitoneal KHE (the most common visceral location) creates symptoms of compression. An abdominal compartment syndrome may develop because of hemorrhage. KHE in the mediastinum may induce hemothorax and acute respiratory distress [29]. KHE also can affect muscles. Bones are rarely involved; pure bony KHE produces multifocal lytic lesions [24,26]. Lesions extending from the soft tissues to bones, creating bony erosion and cortical destruction, simulate a malignancy on radiologic imaging [30]. Although destructive, the course of the bony involvement by KHE is benign. Nevertheless, fractures occur, and, rarely, amputation of a limb has been indicated [24]. Unusual cases of hemorrhagic KHE associated with non-immune hydrops fetalis and intrauterine fetal death have been reported [31,32].

Biopsy is mandatory in all situations to confirm the correct diagnosis. The microscopic features of KHE include a dense cellularity composed of spindled cells creating large, interconnecting nodules and sheets separated by fibrous tissue [6,8,24]. Microthrombi and microhemorrhages are common; mitoses are rare. Slitlike lumina reminiscent of Kaposi sarcoma are noted. The cellular lobules deeply infiltrate the dermis, subcutis, and muscles in superficial KHE and mediastinum or retroperitoneum and muscles in visceral KHE. Endothelial cells lining more mature vessels at the periphery of the lobules stain for von Willebrand's factor and *Ulex europaeus*, whereas perithelial cells stain for smooth muscle actin [6]. The spindled cells in the tumor do not stain for *Ulex europaeus* or von Willebrand's factor. They stain diffusely for common endothelial markers CD31 and CD34 [33]. In some areas, clusters of rounded epithelioid endothelial cells containing hemosiderin granules are observed. Glomeruloid islands are present in the central portion of lobules, and it was hypothesized that the epithelioid and glomeruloid islands might represent areas in which platelet trapping occurs when KMS complicates a KHE [25,33]. Small and large lymphatic channels are seen [6,9,25,34]; they may be either prominent or inconspicuous. Zukerberg and colleagues [6] first described cases of KHE that developed on a lymphatic malformation (called "lymphangiomatosis") in patients without further KMS. A large pathologic study highlighted the lymphatic abnormalities possibly extending beyond the tumor nodules, suggesting that the lymphatic anomaly represents an intrinsic part of the lesion [25]. Immunoreaction with D2-40, a selective marker of lymphatic endothelium, was demonstrated on the lymphatic vessels adjacent to the lobules and on 70% to 90% of the large spindled cells [33]. Vessels in KHE strongly express VEGFR3 [34]. GLUT-1 and Lewis Y antigen (LeY) staining are negative, helping differentiate KHE from infantile hemangioma. Finally, there has been no evidence of HHV8 infection in association with KHE [35], and HHV8 transcripts were not identified in KHE lesions [25]. Cutaneous, noncoagulopathic KHE and KHE with KMS are similar with regard to sex ratio, age at onset, appearance, imaging findings, and pathology.

Treatment of KHE without KMS is disappointing; the lesion rarely involutes completely even when the medical treatment has some effectiveness. No single medical treatment (including systemic corticosteroids, interferon alpha, vincristine, or thalidomide) results in a fully satisfactory outcome. When KMS develops, treatment is lifesaving. Margins of KHE often are poorly defined, so complete excision is seldom possible.

Tufted angioma

TA was described by Wilson Jones in 1989 [11], but it has been reported in the Japanese literature as "angioblastoma of Nakagawa" since 1949. More recent papers underscore the similarity of TA and KHE [36–38]. As in KHE, the definitive diagnosis of TA relies on histologic characteristics. Both sexes are equally affected. Skin lesions in TA often are clinically indiscernible from KHE. Various presentations have been reported [39], including a red stain; multiple ill-defined pink to red macules (often, in fact, a single lesion that is partly superficial with visible islands and partly hidden because of a deep cutaneous location); a red, homogeneous plaque, possibly with lanuginous hairiness and sometimes focal hyperhydrosis [40]; coalescent red papules on a pink macular stain; a solitary infiltrative plaque with concentric rims, ranging in color from deep purple in the center to pink at the edge; a bulging lump; or a massive diffuse infiltration (Fig. 7). Lesions develop anywhere on the skin, including the face and neck.

TA most often is congenital (15%) or appears in early childhood; it develops before 1 year of age in 50% of patients and before 10 years of age in 80% [11]. Adult onset is possible. Congenital cases sometimes regress spontaneously [41–43]. Ishikawa [44] reported on 27 children in the Japanese and non-Japanese literature, plus a personal patient, whose TA regressed spontaneously in less than 2 years. Most TA persist, however. The growth is slow. The lesions vary slightly in size and shape over the years. Patients often experience episodes of local pain that can be soothed by aspirin. KMS may complicate a TA that is congenital or of early onset within the first weeks of life [45], but apparently this complication occurs less frequently with TA than with KHE. Some lesions become fibrous and stiff over the years [46,47]. In one of the authors' cases, a congenital TA of the ankle followed from birth to 23 years, the sclerosing lesion progressed from skin to joint and bone, creating pain and considerable functional difficulties (O. Enjolras, unpublished data).

The authors have found it difficult to distinguish some neonatal cases of plaque-type TA with a large bluish rim from some cases of NICH. The pathology helps differentiate the two. In TA, small tufts of capillaries in a cannonball arrangement extend throughout the dermis, deep to the hypodermis and subcutis. These capillary tufts are irregularly sized and are surrounded by a cleftlike semilunar empty vascular space in close contact with the lobule. Bloodless lymphatic spaces, some with valves, are seen in the dermis. Fibrosis surrounds the capillary tufts. Fibrosis is particularly dense in residual TA after KMS. Cells in the tufts stain weakly for factor VIII–related antigen and strongly for CD34 [37]. Numerous cells are labeled with α-smooth muscle actin. Immunostaining

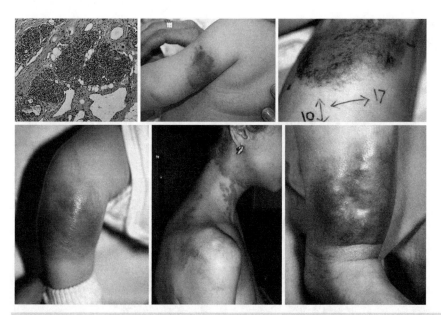

Fig. 7. Various presentations of tufted angioma (*top middle and right, bottom row*). H&S original magnification × 25 (*top left*).

for GLUT-1, the marker for infantile hemangioma, is negative. Some biopsy samples show concurrent features of TA and KHE, with rather large lobules and some spindling of the cellular component, supporting the hypothesis that TA and KHE belong to a single entity [34,47,48]. D2-40 immunostaining of lymphatic channels gave different results in TA and KHE, suggesting that they may reflect two steps in the development of a single entity [48].

As in noncoagulopathic KHE, treatment of TA without KMS often is unsatisfactory. High-dosage oral corticosteroids, interferon alpha, or vincristine may result in some improvement, but complete cure is improbable. Flash-lamp pulsed dye laser (FPDL) induced increased growth in two of the authors' adult cases, both of which were longstanding large pinkish plaque-type TA persisting from infancy (unpublished data). Occasionally, however, FPDL has been reported to be effective. Depending upon the size and site of the TA, surgical excision may be a therapeutic option.

The Kasabach-Merritt syndrome or phenomenon

KMS, a life-threatening complication, is defined by a profound thrombocytopenia and stigmata of coagulopathy including high D-dimers and low fibrinogen levels, engrafting on a pre-existing infantile vascular tumor. Platelet trapping is demonstrated in the tumor. Clinically, the pre-existing lesion suddenly increases in size. It becomes tense, purple, ecchymotic (Fig. 8), warm, and painful, while the platelet count drops rapidly. Risks of KMS include bleeding superficially or within the viscera (intracranial, abdominal, or thoracic),

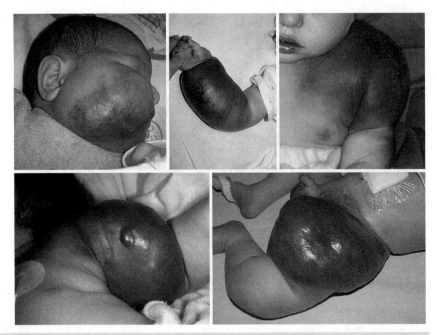

Fig. 8. Various presentations of Kasabach Merritt syndrome.

anemia, cardiac overload, and secondary infection in cases with ulceration of the fragile surface of the tumor.

The tumor can be discovered in utero, where it appears as a solid hypervascularized mass, more extensive and less delineated than a RICH. Large dilated vessels account for some of the heterogeneous appearance on US and MRI. There is a high risk of congestive heart failure or hydrops fetalis. These hemodynamic complications are the consequence of both the high flow with arteriovenous shunting and the severe anemia caused by KMS intralesional bleeding. In one of the authors' patients, the tumor was detected first in the neck during the fourth month of gestation. In congenital KMS, neonatal complications including severe anemia, intracranial hemorrhage, and cardiac failure are potentially lethal within a few days of birth [49].

Analyzing 16 biopsies from a group of 22 patients who had KMS and later 30 biopsies available for 26 of 41 patients who had KMS, the authors concluded that two types of tumors are linked to KMS: KHE and TA. Infantile hemangioma is not implicated [9,34]. Currently, GLUT-1 staining is absolutely indispensable in the pathologic assessment of the biopsy of a patient who has KMS to avoid a misdiagnosis of infantile hemangioma, as occurred in one report when the evaluation was based only on morphologic criteria [50].

The authors [9,34] have observed that

1. The tumor was evident at birth in more than 50% of cases, and there was no female preponderance.

2. When KMS develops in the superficial soft tissues, skin, and muscles, there is no difference in clinical severity or biologic behavior when it engrafts on KHE or TA.
3. Visceral, thoracic, or abdominal KMS had predominantly histologic features of KHE.
4. In some patients, KHE and TA co-existed in the same tumor pathology sample, a finding often noticed in cutaneous locations [41], but only one report points to the coexistence of KHE and TA in a retroperitoneal KHE with KMS [51].
5. Areas of pure lymphatic malformation not intermingled with the spindled cellular component could be found in some pathologic samples.
6. TA was two times more frequent than KHE in cutaneous residual lesions.
7. The lowest platelet count the authors observed was 3000 platelets/mm^3, and the lowest fibrinogen level was 0.2 g/L. During the acute phase, D-dimer levels were high, and soluble complexes of fibrin split products were present to varying degrees.

In a series of 15 biopsy samples of KMS tumors, the authors found features of KHE in 8 patients and features of TA in 5 patients. Two patients had a mainly lymphatic anomaly with slitlike or larger lymphatic vessels lined by thin endothelial cells or presented with a muscular media and valves consistent with lymphatic veins. Uptake of platelets within the tumor was demonstrated by various techniques [52]. Imaging studies often are difficult to evaluate. MRI usually shows a diffuse mass, isointense to muscle on T1 sequences, enhancing after gadolinium injection, and hyper-intense on T2 sequences, with poorly defined margins, prominent peripheral vessels, and homogenous signal abnormalities in most cases, although nonhomogeneous aspects could result from hemosiderin deposits [10].

Treatment of KMP is an emergency when the thrombocytopenia is profound because of a risk of visceral bleeding. Platelet counts as low as 10,000 to 15,000/mm^3 commonly are well tolerated without bleeding for months to years, however. It is noteworthy that platelet infusion amplifies the KM phenomenon. The platelets are consumed quickly inside the tumor, with a short half-life of 1 to 24 hours [53]. After platelet infusion, the lesion becomes more tense, shiny, and purple. Swelling and pain increase along with the risk of visceral hemorrhage risk. Unless the child is actively bleeding, platelets are of no help in the management of KMS, as illustrated by the patient reported by Henley [54] who received 6622 platelet concentrates over 19 months! Platelets are indicated only when a biopsy or excision of the entire tumor is planned. In these cases, platelets must be delivered immediately before the operative procedure [53]. A selective arterial embolization performed a maximum of 24 to 48 hours before surgery can be valuable in decreasing the risk of intraoperative hemorrhage. Occasionally, therapeutic embolization alone was curative. Surgical excision, when technically feasible, immediately cures the hematologic disorder and coagulopathy [55,56]. Surgery rarely is a realistic option, however, because of the size and/or site of the lesion. Thus, medical treatment is undertaken. Monotherapy or bi-modal therapy is advised first to minimize the risk of severe iatrogenic complications, which have caused death in some patients.

The goal of the treatment is first to control the biologic anomalies and then to induce involution of the tumor [57]. As underscored by Blei [58], "no uniformly successful sequence of therapies" can be recommended. Medical treatments include oral corticosteroids (prednisone, 2–5 mg/kg/d, or betamethasone, 0.2 mg/kg/d) or intravenous megadoses of corticosteroids (rarely effective alone), vincristine (1 mg/m^2 by weekly intravenous infusion) alone or with corticosteroids [59], and interferon alpha-2a or alpha-2b (3 million units/m^2/ d subcutaneously) [60–63]. In a subset of patients, an anti–platelet-aggregation treatment combining ticlopidine and aspirin (each, 10 mg/kg/d) was effective [34,64]. In a small number of patients, improvement was reported with other anti–platelet-aggregation drugs (pentoxifylline [65,66], dipyridamole) or antifibrinolytic agents (epsilon-aminocaproic acid or tranexamic acid), usually in combination with either corticosteroids or radiation therapy. Multimodal medical management, simultaneously or as a stepwise regimen, may be necessary for life-threatening cases of KMP. Regimens that have been used include interferon alpha and cyclophosphamide [58]; cyclophosphamide, vincristine, and actinomycin D [67]; interferon alpha and radiotherapy [68]; and corticosteroids, dipyridamole, interferon alpha 2b, and vincristine [62]. A compressive bandage is useful for lesions on the limbs and trunk [61]. It must not be wrapped too tightly to avoid injuring the fragile skin; even small wounds carry a risk of secondary infection and rapidly spreading sepsis because of the background of edema, necrosis, and thrombi. Radiotherapy has been an effective option, often in association with a medical treatment [68–70], but because of the risk of radiation-related complications, specifically long-term diverse malignancies, radiotherapy is considered only for medically uncontrollable situations that cannot be managed by excision or arterial embolization.

The treatment of KMS is discontinued when hematologic alterations normalize and remain stable, regardless of the tumor size. In fact, the tumor may still be rather large and bulging, but its color has faded, and the ecchymotic or inflammatory hue is no longer present. The tumor will continue to shrink over months. Finally, a more or less prominent residuum will be left. In a group of 41 patients, the most common cutaneous residual aspect was a pseudo port-wine stain (in 68% of patients), followed by a sclerodermiform infiltration (in 20%) or telangiectasia and swelling (in 12%) [34]. In all cases biopsy revealed a residual tumor, mostly a TA pattern. Fibrous sequelae also occurred in muscles and joints, impairing mobility. When trunk paravertebral muscles were involved, patients developed scoliosis. Recurrence of KMS in adolescents or adults is rare (one of the authors' unpublished cases has recurred at 15 years, and the patient's profound thrombocytopenia has been uncontrolled despite the use of varied chemotherapeutic agents).

SUMMARY

Significant progress in the diagnosis of infantile vascular tumors has been achieved during the past 2 decades because of improvements in the recognition of clinical characteristics, radiologic features, and histopathologic analysis, as well as the discovery of important immunophenotypic markers such as GLUT-1. These recent advances make it possible to define more clearly the distinct clinical entities with their variable prognoses and to improve the management of lesions that, although histologically benign, infrequently may be lethal because of their invasive potential.

References

[1] Enjolras O, Wassef M, Chapot R. A color atlas of vascular tumors and vascular malformations. New York: Cambridge University Press; 2007.

[2] Boon L, Enjolras O, Mulliken JB. Congenital hemangioma; evidence for accelerated involution. J Pediatr 1996;128(3):329–35.

[3] Enjolras O, Boon LM, Kozakewich HP, et al. Non-involuting congenital hemangioma: a rare cutaneous vascular anomaly. Plast Reconstr Surg 2001;107(7):1647–54.

[4] Berenguer B, Mulliken JB, Enjolras O, et al. Rapidly involuting congenital hemangioma: clinical and histopathologic features. Pediatr Dev Pathol 2003;6(6):495–510.

[5] North PE, Waner M, James CA, et al. Congenital nonprogressive hemangioma. A distinct clinicopathologic entity unlike infantile hemangioma. Arch Dermatol 2001;137(12):1607–20.

[6] Zukerberg LR, Nickoloff BJ, Weiss SW. Kaposiform hemangioendothelioma of infancy and childhood: an aggressive neoplasm associated with Kasabach-Merritt syndrome and lymphangiomatoses. Am J Surg Pathol 1993;17(4):321–8.

[7] Niedt GW, Greco A, Wieczorek R, et al. Hemangioma with Kaposi's sarcoma-like features, report of two cases. Pediatr Pathol 1989;9(5):567–75.

[8] Tsang WYW, Chan JKC. Kaposi-like infantile hemangioendothelioma. Am J Surg Pathol 1991;15(10):982–9.

[9] Enjolras O, Wassef M, Mazoyer E, et al. Infants with do not have "true" hemangioma. J Pediatr 1997;130(4):631–40.

[10] Sarkar M, Mulliken JB, Kozakewich HP, et al. Thrombocytopenic coagulopathy (Kasabach-Merritt phenomenon) is associated with kaposiform hemangioendothelioma and not with common infantile hemangioma. Plast Reconstr Surg 1997;100(6):1377–86.

[11] Wilson-Jones E, Orkin M. Tufted angioma (angioblastoma): a benign progressive angioma, not to be confused with Kaposi's sarcoma or low-grade angiosarcoma. J Am Acad Dermatol 1989;20:214–25.

[12] Mazoyer E, Enjolras O, Bisdorff A, et al. Coagulation disorders in patients with venous malformation of limbs and trunk. A study in 118 patients. Arch Dermatol, in press.

[13] Salameh F, Henig I, Bar-Shalom R, et al. Metastatic angiosarcoma of the scalp causing Kasabach-Merritt syndrome. Am J Med Sci 2007;333(5):293–5.

[14] Malagari K, Alexopoulou E, Dourakis S, et al. Transarterial embolization of liver hemangiomas associated with Kasabach-Merritt syndrome: a case report. Acta Radiol 2007;48(6):608–12.

[15] Krol A, MacArthur CJ. Congenital hemangiomas. Rapidly involuting and noninvoluting congenital hemangiomas. Arch Facial Plast Surg 2005;7(5):307–11.

[16] Picard A, Boscolo E, Khan ZA, et al. IGF-2 and FLT-1/VEGF-R1 mRNA levels reveals distinctions and similarities between congenital and common infantile hemangioma. Pediatr Res 2008;63(3):263–7.

[17] Rogers M, Lam A, Fischer G. Sonographic findings in a series of RICH. Pediatr Dermatol 2002;19(1):5–11.

[18] Konez O, Burrows PE, Mulliken JB, et al. Angiographic features of rapidly involuting congenital hemangioma (RICH). Pediatr Radiol 2002;33(1):15–9.

[19] Baselga E, Cordisco MR, Garzon M, et al. Rapidly involuting congenital haemangioma associated with transient thrombocytopenia and coagulopathy: a case series. Br J Dermatol 2008;158(6):1363–70.

[20] Kassarjian A, Zurakowski D, Dubois J, et al. Infantile hepatic hemangiomas: clinical and imaging findings and their correlation with therapy. AJR 2004;182(3):785–95.

[21] Christison-Lagay E, Burrows PE, Alomari A, et al. Hepatic hemangiomas: subtype classification and development of a clinical practice algorithm and registry. J Pediatr Surg 2007;42: 62–8.

[22] Ritter MR, Dorrell MI, Edmonds J, et al. Insulin-like growth factor 2 and potential regulators of hemangioma growth and involution identified by large-scale expression analysis. Proc Natl Acad Sci U S A 2002;99:7455–60.

[23] Cooper JG, Edwards SL, Holmes JD. Kaposiform hemangioendothelioma: case report and review of the literature. Br J Plast Surg 2002;55(2):163–5.

[24] Mac-Moune Lai F, To KF, Choi PC, et al. Kaposiform hemangioendothelioma: five patients with cutaneous lesion and long follow-up. Mod Pathol 2001;14(11):1087–92.

[25] Lyons LL, North PE, Mac-Moune Lai F, et al. Kaposiform hemangioendothelioma: a study of 33 cases emphasizing its pathologic, immunophenotypic and biologic uniqueness from juvenile hemangioma. Am J Surg Pathol 2004;28(5):559–68.

[26] Deraedt K, Vander Poorten V, Van Geet C, et al. Multifocal kaposiform hemangioendothelioma. Virchows Arch 2006;448(6):843–6.

[27] Gianotti R, Gelmetti C, Alessi E. Congenital cutaneous multifocal kaposiform hemangioendothelioma. Am J Dermatopathol 1999;21(6):557–61.

[28] Gruman A, Liang MG, Mulliken JB, et al. Kaposiform hemangioendothelioma without Kasabach-Merritt phenomenon. J Am Acad Dermatol 2005;52(4):616–22.

[29] Iwami D, Shimaoka S, Mochizuki I, et al. Kaposiform hemangioendothelioma of the mediastinum in a 7-month old boy: a case report. J Pediatr Surg 2006;41(8):1486–8.

[30] Lalaji TA, Haller JO, Burgess RJ. A case of head and neck kaposiform hemangioendothelioma simulating a malignancy on imaging. Pediatr Radiol 2001;31(12):876–8.

[31] Anai T, Miyakawa I, Ohki H, et al. Hydrops fetalis caused by Kasabach-Merritt syndrome. Acta Paediatr Jpn 1992;34(3):324–7.

[32] Martinez AE, Robinson MJ, Alexis JB. Kaposiform hemangioendothelioma associated with nonimmune fetal hydrops. Arch Pathol Lab Med 2004;128(6):678–81.

[33] Debelenko LV, Perez-Atayde AR, Mulliken JB, et al. D2-40 immunohistochemical analysis of pediatric vascular tumors reveals positivity in kaposiform hemangioendothelioma. Mod Pathol 2005;18(11):1454–60.

[34] Enjolras O, Mulliken JB, Wassef M, et al. Residual lesions after Kasabach-Merritt phenomenon in 41 patients. J Am Acad Dermatol 2000;42(2):225–35.

[35] Vin-Christian K, McCalmont TH, Frieden IJ. Kaposiform hemangioendothelioma. An aggressive, locally invasive vascular tumor that can mimic hemangioma of infancy. Arch Dermatol 1997;133(12):1573–8.

[36] Kh Cho, Sim SH, Park KC, et al. Angioblastoma (Nakagawa): is it the same as tufted angioma? Clin Exp Dermatol 1991;16(2):110–3.

[37] Okada E, Tamura A, Ishikawa O, et al. Tufted angioma (angioblastoma), case report and review of 41 cases in the Japanese literature. Clin Exp Dermatol 2000;25(8): 627–30.

[38] Igarashi M, Oh-I T, Koga M. The relationship between angioblastoma (Nakagawa) and tufted angioma. J Dermatol 2000;27(8):537–42.

[39] Herron MD, Coffin CM, Vanderhooft SL. Tufted angiomas: variability of the clinical morphology. Pediatr Dermatol 2002;19(5):394–401.

[40] Mulliken JB, Enjolras O. Congenital hemangiomas and infantile hemangioma: missing links. J Am Acad Dermatol 2004;50(6):875–82.

[41] Lam WY, Mac-Moune Lai F, Look CN, et al. Tufted angioma with complete regression. J Cutan Pathol 1994;21(5):461–6.

[42] Satter EK, Graham BS, Gibbs NF. Congenital tufted angioma. Pediatr Dermatol 2002;19(5):445–7.

[43] Browning J, Frieden IJ, Baselga E, et al. Congenital self-regressing tufted angioma. Arch Dermatol 2006;142(6):749–51.

[44] Ishikawa K, Hatano Y, Ichikawa H, et al. The spontaneous regression of tufted angioma. A case of regression after two recurrences and a review of 27 cases reported in the literature. Dermatology 2005;210(4):346–8.

[45] Enjolras O, Wassef M, Dosquet C, et al. Syndrome de Kasabach-Merritt sur angiome en touffes congénital. Ann Dermatol Venereol 1998;125(4):257–60.

[46] Catteau B, Enjolras O, Delaporte E, et al. Angiome en touffes sclerosant. A propos de 4 observations aux membres inférieurs. Ann Dermatol Venereol 1998;125(10):682–7.

[47] Chu CY, Hsiao CH, Chiu HC. Transformation between kaposiform hemangioendothelioma and tufted angioma. Dermatology 2003;206(4):334–7.

[48] Arai E, Kuramachi A, Tsuchida T, et al. Usefulness of D2-40 immunochemistry for differentiation between kaposiform hemangioendothelioma and tufted angioma. J Cutan Pathol 2006;33(7):492–7.

[49] Raman S, Ramanujam T, Lim CT. Prenatal diagnosis of an extensive haemangioma of the fetal leg. J Obstet Gynaecol Res 1996;22(4):375–8.

[50] Alvarez-Mendoza A, Lourdes TS, Ridaura-Sanz C, et al. Histopathology of lesions found in Kasabach-Merritt syndrome: review based on 13 cases. Pediatr Dev Pathol 2000;3(6): 556–60.

[51] Brasanac D, Janic D, Boricic I, et al. Retroperitoneal kaposiform hemangioendothelioma with tufted angioma–like features in an infant with Kasabach-Merritt syndrome. Pathol Int 2003;53(9):627–31.

[52] Seo SK, Suh JC, Na GY, et al. Kasabach-Merritt syndrome: identification of platelet trapping in a tufted angioma by immunochemistry technique using a monoclonal antibody to CD61. Pediatr Dermatol 1999;16(5):392–4.

[53] Mulliken JB, Anupindi S, Ezekowitz RAB, et al. Case 13-2004: a newborn girl with a large cutaneous lesion, thrombocytopenia and anemia. N Engl J Med 2004;350:1764–75.

[54] Henley JD, Danielson CF, Rothenberger SS, et al. Kasabach-Merritt syndrome with profound platelet support. Am J Clin Pathol 1993;99(5):628–30.

[55] Velin P, Dupont D, Golkar A, et al. Syndrome de Kasabach-Merritt néonatal guéri par excision chirurgicale complète de l'angiome. Arch Pediatr 1998;5(3):295–7.

[56] Drolet BA, Scott LA, Esterly NB, et al. Early surgical intervention in a patient with Kasabach-Merritt syndrome. J Pediatr 2000;138(5):756–8.

[57] Lanau Arilla MP, Garcia Erce JA, Torres Gomez M, et al. Tratamiento del sindrome de Kasabach-Merritt. Sangre 1998;4(3):218–22.

[58] Blei F, Karp N, Rofsky N, et al. Successful multimodal management for kaposiform hemangioendothelioma complicated by Kasabach-Merritt phenomenon. Pediatr Hematol Oncol 1998;15(4):295–305.

[59] Haisley-Royster C, Enjolras O, Frieden IJ, et al. Kasabach-Merritt phenomenon: a retrospective study of treatment with vincristine. J Pediatr Hematol Oncol 2002;24(6):459–62.

[60] Ezekowitz RA, Mulliken JB, Folkman J. Interferon alfa-2a therapy for life-threatening hemangiomas. N Eng J Med 1992;326(22):1456–63.

[61] Sarihan H, Mocan H, Abeys M, et al. Kasabach-Merritt syndrome in infants. Panminerva Med 1998;40(2):128–31.

[62] Wananukul S, Nuchprayoon I, Seksarn P. Treatment of Kasabach-Merritt syndrome: a stepwise regimen of prednisolone, dipyridamole and interferon. Int J Dermatol 2003;42(9): 741–8.

[63] Harper L, Michel JL, Enjolras O, et al. Successful management of retroperitoneal kaposiform hemangioendothelioma with Kasabach-Merritt phenomenon using alpha-interferon. Eur J Pediatr Surg 2006;16(5):369–72.

[64] Lopez-Gutierrez JC, Patron Romero M. Hemangioendothelioma kaposiforme toracico. Cuatro casos con evolucion variable. Ann Pediatr 2005;63(1):72–6.

[65] De Prost Y, Teillac D, Bodemer C, et al. Successful treatment of Kasabach-Merritt syndrome with pentoxifylline. J Am Acad Dermatol 1991;25(5):854–5.

[66] De la Hunt MN. Kasabach-Merritt syndrome: dangers of interferon and successful treatment with pentoxifylline. Pediatr Surg 2006;41(1):e29–31.

[67] Hu B, Lachman R, Phillips J, et al. Kasabach-Merritt syndrome–associated kaposiform hemangioendothelioma successfully treated with cyclophosphamide, vincristine and actinomycin D. J Pediatr Hematol Oncol 1998;20(6):567–9.

[68] Hesselmann S, Micke O, Marquardt T, et al. Case report: Kasabach-Merritt syndrome: a review of the therapeutic options and a case report of successful treatment with radiotherapy and interferon alpha. Br J Radiol 2002;75(890):180–4.

[69] Mitsuhashi N, Furuta M, Sakurai H, et al. Outcome of radiation therapy for patients with Kasabach-Merritt syndrome. Int J Radiat Oncol Biol Phys 1997;39(2):467–73.

[70] Miller JG, Orton Cl. Long term follow-up of a case of Kasabach-Merritt syndrome successfully treated with radiotherapy and corticosteroids. Br J Plast Surg 1992;45(7):559–61.

Management of Childhood Psoriasis

Kelly M. Cordoro, MD

University of California, San Francisco, 1701 Divisadero Street, Box 0316, San Francisco, CA 94115, USA

EDITORIAL COMMENT

Psoriasis in the pediatric setting is a very common yet challenging dermatologic disorder. Infants and children with psoriasis may have an extremely heterogenous presentation and clinical course, which may differ from that in adults. In this article, pediatric dermatologist Dr. Kelly Cordoro masterfully reviews the clinical presentation of psoriasis in the pediatric population and highlights unique features of affected children. She provides the reader with very comprehensive and practical management strategies for the young patient, as well as some very useful Tables that contain guidelines for monitoring systemic therapies. This article provides an excellent review for the experienced clinician, and is an outstanding resource for the new dermatologist with less clinical experience. I anticipate you will enjoy this article as much as I have.

P soriasis is not rare in children. Diagnosis is usually clinical and based on recognition of classic clinical features; however, presentations in children are quite variable and may differ greatly from adults in characteristic morphology, distribution, and natural history. Psoriasis can be a life-altering disease with a potentially profound impact on physical, emotional and social functioning and overall quality of life [1]. Fortunately, the majority of cases are mild and managed adequately with topical medications. The true challenge exists in treating the subset of children who present with severe, rapidly evolving, debilitating, life-altering or life-threatening disease. It is these patients whose management represents a merging of the art and science of dermatology: the science derives from an understanding of the specific mechanisms, clinical utility, benefits, and toxicities of available treatments; the art is in the effective and novel application of such treatments alone and in combination. This article is designed to arm the clinician with such information, including the basic principles and advanced practices necessary to treat mild and severe psoriasis in children.

E-mail address: cordorok@derm.ucsf.edu

0882-0880/08/$ – see front matter
doi:10.1016/j.yadr.2008.09.009

EPIDEMIOLOGY, PATHOPHYSIOLOGY AND CLINICAL FEATURES

The unique clinical features, epidemiology, and genetic basis of childhood psoriasis have been recently comprehensively reviewed [2–8]. Although true estimates of the incidence in children are hampered by the overlapping clinical features between psoriasis and other common childhood papulosquamous eruptions, available data suggest that greater than one-third of patients present in the first two decades of life [8,9]. Up to 27% present by age 2, when psoriatic diaper eruption is included [4,7,10]. The actual incidence of children with so-called "napkin psoriasis" who eventually develop typical psoriasis is unknown. Neville and colleagues [11] reported 17% of 71 patients with psoriasiform napkin dermatitis diagnosed in the first year of life had various forms of psoriasis on review up to 13 years later. Infants presenting with a confluent eruption in the diaper area with disseminated lesions exhibiting psoriasiform morphology and a positive first-degree family history of psoriasis are at greater risk [11–13]. Psoriasis represents approximately 4% of all dermatoses presenting in patients less than 16 years old [14]. Substantiated data on epidemiology, natural history, and response to treatment is scarce, likely in large measure because of inexact terminology and lack of standardized classification schemes. The exact etiology of psoriasis remains elusive; however, an immunologic pathogenesis [15] modified by environmental factors in genetically predisposed individuals is suggested and well supported [8,16–20].

The genetic basis of the disease has been convincingly established by epidemiologic and twin study data [7,21], as well as linkage analysis revealing at least nine psoriasis-susceptibility loci on several chromosomes [22]. PSORS 1, localized to the region of the major histocompatibility complex on chromosome 6p21.3 has been identified as the major genetic determinant of early onset psoriasis, especially the guttate phenotype. Sequence and haplotype analysis suggest that HLA-Cw6 is the PSORS1-risk allele that confers susceptibility to early-onset psoriasis [2,23–26].

Pathogenesis of psoriasis is complex. The relative contributions of T-lymphocytes, keratinocyte defects [27,28], innate and adaptive immune responses, cell signaling pathways, and proinflammatory and angiogenic cytokines [29] to the development and maintenance of psoriasis remain to be definitively established. Good evidence exists linking specific antigen-driven [15,30] proliferation and abnormal differentiation of keratinocytes in response to streptoccal superantigens [31], especially in children.

Childhood psoriasis in most cases presents as in adults, with plaque-type being most common. The relative frequency of particular morphologies and the pattern of distribution and symptoms can be very distinct and differ from that in adults (Box 1). For example, annular and serpiginous forms are common (Figs. 1–3), involvement of the face and anogenital region is typical (Figs. 4 and 5), and pruritus is often a feature of childhood psoriasis [2]. In the largest case series of childhood psoriasis published to date, Morris and colleagues [7] reviewed the distribution, morphology, and family history of 1,262 consecutive

Box 1: Clinical variants and distributions of psoriasis in children

Plaque: most frequent, often smaller, thinner and less scaly than in adults [2]. Includes scalp, face, trunk, extremities, and anogenital (perianal, psoriasiform vulvitis and balanitis)

Guttate

Annular/figurate/arcuate/serpiginous

Eczema-psoriasis overlap (eczematous psoriasis or psoriasiform eczema)

Papulosquamous (discrete papules admixed with typical scaly patches and plaques)

Papular

Follicular

Scalp: diffuse plaque, tinea/pityriasis amiantacea, dermatitis erythema nuchae

Inverse: flexures, intertriginous

Facial: periorbital, perioral, angular cheilitis

Nails: pits, oil drops, onycholysis, subungual hyperkeratosis, onychodystrophy (up to 40% of children with psoriasis) [10]

Linear/Blaschkoid

Anogenital

Psoriatic diaper rash

Interdigital web spaces

Psoriatic arthropathy: peak of onset in childhood is between ages 9 and 12 [2]

Pustular (rare)

Localized:

Acrodermatitis Continua of Hallopeau (digits and nails)

Palmoplantar pustulosis

Plaque psoriasis studded with surface pustules

Generalized:

von Zumbusch (more common in infancy)

Annular variant with peripheral pustules (common in older children)

Erythrodermic (rare)

Data from Refs. [2,3,7,8,10,203,210].

pediatric psoriasis patients presenting to a tertiary referral pediatric dermatology department over 14 years. Ages ranged from 1 month to 15 years, equal sex distribution was noted, and a positive family history identified in 71%. Of the patients, 16% were less than 1 year of age, and 27% less than 2 years of age. In all patients, plaque type was most common, followed by psoriatic diaper rash with dissemination (particularly in children less than 2 years of age,

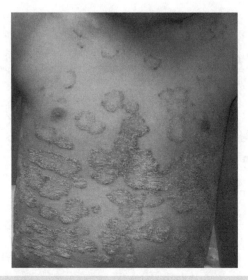

Fig. 1. Annular pustular psoriasis.

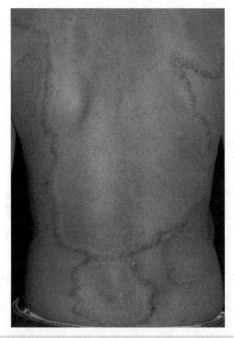

Fig. 2. Annular psoriasis. (*Courtesy of* Amy J. Nopper, MD, Kansas City, MO.)

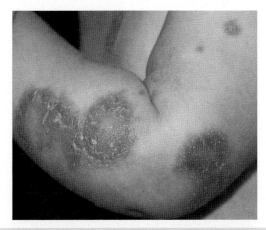

Fig. 3. Annular psoriasis. (*Courtesy of* Ilona J. Frieden, MD, San Francisco, CA.)

defined as bright, well marginated "glazed" erythematous diaper rash followed by an explosive and widespread dissemination of small psoriasis-like lesions; Figs. 6 and 7), scalp, anogenital, and guttate types. When psoriatic diaper rash was excluded, the most common presentations in children less than 2 years old were plaque type, scalp, guttate, and facial, while in children greater than 2, plaque, scalp, anogenital, and guttate psoriasis were most commonly observed. All other clinical variants of psoriasis were represented in all age groups, with the exception of linear and erythrodermic forms, which were not identified in any child less than 2 [7]. Several recent reviews detail the

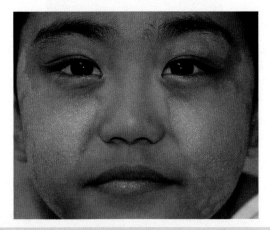

Fig. 4. Facial plaque psoriasis. (*Courtesy of* Ilona J. Frieden, MD, San Francisco, CA.)

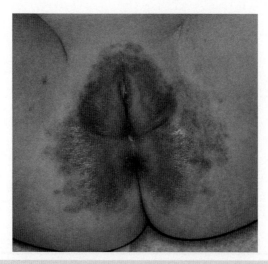

Fig. 5. Anogenital psoriasis. (*Courtesy of* Ilona J. Frieden, MD, San Francisco, CA.)

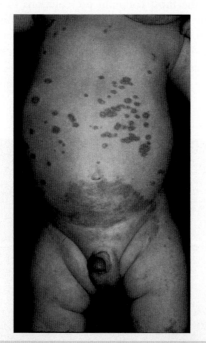

Fig. 6. Psoriatic diaper rash with dissemination. (*Courtesy of* Kenneth E. Greer, MD, Charlottesville, VA.)

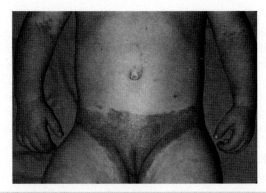

Fig. 7. Psoriatic diaper rash with dissemination. (*Courtesy of* Kenneth E. Greer, MD.)

unique clinical aspects of childhood psoriasis and serve as excellent clinical references [2,7,8].

EXTRACUTANEOUS ASSOCIATIONS

Psoriasis is an inflammatory disease characterized by a dysregulated immune system. As knowledge related to its pathophysiology and genetic basis has exploded, it is clear that psoriasis should not be viewed as an isolated skin disease but rather as a group of diseases of the skin and joints, associated in some cases with extracutaneous and extra-articular manifestations [32]. Prevalence estimates of psoriatic arthritis in all psoriasis patients are a matter of considerable debate and range in the literature from 5% to 40% [33]. Data collection to clarify the prevalence of psoriatic arthritis in children, as in adults, is hampered by the lack of universally accepted diagnostic and classification criteria. Nail pitting, dactylitis, and enthesitis are clinical signs suggestive of psoriasis and may serve as markers of psoriatic arthritis versus other juvenile idiopathic arthritides [34]. A large clinical and epidemiologic study from Spain detected a significantly increased risk for joint involvement in patients of all ages with erythrodermic, generalized pustular, and intertriginous (inverse) psoriasis, as well as in patients with psoriatic nail involvement [35]. Correlation between the severity of the skin disease and the arthritis is usually poor [33].

Internet-savvy parents often ask whether there is an increased risk of cancer in their affected child. Although significantly higher rates of nonmelanoma skin cancer and lymphoma have been reported in patients with psoriasis, the relative contributions of disease severity, systemic medications, phototherapy, and other independent risk factors or a combination thereof remain to be clearly defined by additional studies [36]. New data from a cross-sectional study suggest a possible link between psoriasis and the metabolic syndrome [37,38]. The findings do not imply causality one way or another but do indicate that the management of psoriasis should encompass a multidisciplinary approach and may be enhanced by treatment of coexistent diabetes, obesity, dyslipidemia, and hypertension. Early work suggested a relationship between psoriasis, ankylosing spondylitis, sacroiliitis, peripheral arthropathy, and inflammatory bowel disease because of common genetic factors [39]. A statistically significant association between psoriasis and Crohn disease has been proven [32]. SAPHO (synovitis, acne, pustulosis, hyperostosis, osteitis) represents a chronic, recurrent multifocal osteomyelitis associated with aseptic neutrophilic dermatoses, including pustular psoriasis, Sweet syndrome, and pyoderma gangrenosum [40].

ENVIRONMENTAL TRIGGERS

Precipitating factors are more common in childhood compared with adult-onset psoriasis. Trauma (via Koebner phenomenon), infections (pharyngeal and perianal Lancefield group A beta hemolytic streptococci in particular) [30,31], drugs [41], and stress have been frequently implicated in initiation and exacerbation of early onset psoriasis [2]. High carriage rates of the Cw6 allele in patients with streptococcal-associated guttate psoriasis compared with controls have been documented [42]. The risk of future psoriasis in children after an episode of acute guttate psoriasis has not been adequately determined with longitudinal studies. A small follow-up study of 15 patients who suffered an episode of acute guttate psoriasis a minimum of 10 years earlier reported development of psoriasis in five of the patients, suggesting a probability of 33% [43].

APPROACH TO MANAGEMENT

One of the most important aspects of optimal management of childhood psoriasis is educating the patient (if age-appropriate) and the family and providing supportive and educational resources. Psoriasis is a chronic disease with periods of remission and exacerbation, and with the exception of guttate flares clearly linked to recent infection, is likely to be an ongoing process requiring frequent office visits and consistent use of topical and perhaps systemic and phototherapy. Complete clearance of psoriasis may be unrealistic and recurrence is expected; thus, emphasis of control versus cure sets realistic expectations for treatment and is likely to enhance compliance. Medical treatment remains a challenge and primarily anecdotal, as most therapies are neither studied nor approved for use in children. Depending on the individual case presentation and comorbidities, the most effective approach is multidisciplinary and includes the dermatologist, pediatrician, rheumatologist, and other subspecialists as the need arises.

The choice of treatment is determined by disease morphology, distribution, severity, the presence of comorbidities such as psoriatic arthropathy, and patient age and preference as related to quality of life and level of social, emotional, or functional disability. The treatment plan must be in line with the perceptions and attitudes of the patient and parents, as willingness to comply with the regimen is based on the level of agreement between doctor and the patient and family. Stay mindful of the actual practicality of a proposed regimen in terms of ease of use, accessibility, risk-to-benefit ratio, cost, and individual perceptions of disease. Patients may vary in their expectations from desire for total clearance to maintenance of an aesthetically acceptable level of control. Extent does not necessarily equate to severity, as a patient with involvement of 2% body surface area (BSA) in a public location, such as the face, or a private location, such as the genitals, may be equally psychosocially debilitated as a patient with greater than 30% BSA of involvement. The reverse is also true: a patient with greater than 30% BSA, if covered by clothing, may perceive no effects on quality of life whatsoever. Ask the patient how much they are bothered by their psoriasis and approach treatment accordingly.

HISTORY AND PHYSICAL EXAMINATION

A review of possible triggers, disease associations as discussed above, and the patient's expectations provide the foundation upon which to base early investigations and a therapeutic plan of attack. Elicit a history of exposure that may have initiated the psoriasis via an isomorphic response, including physical, chemical, thermal, surgical, or inflammatory trauma. Screen via history, physical examination, and appropriate studies as indicated for recent or current pharyngeal, perianal, or other infection, including risk factors for HIV [44,45]. While β-blockers and lithium are more common offending agents in adults, antimalarials and recent withdrawal of oral or topical corticosteroids have been implicated in some childhood cases. Inquire about the emotional impact of the disease, as the importance of psychologic stress and lack of social support has recently been emphasized as an influence on the course of psoriasis in children [2]. Important historical aspects that will affect the choice of therapy include presence of comorbid conditions, particularly photosensitive conditions such as polymorphous light eruption and connective tissue disease. Assess the risk for metabolic syndrome in the patient and family by documenting a personal or family history of obesity, diabetes, hypertension and dyslipidemia. These factors not only affect choice of therapy and monitoring parameters but also aim to encompass the desired comprehensive, multidisciplinary approach to children with psoriasis. Written and photographic documentation of body surface area of involvement, precise morphology, distribution, joint involvement, and functional limitations allows precise categorization of disease and aids in management decisions and subsequent assessments of response to therapy.

MANAGEMENT PRINCIPLES: TOPICAL THERAPIES

Compliance is the key to good outcomes, so start simple if possible. Highly complex and elaborate regimens may be appropriate in carefully selected motivated patients and parents but in the more common context of a busy household with working parents and multiple children, simplicity is preferable and will enhance adherence to the regimen. The regimen can be supplemented as necessary at future visits. Do not over-promise and under-deliver. A simple regimen can still be aggressive and proves to the patient and the parents that improvement is possible. Ointment formulations tend to have greater efficacy than creams but some patients, particularly adolescents, find them objection-able. In an effort to increase compliance, prescribe whichever vehicle the patient finds preferable [46]. Monotherapy may be effective for limited, focal or mild disease. In cases where multiple medications are necessary, the number of agents that must be applied can be reduced by compounding compatible agents (see below). Pharmacies are becoming more and more resistant to compounding because of time and expense, but research the local and surrounding community and keep a list of pharmacies willing to compound to provide to your patients. Combination, rotational and sequential therapy as introduced by Menter, Weinstein and White, and Koo, respectively, are time honored methods to improve overall efficacy while reducing toxicity of the chosen therapies [47]. Although originally described within the context of systemic therapy, these concepts are readily applied to the use of topical therapy as well. Topical medications can be combined with other topicals, phototherapy, and systemic therapy, the key aspects of which are discussed within the relevant sections below. Carefully consider the area and frequency of application and prescribe appropriate quantities of medication accordingly (Table 1).

Corticosteroids

Corticosteroids remain among the first line agents in the topical treatment of psoriasis in all age groups. They have anti-inflammatory and antiproliferative properties and when applied to psoriasis will reduce erythema, scaling, and pruritus [48]. They range in potency from very weak Class VII agents to su-per-potent Class I agents as ranked by the Stoughton-Cornell vasoconstriction classification [49]. Delivering the steroid to the involved skin in a convenient, tolerable, safe, and efficacious manner requires selection of a vehicle well suited to the site-specific qualities. Features such as the presence of hair (scalp), moisture (intertriginous zones), occlusion (axillae, diaper area, gluteal cleft), and the thickness of the skin and the psoriasis all contribute to the choice of a vehicle. A variety of vehicles are available to choose from, including powders, sprays, lotions, solutions, creams, emollient creams, ointments, gels, tape, and foam. The patient's and parent's preferences should be factored in as appropriate in an effort to enhance compliance. Recommend application of thick, greasy ointments at nighttime and reserve more cosmetically acceptable creams, lotions, and solutions for daytime use. In general, thin and intertriginous skin areas respond to lower potencies and thick hyperkeratotic areas, such as the palms and soles (Fig. 8), require high potency agents. Infants have a large BSA, which increases the chance of systemic absorption and adverse events, such as adrenal suppression [50]. Only the mildest topical corticosteroids should be used in the diaper area. If higher potency agents are required in high-risk areas, limit their use to short bursts and then reduce the potency or the frequency or both. In general, very high potency agents should be avoided in children if possible or used sparingly in combination or rotation with steroid-sparing alternatives, such as coal tar, anthralin, calcipotriene, and topical calcineurin inhibitors. The judicious use and creation of novel compounds and combination regimens will reduce the frequency of side effects of the topical steroid, such as skin atrophy, striae, telangiectasia, acneiform eruptions, and adrenal suppression, while still achieving adequate efficacy [47]. One such regimen includes application of a topical steroid twice daily for 2 weeks, followed by application on weekend days only [51]. This regimen is often a lead-in to substitution of the weekday topical steroid with calcipotriene ointment (calcipotriene twice daily on weekdays and topical steroid twice daily on weekends) and represents a combination and sequential regimen [47]. An ointment combination of calcipotriene hydrate and betamethasone dipropionate (Taclonex) is Food and Drug Administration (FDA)-approved and indicated for the topical treatment of psoriasis vulgaris in adults; it is discussed in more detail below. Combinations such as this allegedly decrease the occurrence of tachyphylaxis, the phenomenon defined as loss of efficacy with prolonged use of a drug. Whether tachyphylaxis truly exists or represents poor adherence to the regimen is debatable (see Table 1) [52].

Coal tar

Crude coal tar is prepared as a condensation product from the carbonization of coal and is a complex mixture of as many as 10,000 substances [53], of which only about half are identified (Fig. 9) [54]. This diverse compound has antipsoriatic, antiseborrheic, antipruritic, and keratolytic effects [55]. The mechanism of action is largely unknown, but enzyme inhibition, antimitotic actions [56], and suppression of DNA synthesis [57] have been identified. Treatment of psoriasis with crude coal tar was popularized by Goeckerman in 1931 at the Mayo Clinic, where he successfully used coal tar in ointment and bath form in combination with ultraviolet light (Goeckerman regimen). This regimen remains a standard treatment for psoriasis in day-care treatment centers throughout the world and is useful in adults and children [53,58]. Liquor carbonis detergens (LCD) used in concentrations from 0.5% to 20% is a modified coal tar prepared by extracting coal tar with alcohol and emulsifying with polysorbate 80 [54]. LCD is less clinically active but is yellow-brown rather than black and rubs almost invisibly into the skin with a faint residual odor. LCD has largely replaced crude coal tar in the outpatient setting, given its better cosmetic acceptability (Fig. 10), and can be compounded in an ointment, cream, or solution vehicle. Tar is an effective adjunctive treatment for childhood psoriasis that can be used alone topically or as a bath, in compounded form with other medications such as corticosteroids, lactic and salicylic acid, or with ultraviolet (UV) irradiation. Ultraviolet irradiation (UVA > UVB) following the application of tar profoundly enhances suppression of DNA synthesis within psoriatic plaques [59].

Crude coal tar has been demonstrated to have comparable long-term efficacy to calcipotriene ointment, although calcipotriene produces faster initial responses and is more cosmetically acceptable. Both agents can produce local irritation, and there is no statistically significant difference in relapse rates [60]. Tar is supplied in a variety of topical formulations and shampoos, and its relatively low cost compared with other topical agents is an advantage in the

Table 1
Topical therapies

Medication	Mechanism of action	FDA data	Clinical utility	Strength of evidence	Adverse effects (AE)/ Contraindications (CI)
Corticosteroids	Anti-inflammatory and antiproliferative [48]	Approved for psoriasis: Adult, yes; Pediatric, yes (minimum age of approval depends on specific agent) Pregnancy category C	All psoriasis variants; all sites of involvement (vary potency and frequency according to site of application- see text)	B	AE: acneiform eruptions, skin atrophy, striae, secondary infection CI: hypersensitivity to preparation; local viral, fungal, or bacterial infections
Anthralin (dithranol)	Antiproliferative/anti-inflammatory [66]; Activates JNK pathway involved in regulation of cell proliferation and apoptosis [67]	Approved for psoriasis: Adult, yes; Pediatric, no Pregnancy category C	Plaque psoriasis: scalp, trunk, extremities, nail psoriasis	B	AE: staining, irritation, contact dermatitis [211] CI: erythroderma; generalized pustular psoriasis

Coal tar/LCD	Largely unknown Enzyme inhibition and antimitotic actions [56]; suppression of DNA synthesis [57]	Approved for psoriasis: Adult, yes; Pediatric, no Pregnancy category C	Plaque psoriasis: Scalp, face, trunk, extremities, flexures palms/soles [212]	C	AE: folliculitis, irritant/allergic contact dermatitis, photosensitivity; pustular or erythrodermic reactions if used on acutely inflamed psoriasis [53] CI: Inflamed, erythrodermic or generalized pustular psoriasis; hypersensitivity to coal tar; photosensitivity; presence of folliculitis or acne vulgaris
Calcipotriene	Stimulates epidermal differentiation and inhibits epidermal proliferation [73,74]	Approved for psoriasis: Adult, yes; Pediatric, no Pregnancy category C	Plaque and pustular psoriasis: Trunk, extremities, scalp	C	AE: Irritation, hypercalcemia in excessive dosages [81] CI: Disorders of calcium metabolism

(continued on next page)

Table 1
(continued)

Medication	Mechanism of action	FDA data	Clinical utility	Strength of evidence	Adverse effects (AE)/Contraindications (CI)
Taclonex (calcipotriene hydrate and betamethasone dipropionate)	As per topical corticosteroids (anti-inflammatory, antipruritic, and vasoconstrictive) and calcipotriene (Stimulates epidermal differentiation and inhibits epidermal proliferation)	Approved for psoriasis: Adult, yes; Pediatric, no Pregnancy category C	Plaque psoriasis: Avoid face, axillae and groin	No evidence in children	AE: Irritation, folliculitis, atrophy CI: Disorders of calcium metabolism; erythrodermic, exfoliative and pustular psoriasis
Tazarotene	Restores normal epidermal differentiation and proliferation and reduces epidermal inflammation [82]	Approved for psoriasis: Adult, yes; Pediatric, no (approved for acne in children aged 12 and older) Pregnancy category X	Plaque psoriasis: Trunk, extremities, palms/soles, nail psoriasis	C	AE: Irritation CI: Pregnancy
Calcineurin inhibitors	Inhibit production of IL-2 and subsequent T-cell activation/proliferation [87]	Approved for psoriasis: Adult and pediatric: no Pregnancy category C	Face, flexures, anogenital	C	AE: Skin burning, stinging and pruritus CI: [Based on FDA warnings: Children < 2 (pimecrolimus and tacrolimus 0.03% and 0.1%); Children < 15 y/o (tacrolimus 0.1%)]

Abbreviations: IL, interleukin; JNK, c-jun-N-terminal-kinase signal transduction pathway; LCD, liquor carbonis detergens.

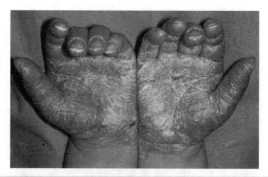

Fig. 8. Palmar psoriasis. (*Courtesy of* Kenneth E. Greer, MD.)

long-term treatment of psoriasis. Some patients and parents may find the brown-yellow color, odor, and potential for phototoxicity unacceptable, thereby creating issues with long-term compliance. Unfortunately, attempts at improving the cosmetic acceptability of coal tar have consistently resulted in products of inferior quality and efficacy [54]. Education regarding the excellent safety profile and place in therapy as a steroid-sparing adjunct may increase tolerance and compliance of this excellent and underutilized topical therapy.

Side effects of tar are primarily cutaneous and include folliculitis, irritant and allergic reactions, photosensitivity, and induction of pustular or erythrodermic reactions if used on acutely inflamed psoriasis [53]. Long-term industrial or occupational exposure to tar and animal studies have demonstrated cutaneous carcinogenicity [61] potentiated by ultraviolet radiation. Large series and epidemiologic studies in human beings, however, have not definitively shown an increase in skin cancer above the expected incidence for the general population from the use of therapeutic tar with or without ultraviolet radiation [54,61–63].

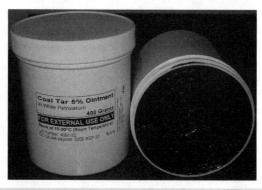

Fig. 9. Crude coal tar (5% in petrolatum).

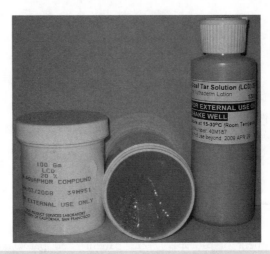

Fig. 10. LCD compounded in an ointment base and as a lotion. Note the lighter color versus crude coal tar.

Anthralin

Chrysarobin is a natural substance derived from the araroba tree of South America. It has been used to treat psoriasis for nearly 100 years [64]. Anthralin (dithranol), a synthetic version, was first synthesized in 1916 and is well established as an effective topical treatment for psoriasis. It has been used successfully as part of the Ingram regimen (anthralin, tar baths, and ultraviolet irradiation) for over 30 years [65]. Negligible systemic absorption is responsible for its excellent safety profile and ease of use, especially in children. Anthralin is a potent anti-inflammatory and antiproliferative agent [66] thought to be a result, in part, of effects on mitochondrial deoxyribonucleic acid and on various enzyme systems [64]. Recent studies demonstrate potent effects on keratinocytes and mononuclear cells through induction of lipid peroxidation and JNK activation, a stress-induced signal transduction pathway important in the regulation of cell proliferation and apoptosis [67]. Anthralin therapy can be combined with other topical treatments or UVB, as in the Ingram regimen.

Outside of psoriasis day-care treatment facilities, its use has been limited because of staining and irritation, which result in poor patient tolerance and compliance. Novel regimens using shorter contact times have resulted in more widespread clinical use and patient acceptability. Short contact therapy (SCT) describes 0.1% dithranol cream applied daily for 10 to 30 minutes to all parts of the body, including scalp and flexures. The starting concentration is increased slowly every other day up to 3% to 4% until a mild irritation develops. The dose is then held constant and application repeated daily for 30 minutes until clear. Petroleum jelly applied to perilesional skin serves to protect it from irritation. This regimen, applied after a single initial application of 5% salicylic acid for removal of thick scales, effectively cleared plaques in 47 of 58

(81%) pediatric psoriasis patients aged 2 to 15 years [68]. A variant of SCT, termed "minutes" therapy, uses the same principle of increasing concentrations of dithranol applied to the skin and left in place for 10 to 20 minutes daily [69]. Alternatively, very low concentrations (0.1%) compounded with a gentle keratolytic (17% urea) can be applied twice daily to mild-to-moderate psoriasis for 6 to 12 weeks with excellent effect, as demonstrated in 34 children aged 3 to 16 years who showed a mean improvement of 70% after 6 weeks [70]. For best results, maintain a slight irritation of the skin. Lower concentrations or less contact time should be maintained on more sensitive sites, such as genital skin. Tar inactivates anthralin, so the two agents should not be used simultaneously. Refer to the manufacturer package insert on individual formulations for instructions on proper medication removal.

Calcipotriene

Calcipotriene (calcipotriol) is an analog of vitamin D3 that has been proven safe and effective in adults with psoriasis. It is an efficient nonsteroidal alternative in the treatment of psoriasis and has utility as monotherapy, as well as in novel sequential and rotational combinations with topical steroids [71]. In adult clinical trials, its efficacy was demonstrated to be comparable to or better than class II corticosteroid ointments and anthralin and preferred cosmetically over the latter [72]. Its utility in the treatment of psoriasis is derived from its anti-inflammatory effects, as well as induction of keratinocyte differentiation and inhibition of epidermal proliferation [73,74]. Regimens combining calcipotriene and superpotent topical steroids, such as once daily use of each, are steroid-sparing and superior in efficacy to twice daily monotherapy with either agent [75]. Another novel and effective, steroid-sparing regimen includes twice daily use of calcipotriene Monday through Friday, followed by twice daily application of topical steroid Saturday and Sunday [76]. An ointment combination of calcipotriene hydrate and betamethasone dipropionate (Taclonex) is FDA-approved and indicated for the topical treatment of psoriasis vulgaris in adults. As with calcipotriene monotherapy, the maximum weekly dose should not exceed 100 g, and treatment of more than 30% body surface area or use on the face, axillae or groin is not recommended. The safety and efficacy in pediatric patients has not been established, but anecdotally this product is used successfully in children and has the advantage of once daily dosing; however, the exorbitant cost is a disadvantage. Treatment with calcipotriene on weekdays and the combination product on weekends is proven to be effective and safe [77]. Calcipotriene destabilizes in the presence of salicylic acid, ammonium lactate, and hydrocortisone valerate 0.2% ointment and thus should not be used at the same time as or compounded with these molecules [72].

Calcipotriol ointment has been shown to be effective, well tolerated, and safe in children with psoriasis. In 1996, a multicenter, prospective, uncontrolled, open label trial of calcipotriol ointment, applied twice daily for up to 8 weeks in 66 children aged 2 to 14 with stable plaque psoriasis involving less than 30% BSA on the trunk and extremities, showed statistically significant reductions in mean Psoriasis Area Severity Index (PASI) scores compared with baseline. Marked improvement or clearance as assessed by the investigator or the patient was achieved in greater than 60% of patients. Local irritation was the most common adverse event and there was no significant change in hematologic or biochemical laboratory parameters, including serum ionized calcium. The study also suggested that use of up to 45 g per week per square meter [2] in children does not seem to influence serum ionized calcium levels [14]. A year later, a multicenter, prospective, double-blind, randomized, vehicle-controlled, parallel group trial compared calcipotriol ointment 50 µg/g to the ointment vehicle applied twice daily for up to 8 weeks in 77 children aged 2 to 14 years (mean age 10) with mild to moderate stable plaque psoriasis involving less than 30% BSA. Statistically significant reductions in redness, scaliness, and investigator's overall assessment, but not thickness or PASI score, were found in the calcipotriol group versus the vehicle group. Lesional and perilesional irritation were similar in both groups and no serious adverse events were documented, including laboratory parameters relating to calcium and bone metabolism [78]. More recently, Choi and colleagues [79] reported successful use of calcipotriene and emollients twice daily in a 6-month-old child with plaque and pustular morphology refractory to topical steroids. Travis and Silverberg reported a male infant, 2 months of age, with erythrodermic psoriasis refractory to topical corticosteroids. Calcipotriol ointment applied twice daily resulted in 90% resolution after 1 month of treatment and 100% at 7 months of age. Dosages exceeded 200 g during the first month of treatment. Laboratory testing for calcium metabolism was normal during the course of therapy [80].

Local side effects of calcipotriene are primarily limited to cutaneous irritation. Adverse effects of topical calcipotriol on systemic calcium homeostasis in adult patients with chronic plaque psoriasis have been evaluated and is related to dose-per-unit body weight of the patient [81]. Systemic calcipotriol toxicity is similar to vitamin D toxicity and can result in hypercalcemia, hypercalciuria, and subsequent renal calculi if usage exceeds greater than 100 g per week of the standard 50 µg/g formulation [81]. This figure has not been determined definitively in children, but the results of a multicenter, prospective, uncontrolled, open label trial of calcipotriol ointment applied twice daily for up to 8 weeks in 66 children aged 2 to 14 with stable plaque psoriasis involving less than 30% BSA suggest that use of up to 45 g per week per square meter [2] in children does not seem to influence serum ionized calcium levels [14].

Tazarotene

Tazarotene (Tazorac) is a third-generation topical retinoid, FDA-approved for once daily treatment of psoriasis in adults aged 18 and older and acne vulgaris in patients aged 12 and above. It is supplied as 0.05% and 0.1% gel and cream with minimal systemic absorption and rapid elimination. Similar to other retinoids, tazarotene restores normal epidermal differentiation and proliferation and reduces epidermal inflammation [82]. Topical treatment of plaque psoriasis with tazarotene normalizes markers of differentiation, such as keratin 16, involucrin, keratinocyte transglutaminase, epidermal growth factor receptor, and reduces dermal and epidermal expression of inflammatory markers, such as intracellular adhesion molecule 1 in parallel to clinical improvement [82]. It is neither sensitizing nor phototoxic [83], but dose-related skin irritation is common and often necessitates combination with a topical steroid applied at the same or different time of day to decrease irritation and improve overall efficacy [84].

Therapeutic effects of tazarotene are sustained for up to 3 months after discontinuation of a 2 to 3 month treatment regimen [83]. Short contact (10–60 minutes per day, then wash off), alternate day or weekly applications are potential ways to include this useful agent in sequential and rotational regimens. Effectiveness of tazarotene for nail psoriasis has been demonstrated clinically in adults [85] and children [86]. A 6-year-old female with fungal culture and microscopy-negative onychodystrophy of all fingernails, refractory to systemic and topical anti-fungal drugs and steroids, was treated with tazarotene 0.05% gel applied once daily to the affected nail plates, nail folds, and periungual skin without occlusion for 8 weeks. The hyperkeratosis improved, fragility disappeared, and normal nail growth resumed. The pitting remained unchanged and local irritation during the first week was the only side effect. The duration of response was not reported [86].

Topical calcineurin inhibitors

Tacrolimus and pimecrolimus are nonsteroidal immunomodulating macrolactams that work by blocking the enzyme calcineurin, ultimately inhibiting the downstream production of IL-2 and subsequent T-cell activation and proliferation [87]. Both topical agents are currently FDA-approved for second-line intermittent treatment of atopic dermatitis in patients aged 2 years and older (pimecrolimus and tacrolimus 0.03%) and aged 15 and older (tacrolimus 0.1%). These agents are particularly attractive steroid alternatives for use on facial and intertriginous sites, given their anti-inflammatory properties devoid of the side effects associated with topical steroids, such as atrophy, striae, telangiectasia, periorificial dermatitis, and ocular toxicity. Recent studies have documented the safety and utility of tacrolimus and pimecrolimus for the treatment of intertriginous and facial psoriasis in adults [88–96] and children [97–101].

In a pilot, single-center, open-label clinical trial in 11 subjects aged 6 to 15 years with mild to severe psoriasis, 0.1% tacrolimus ointment applied twice daily to facial and intertriginous sites for up to 180 days resulted in excellent improvement in 88% and complete clearing in 12%. The most significant improvement occurred within the first month and the only adverse event noted during the study was significant pruritus in one patient who ultimately dropped out [99]. A retrospective case study evaluated the efficacy of tacrolimus ointment for inverse psoriasis in 13 subjects aged 22 months to 16 years. Twelve patients (treated with 0.1% ointment) cleared within 2 weeks of initiating treatment and had no adverse effects. One patient (treated with 0.03%) failed to respond to therapy and experienced burning and irritation at the application site, which altered compliance [101]. Pimecrolimus cream 1% applied twice daily in combination with narrowband (NB)-UVB was reported to clear severe facial and digital plaque psoriasis complicated by pseudo-ainhum type restrictions in a 5-month-old female [97]. Other sites treated successfully by pimecrolimus include the penis in a 9-year-old male [98] and periorbital and anogenital plaques in a 10-year-old female [100].

Tacrolimus and pimecrolimus are effective, safe and well-tolerated therapeutic options for thin patches and plaques of psoriasis at sites more sensitive to the long-term adverse effects of topical steroids, such as the face, flexures, and anogenital region. In practice, calcineurin inhibitors provide a valuable option for use within the context of sequential and rotational regimens, including topical steroids, calcipotriene, tar, and anthralin.

Salicylic acid

Salicylic acid is a useful adjunctive keratolytic agent for very thick localized plaques. It is supplied individually as shampoo and as a 6% gel or can be compounded with topical corticosteroids, which enhances penetration of the steroid [102]. Salicylic acid should be used sparingly and with caution in the pediatric population because of the risk of percutaneous salicylate intoxication [103]. Limit the concentration to 6% and application to very small, thick, focal plaques, such as those arising on the scalp, palms, and soles. Restrict the use of salicylic acid to children older than 6 years and adolescents, and avoid its use altogether in infants and younger children.

Emollients

Liberal application of bland emollients is often effective for mild psoriasis and always plays an adjunctive role, particularly in winter when low humidity and lack of sunlight initiate predictable flares. Emollients are antipruritic, mildly desquamative, relatively inexpensive and well tolerated by almost all patients [48]. Emollient vehicles should be selected on an individual basis based on tolerability, ease of application and patient preference.

MANAGEMENT PRINCIPLES: SYSTEMIC THERAPY

The three most commonly used systemic treatments for psoriasis in children, as in adults, are acitretin, methotrexate, and cyclosporine. None are FDA-labeled for this indication in children and none have undergone the scrutiny of randomized, controlled trials in the pediatric population. Accumulated data regarding the utility, benefits, and risks of these agents for treatment of psoriasis derives largely from long-term use in children with disorders of cornification (retinoids), juvenile rheumatoid arthritis (methotrexate), and transplanted organs (cyclosporine). For enhanced therapeutic effect and reduced toxicity of the individual agent, systemic therapies may be used in combination with topical therapies and in more severe cases with each other and with phototherapy [104]. Caution is advised, as toxicities may be cumulative and the individual agent must be carefully considered before combining it with another systemic agent. If long-term systemic treatment is anticipated, rotation of individual agents from one to another after a period of time results in reduced overall cumulative dose of each agent [47]. Treatment with systemic agents is typically reserved for severe, refractory, widespread or incapacitating disease, pustular (Fig. 11) or erythrodermic forms, and psoriatic arthropathy. Phototherapy is an excellent and safe treatment in children with diffuse plaque, guttate, and pustular psoriasis and is considered before systemic therapy in many cases (see "Phototherapy" section, below). Within the conceptual framework of a sequential, three-phase approach to psoriasis management (clearing, transition, and maintenance), one selects appropriate therapies for each phase and proceeds accordingly, limiting undue exposure for long periods of time to any individual agent [105,106]. One example of the sequential therapy concept in a patient with severe psoriasis, as formally introduced by Dr. John Koo, is to initially gain control and clear the psoriasis with a systemic agent, such as cyclosporine (clearing phase). Next, a second agent, such as acitretin, is added with the goal of eventually discontinuing the first agent (transition phase). Finally, the first agent (cyclosporine, in this example) is gradually tapered off and the second agent (acitretin, in this example) is continued for maintenance (maintenance phase) (Table 2) [105].

Retinoids

Retinoids are natural and synthetic compounds that possess vitamin-A activity. They exert physiologic effects on cellular metabolism, epidermal differentiation, and apoptosis by binding to nuclear receptors and activating target genes

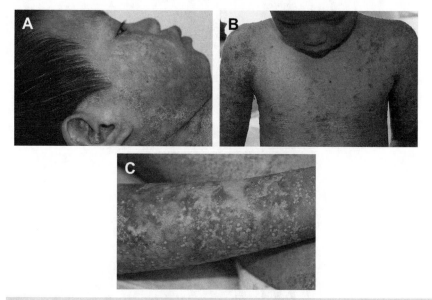

Fig. 11. Generalized pustular psoriasis involving the face (A), trunk (B), and extremities (C).

Table 2
Systemic therapies

Medication	Mechanism of action	FDA data	Clinical utility	Strength of evidence	Adverse effects (AE)/ Contraindications (CI)
Methotrexate	Folic acid antagonist: inhibits DHFR and DNA synthesis [127]	Approved for psoriasis: Adult, yes; Pediatric, no Pregnancy category X	Severe plaque, pustular and erythrodermic psoriasis	C	AE: Nausea, vomiting, diarrhea, headache, hepatotoxicity, interstitial pneumonitis, bone marrow suppression, fetal death/malformation, photosensitivity, treatment-emergent lymphoma [213] CI: Pregnancy, breastfeeding, alcoholism, liver disease, pre-existing blood dyscrasias, immunodeficiency syndromes, impaired kidney function

Acitretin	Effects on cellular metabolism, epidermal differentiation and apoptosis via binding to nuclear receptors and activating target genes [107]	Approved for psoriasis: Adult, yes; Pediatric, no Pregnancy category X	Severe pustular and erythrodermic >> plaque psoriasis	C	AE: Mucocutaneous: cheilitis, xerosis, conjunctivitis, palmoplantar desquamation and fragility. Liver enzyme elevations; hyperlipidemia. Rare skeletal hyperostosis and calcification of ligaments. CI: Impaired liver or kidney function; chronic abnormally elevated blood lipids; concurrent use of tetracyclines or additional vitamin A derivatives
Cyclosporin	Immunosuppressive via inhibition of T-lymphocytes and suppression of IL-2 and interferon-gamma production [148]	Approved for psoriasis: Adult, yes; Pediatric, no Pregnancy category C	Severe pustular and plaque psoriasis.	C	AE: Hypertension, hyperlipidemia, nephrotoxicity, hyperkalemia, hypomagnesemia, gingival hyperplasia, nausea CI: Acute infections, active malignancies, hypertension, impaired renal function, phototherapy

Abbreviation: DHFR, dihydrofolate reductase.

[107]. Acitretin, the active metabolite of etretinate, is a second-generation aromatic retinoid that replaced etretinate in 1998 and is FDA-approved for the treatment of severe psoriasis in adults. Acitretin is not immunosuppressive and has no formal restrictions on duration of therapy, making it useful for intermittent rescue therapy in children with generalized pustular flares or longer term maintenance of older children with pustular, erythrodermic, or severe plaque psoriasis as monotherapy or in combination with other agents, such as topicals and NB-UVB phototherapy [108,109]. Reports in children as young as 6 months indicate that pustular forms respond more favorably to retinoids than erythrodermic and plaque forms, and time to response may be as little as 3 weeks [108,110,111]. Treatment should be initiated and maintained at dosages at or below 0.5 mg/kg to 1 mg/kg per day to limit short- and long-term toxicities. Acitretin is available in 10-mg and 25-mg gelatin capsules and oral administration with milk or fatty foods enhances absorption [107]. Patients should avoid concomitant intake of supplements containing greater than 5,000 IU of Vitamin A while taking retinoids. The potent teratogenicity of the retinoids is well known to dermatologists and use in females of childbearing potential proceeds with extreme caution. Pregnancy must be avoided while on systemic retinoids and for 3 years following discontinuation of acitretin because of the potential for irreversible esterification of acitretin to etretinate with ingestion of ethanol, inadvertently available to children as an ingredient in cough syrup, over-the-counter medications, and recipes [104]. Isotretinoin, despite debatable efficacy compared with acitretin, clears from the system in 1 month [107] and, therefore, is a rational substitute for acitretin in cases of pustular psoriasis in adolescent and teenage females, provided appropriate contraceptive counseling and control measures are in place [112].

There are convincing data from long-term clinical follow-up of patients with disorders of cornification that oral retinoids are safe in children but do require monitoring as in adults (Table 3) [113]. Associated toxicity is primarily limited to mucocutaneous effects and minor reversible alterations in liver enzymes and lipids, rarely necessitating cessation of therapy [113,114]. Brecher and Orlow [114] reviewed the dermatologic literature and detailed the evidence relating to the efficacy and toxicity of systemic retinoids used in children for acne, psoriasis, and disorders of cornification. The most common side effects observed were reversible, treatable, and dose-dependent mucocutaneous alterations such as cheilitis (Fig. 12), xerosis, skin fragility, epistaxis and blepharoconjunctivitis. More apparent in patients on etretinate and acitretin specifically are diffuse hair thinning, brittle nails, and palmoplantar and fingertip desquamation and fragility (Figs. 13 and 14). Serious ocular toxicity, including corneal opacities, papilledema, cataracts, and abnormal retinal function are very rare in children and typically reversible. These are thought to result primarily from xerosis and diminished Meibomian gland secretion, as well as interference by the retinoids with steps in the rhodopsin cycle [115]. Transient hyperlipidemia, particularly hypertriglyceridemia, occurs in up to 25% of patients and is dose-dependent and reversible upon dose reduction or discontinuation [116].

Table 3
Drug monitoring

Drug	Baseline	Follow-up	Miscellaneous
Methotrexate [104,128,130]	CBC/platelets Liver function Renal function Hepatitis A/B/C; HIV (if at risk)	CBC, platelets, liver function 7 days after test dose, then: weekly for 2–4 weeks and after each dose increase, then every 2 weeks for 1 month and every 2–3 months while on stable doses Renal function every 6–12 months	Liver enzymes transiently rise after MTX dosing; obtain labs 5–7 days after the last dose [126,128] Liver biopsy: no standard recommendations; see text CXR if respiratory symptoms arise [130,131]
Retinoids [107,113,114,131]	CBC/platelets Liver function Renal function Fasting lipid profile Pregnancy testing per FDA prevention program guidelines	Liver function and lipid profile after 1 month of treatment and with dose increases, then every 3 months Monthly pregnancy test	Baseline skeletal survey if long-term treatment anticipated: X-rays of all four limbs and spine, repeated yearly or as symptoms arise Ophthalmologic examination if symptoms arise
Cyclosporine [104,131,214]	Blood pressure × 2 Renal function Urinalysis w/micro Fasting lipid profile CBC/platelets Liver function Magnesium Potassium Uric acid if at risk for gout HIV if at risk	Blood pressure every visit Every 2 weeks for 1–2 months, then monthly: renal function, liver function, lipids, CBC, Mg+, K+, uric acid	Whole-blood CSP trough level if inadequate clinical response or concomitant use of potentially interacting medications (see text) If creatinine increases > 25% above baseline, reduce dose by 1 mg/kg per day for 2–4 weeks and recheck. Stop CSP if Cr remains > 25% above baseline; hold lower dose if level is within 25% of baseline [131]

Abbreviations: CBC, complete blood count; Cr, creatinine; CSP, cyclosporine; CXR, chest X-ray; MTX, methotrexate.
Data from Refs. [104,107,113,114,126,128,130,131,214].

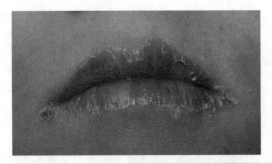

Fig. 12. Retinoid effect: chelitis, xerosis, and peeling of the lips in a patient taking acitretin.

Triglyceride levels in excess of 1,000 mg/dL increase the risk of eruptive xanthoma and pancreatitis, thus frequent monitoring while on therapy is recommended. Transient elevations of lipids during short courses of retinoid therapy are unlikely to affect long-term cardiovascular risk [117]. Mild, transient alterations in liver transaminases may occur in up to 15% of patients and generally return to normal despite continued therapy. There is no evidence linking chronic retinoid use with hepatotoxicty and acute hepatitis has never been reported in a child [114].

Chronic vitamin A toxicity is associated with premature epiphyseal closure, hyperostosis resembling diffuse idiopathic skeletal hyperostosis (DISH), calcification of anterior spinal ligaments, formation of periosteal bone, and effects on bone mineral density [118]. Synthetic retinoids can produce similar changes but exhaustive reviews of the literature reveal conflicting reports [114,119]. While bone abnormalities from short courses of retinoids in low doses (1 mg/kg per day or less), such as those employed for psoriasis, are rare in children, long-term consequences, including decreased bone mineral density, hyperostosis,

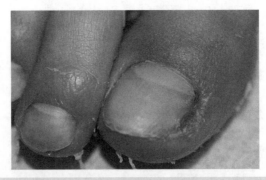

Fig. 13. Retinoid effect: distal toe desquamation and erythema in a patient taking acitretin. Note granulation tissue on the medial aspect of the first digit.

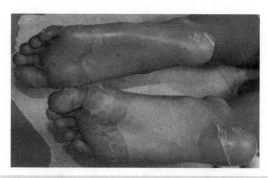

Fig. 14. Retinoid effect: diffuse plantar desquamation and erythema in a patient taking acitretin.

and ligamentous calcification have been identified and continue to be investigated in high dose, long-duration scenarios, such as in the treatment of disorders of cornification [107,113,115,118,120,121]. In almost all cases, adverse effects including the most feared in children, premature epiphyseal closure, are reported in children on long-term, high-dose therapy [114,122,123]. In a recent 25-year follow-up study of 23 patients on long-term retinoid therapy for disorders of cornification, only one patient developed DISH after 25 years of therapy [124]. Furthermore, up to 65% of a population of patients less than 20 years old were shown to have asymptomatic anterior spinal osteophytes in the absence of exposure to retinoids or vitamin A [125]. Halverstam and Lebwohl's recent review of the incidence of abnormal radiographic findings in patients on long-term, low-dose acitretin or etretinate also revealed conflicting data, suggesting that available evidence does not substantiate a clear link between radiologic skeletal abnormalities and this therapeutic subset [119]. Back pain, myalgias, arthralgias and, in rare cases, elevated CPK, are a fairly common phenomenon associated with early retinoid therapy and are more frequent in physically active patients. The mechanism is unknown and a causal relationship to the retinoid is unproven. The process is benign and transient in almost all cases and does not require cessation of therapy [114]. In children anticipated to be on long-term retinoid therapy, baseline and serial or symptom-driven radiologic evaluation of the long bones and spine and close monitoring of growth parameters is appropriate.

Methotrexate

Methotrexate has been used for psoriasis since the 1950s and remains the most widely prescribed drug for severe psoriasis worldwide [126]. It is a folic acid analog that reversibly inhibits dihydrofolate reductase, resulting in interference with DNA synthesis and effects on T-cells [126,127]. Methotrexate lacks FDA approval for use in children other than for cancer chemotherapy and polyarticular-course juvenile rheumatoid arthritis, but is widely and successfully used off-label for a large number of inflammatory and autoimmune conditions, including psoriasis [128–131]. Studies documenting the safety and efficacy of methotrexate in pediatric psoriasis are limited to small series and case reports. Thus, its use is reserved for severe, recalcitrant, extensive disabling disease or psoriatic arthritis, and erythrodermic and generalized pustular forms unresponsive to topical and phototherapy. In children, 0.2 mg/kg to 0.7 mg/kg per week is the recommended therapeutic dose range [130]. In nonemergent situations, a test dose of 1.25 mg to 5 mg followed in 1 week by laboratory monitoring is recommended to detect early toxicity. Regular dosing commences 1 week after the test dose if laboratory results are normal. Conservative dose escalations of 1.25 mg to 5 mg per week are advised until therapeutic effect is obtained, followed by a slow taper to a beneficial maintenance dose. Methotrexate is supplied as 2.5-mg scored tablets that can be split or crushed and given with non-milk food [132] and an injectable preparation (2.5 mg/mL and 25 mg/mL, supplied in 2-mL vials) that can be given orally [127]. Parenteral administration (intravenously or intramuscularly) is advised if adequate oral dosing is ineffective, as the absorption spectrum among individuals can vary substantially [133].

Available evidence regarding the safety and efficacy in pediatric patients with psoriasis is limited to small series and sporadic case reports [129,130,134,135]. Methotrexate was used successfully in seven children aged 3 to 16 years with erythrodermic, generalized pustular psoriasis, or psoriatic arthropathy. Oral dosage ranged from 0.2 mg/kg to 0.4 mg/kg per week for an average of 8 weeks, with no detectable biochemical or hematologic abnormalities. Nausea and vomiting was ameliorated by folic acid supplementation [129]. Dogra and colleagues [134] reported a 4-year-old boy with greater than 40% BSA plaque/pustular psoriasis treated successfully with 0.3 mg/kg per week (5 mg) taken orally. The disease was controlled by week 5 and methotrexate was tapered and discontinued by 12 weeks, followed by a 6-month remission characterized by patchy focal lesions treated with tar and topical steroids. Two flares within the subsequent 14 months were responsive to repeat treatment with methotrexate for 8 to 11 weeks. No laboratory abnormalities were detected. The short duration of active systemic treatment reported by these investigators supports the role of methotrexate in gaining control in the acute phases or flares of the disease, followed by transition to more conventional topical or light-based maintenance regimens. Methotrexate can be used in a sequential regimen with UVB (broadband or narrowband) in an effort to decrease total overall dose and potential toxicity. One method is to initially control and clear the psoriasis with methotrexate, followed by a transition phase of methotrexate/UVB overlap and eventual discontinuation of the methotrexate, with UVB remaining as maintenance therapy.

In children, the bulk of the long-term safety data regarding methotrexate is derived from the rheumatologic literature where the drug is in widespread use for juvenile rheumatoid arthritis [136]. Side effects, both short and long term, are observed in children taking methotrexate for psoriasis but are much less frequent and severe, particularly pulmonary and hepatotoxicity [130,131,136]. Adult use may be associated with greater frequency and severity of side effects because of the comorbidities and concurrent medications used in the vast majority. Regardless of age, methotrexate is associated with a substantial number of potential side effects and drug interactions and requires vigilant clinical and laboratory monitoring (see Table 3) [128,130,131]. The list of drugs that interact with methotrexate with potential to increase its toxicity is vast, and the prescribing physician should consult this list before initiation of therapy [104,128]. Of particular relevance in children are the nonsteroidal anti-inflammatory drugs (NSAIDs) [137,138] and the antibiotic trimethoprim- sulfamethoxazole (TMP-SMX) [139].

Nausea and appetite suppression are the most common side effects encountered during therapy, while vomiting and diarrhea are less frequent but necessitate dose reductions or cessation of therapy. Pulmonary toxicity is extremely rare in children [136] but can present as acute, idiosyncratic pneumonitis early in the course of treatment or chronically as pulmonary fibrosis [104,128]. Bone marrow toxicity is the most serious and potentially life-threatening short-term side effect and can occur early (first 4–6 weeks) in the course of treatment [128,140]. Risk factors for marrow toxicity are often absent in children and include drug interactions, especially TMP-SMX and NSAIDS, renal disease, advanced age, and concurrent major illness. Hepatotoxicity is the most common long-term adverse effect in adults but is rarely encountered in children, probably because of the absence of pre-existing risk factors, such as diabetes, obesity, and alcoholism, as well as exposure to lower cumulative doses. Patients supplemented with folic acid have increased tolerability and substantially reduced risk of pancytopenia, nausea, macrocytic anemia, and liver enzyme elevations without alteration of efficacy [136,141–146].

Currently there is no reliable, specific, noninvasive screening and monitoring test to detect the presence and severity of hepatic fibrosis, despite recent investigations into alternatives to biopsy, such as ultrasound, MRI, dynamic scintigraphy, and measurement of the aminoterminal peptide of type III procollagen (PIIINP), produced during the synthesis of type III collagen. PIIINP in particular, although highly popular in Europe, is not organ-specific and may be raised in children in the absence of pathology [126]. Liver enzymes predictably rise in the days following methotrexate administration and are a poor marker of hepatic fibrosis [126]. Despite substantial controversy, liver biopsy remains the gold standard for accurate diagnosis of fibrosis and cirrhosis, and current American Academy of Dermatology monitoring guidelines suggest an early liver biopsy in patients with risk factors as noted above, and subsequent biopsy for all patients at a cumulative dose of 1.5 g and every 1 g to 1.5 g thereafter [147]. Although no specific monitoring guidelines exist for pediatric patients, general consensus and expert opinion suggests that baseline and monitoring liver biopsies are not required in the absence of clinical or laboratory evidence of pathology and cumulative doses less than 1.5 g [130,131].

Cyclosporine

Cyclosporine is a noncytotoxic drug whose immunosuppressant effects result from specific and reversible inhibition of immunocompetent T-lymphocytes and suppression of IL-2 and interferon-gamma production [148]. It is FDA-approved for severe, recalcitrant psoriasis in nonimmunocompromised adults in oral dosages up to 4 mg/kg per day and for prevention and treatment of transplant rejection in children older than 6 months of age. Although there is good clinical experience in refractory childhood atopic dermatitis [149–151] and psoriasis, it remains unapproved for these indications and its use is limited by the risk of nephrotoxicity, hypertension and immunosuppression. Close laboratory (see Table 3) and blood pressure monitoring before and throughout the treatment period is required to detect dose-related side effects that are typically easily controlled by appropriate dose modification. Cyclosporine usage is limited by restrictions on maximum dosing (4 mg/kg per day United States guidelines and 5 mg/kg per day internationally) and duration (1–2 years) [104,152–154]. Children may require higher doses than that recommended for adults because children have a higher BSA in relation to body weight than do adults, and therefore dose calculations based on mg/kg rather than on BSA may result in lower efficacy. Furthermore, the pharmacokinetics of cyclosporine are age-dependent. Children show reduced oral absorption, more rapid clearance, and a greater volume of distribution at steady state [154]. Cyclosporine is extensively metabolized in the liver and plasma concentrations may be affected by inducers or competitive inhibitors of hepatic enzymes, particularly cytochrome P450 isoenzyme CYP3A4. Dosage adjustments are based on monitoring of clinical response, serum creatinine levels, and blood pressure. There is no clear conclusion from the adult literature as to the necessity for therapeutic monitoring of cyclosporine trough levels during short-term treatment of psoriasis [155,156]. Circulating cyclosporine levels do not reliably correlate with clinical response and therefore do not reliably guide dosing in adults [156]. Given differences in metabolism in children and, in cases where concomitant medications are likely to interact with cyclosporine, monitoring of trough cyclosporine levels in whole blood in an effort to guide dosing and avoid preventable toxicity or lack of efficacy is reasonable. Sequential therapy (addition of a second agent, such as acitretin) in select situations allows reduced total dose and duration of both medications in an effort to maximize effect and minimize toxicity [105]. Simultaneous administration of phototherapy with cyclosporine is best avoided because of the well-documented risk of squamous cell carcinoma. In select cases of severe or refractory disease, cyclosporine can be used to achieve initial clearing followed by phototherapy for maintenance. Cyclosporine (Neoral) is available as 25-mg and 100-mg soft gelatin capsules and as a clear yellow liquid supplied in 50-mL bottles containing 100 mg/mL.

Review of available data in refractory childhood psoriasis reveals use in children as young as 11 months for severe refractory plaque and pustular psoriasis, with dosages ranging from 1.5 mg/kg to 5 mg/kg per day for 6 weeks up to 2 years [153,154,157–159]. Adjuvant therapy with topical steroids, vitamin

D3 ointments, coal tar preparations, or anthralin was used in the majority of children and acitretin was used adjunctively in a minority [153]. Treatment was generally but not universally effective but well tolerated and devoid of significant adverse effects, including hypertension and nephrotoxicity. Onset of effect is rapid (4–8 weeks) and gradual tapering should start after a 1- to 3-month period of stability and adjusted according to clinical response. Rebounds during taper or after withdrawal are not uncommon. Side effects common to high-dose usage in transplant populations, such as nausea, diarrhea, myalgias, arthralgias, headache, paresthesias, gingival hyperplasia, and hypertrichosis are rarely encountered in children treated for psoriasis [153]. The risk of malignancy, skin cancer, and lymphoproliferative disorders as observed in the transplant population are a concern in children; however, evidence suggests that risk is minimal if using 5 mg/kg per day or less in patients who are not on concomitant immunosuppressive medications [160]. Vaccination may be less effective and live attenuated vaccines must be avoided during treatment. In carefully selected and closely monitored patients, cyclosporine can produce relatively rapid clinical effects and can be effectively combined with topical and systemic therapies to increase efficacy and decrease toxicity.

PHOTOTHERAPY

Ultraviolet light has been used safely and effectively to treat psoriasis, even before Dr. Goeckerman popularized UVB phototherapy in 1925 [161]. Phototherapy is appropriate for carefully selected patients with refractory disease, diffuse (>15%–20% BSA) involvement, or focal debilitating palmoplantar psoriasis. Three main types of therapeutic light options exist: broadband UVB (BB-UVB, 290 nm–320 nm), narrowband UVB (NB-UVB, 311 nm–313 nm) and UVA (320–400 nm). BB-UVB encompasses the most biologically active radiation in sunlight, and therapeutic exposure inhibits DNA synthesis and epidermal keratinocyte proliferation and induces T-cell apoptosis and immunosuppressive and anti-inflammatory cytokines [162,163]. Starting dose was conventionally based upon determination of the minimal erythema dose (MED) but this is cumbersome and impractical in children; therefore, starting and incremental dosing is based on Fitzpatrick skin type per established protocols [164–166]. Importantly, dosing protocols differ and are not interchangeable for BB-UVB and NB-UVB sources and between equipment from different manufacturers. Phototherapy encompasses the art and science of medicine, as there is no "one size fits all" approach and dosing modifications must be based at each visit on careful assessment of the individual patient's response to the previous session and the overall clinical situation. Delivery of ultraviolet radiation in Joules or milliJoules is akin to delivery of medications in grams or milligrams; there requires consideration of a multitude of factors related to the patient, the disease, and the risk-benefit ratio of the treatment when deciding the best therapeutic plan. Phototherapy can be conceptualized as proceeding in two phases: clearing (weekly sessions vary from two to five, according to wavelength used and individual factors, and dose is increased at each visit according to individual protocol in the absence of adverse effects or missed treatments) and maintenance (dose is held from clearing phase and frequency of treatment sessions are gradually decreased) [167]. A "standard" course consists of 30 treatments administered three times per week, but the number of weekly sessions may vary depending on individual factors and feasibility.

UVB

Guttate psoriasis responds best to UVB light but plaque psoriasis in children tends to be thinner and will respond to higher doses and longer duration of treatment. Age, duration, and extent of disease have little to no relationship to cumulative clearance dose, number of sittings, or duration of therapy [168]. Treatment is given up to five times weekly in motivated adults, but for practical reasons it is limited to two to three times weekly in children. Fifty percent to 88% of patients achieve clearance or near clearance after 15 to 20 treatments, including those with skin type V [162,165,168]. Short-term side effects of UVB phototherapy are usually mild and consist of xerosis, erythema, pruritus, and photoactivation of herpes simplex virus. Long-term effects include premature photoaging and cutaneous carcinogenesis [169].

One of the greatest advances in phototherapy for psoriasis is the use of selective UVB wavelengths based on early work that defined 296 nm to 313 nm as the therapeutic action spectrum for psoriasis, with 313 nm being less erythemogenic at therapeutic doses than other wavelengths in the UVB range [163,170–173]. Centered on 311 nm to 313 nm, NB-UVB is safe and effective for a number of photoresponsive dermatoses in children, including psoriasis across skin types I to V [166,168], and has become the light treatment of choice for children [164]. Dosing is started at a percentage (50%–80%) of the predetermined MED established by phototesting or, more commonly in children, by Fitzpatrick skin type. Increases in dose and duration are based on the protocol per skin type and adjusted based on clinical response and presence of adverse effects, such as erythema and pruritus [167]. Early studies looking at the ideal frequency of NB-UVB treatments in adults showed that clinical effects are obtained at two to three treatments per week [174,175]. In practice, children typically are treated twice weekly on nonconsecutive days and starting, incremental, and maintenance dosing parameters must be tailored to the individual patient. However, in regions where a formal phototherapy center staffed with trained personnel is not available, reference resources containing protocols can be helpful [176].

The clinical benefit of NB-UVB for moderate to severe psoriasis is proven in adults [162,163,177] and children across all skin types [164,166,168,169]. Treatment with NB-UVB rapidly depletes infiltrating T cells from psoriatic plaques and results in faster clearance, less erythema, and longer remission versus BB-UVB [164]. Interestingly, verbal reports from patients regarding whether their psoriasis improves or not in response to sunlight do not correlate with their actual response to NB-UVB phototherapy [178], and treatment should not be withheld because a patient is presumed a sunlight "nonresponder"

[179]. Topical therapies, such as calcipotriene [180], tazarotene [181], and anthralin [182] combined with NB-UVB will enhance the efficacy of both modalities and decrease the overall exposure to UV radiation. Calcipotriene should be applied after phototherapy, because if applied thickly it absorbs UV light and in turn is degraded by UV light [183]. The combination of acitretin with NB-UVB (RE-NB-UVB) appears to have synergistic effects and may decrease the time to clearance and the overall exposure to both modalities [104,184]. RE-NB-UVB is effective and well tolerated in severe generalized pustular psoriasis in children and may be used within the context of a sequential regimen, as maintenance therapy after the acute toxic stage is controlled with low-dose cyclosporine (Fig. 15) [108,185]. The acute dose-dependent side effects of NB-UVB are erythema, burning, pigmentation, and rare transient lesional blistering [186,187]. The widespread use of suberythemogenic regimens in children minimizes these risks. Long-term safety data for NB-UVB is unavailable, including the precise risks relevant to children, such as photoaging and skin cancer [188]. As with all treatments in children, the potential benefit must be weighed against the risks of other systemic therapies and the severity of the disease in the individual patient.

UVA

Photochemotherapy (psoralen plus ultraviolet A or PUVA) is based on the interaction between UVA radiation and psoralen, a photosensitizing chemical. In

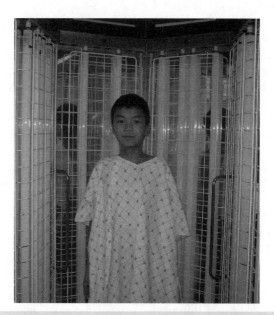

Fig. 15. 11-year-old boy in a NB-UVB phototherapy unit. This patient is treated with RE-NB-UVB for maintenance of annular pustular psoriasis after being initially cleared with cyclosporine.

children less than 12, oral PUVA proceeds with extreme caution and its use is restricted to psoriasis and phototherapy centers staffed by well-trained, experienced physicians and nurses [167]. Many investigators consider oral psoralen relatively contraindicated in children less than 12 [10] and prefer topical PUVA because of the many short- and long-term toxicities associated with psoralen ingestion (nausea, vomiting, headache, hepatotoxicity, generalized photosensitization requiring 24 hours of photoprotection, ocular toxicity, acute risk of burning, and long-term risk of skin cancer) [189,190]. Although considered by many to be safer than oral PUVA, bath PUVA lacks long-term carcinogenicity data and therefore evidence is insufficient to deem this modality totally safe [191]. In centers where oral PUVA is administered to children, the drug is limited to those weighing greater than 100 pounds, is given 90 minutes before UVA exposure, and the child is given the last appointment of the day, which provides a window of safety after treatment as the sun will be down and risk of inadvertent additional exposure is nil [167]. Studies comparing NB-UVB and PUVA show fairly comparable efficacy, with PUVA being slightly more effective [172,192]. In children, NB-UVB is more convenient and may be less carcinogenic [172], and given the downsides of using psoralens in children and adults, NB-UVB is now considered first-line phototherapy [32]. One remaining and important utility of topical PUVA in children is for the treatment of recalcitrant hand and foot psoriasis [193].

BIOLOGICS

The complex molecular mechanisms underlying the pathogenesis of psoriasis are becoming increasingly clear. As such, targeted therapies aimed at specific components of the inflammatory cascade, such as tumor necrosis factor (TNFα), are gaining popularity and are in widespread use among adults with psoriasis and psoriatic arthritis. The United States FDA has approved three TNFα inhibitors for the treatment of psoriasis and psoriatic arthritis in adults: etanercept, a fully human fusion protein of TNF receptor II bound to the Fc component of human IgG1; infliximab, a chimeric monoclonal antibody; and adalimumab, a fully human monoclonal antibody. Of these, etanercept has the most significant published literature and FDA approval for use in children (ankylosing spondylitis and psoriatic arthropathy for children 2 years and older and juvenile rheumatoid arthritis in children 4 years and older) to substantiate recommendations for its use in the pediatric population [194–197]. Infliximab is widely and successfully used in the treatment of pediatric patients with juvenile chronic arthritis and inflammatory bowel disease. Although further investigation is warranted, infliximab appears promising for the treatment of refractory plaque and generalized pustular psoriasis in children [198–200]. Critical evaluation of the potential risk of the anti-TNF agents in children with psoriasis is difficult because of the small number of children treated and the short follow-up period. No specific guidelines exist for dosing and laboratory monitoring in pediatric patients. Enthusiasm for the efficacy, short-term safety, and ease of use of these agents in children is reasonably tempered by concerns about the risk of infection, lymphoma, demyelinating disorders, and cost [201].

MISCELLANEOUS THERAPIES

Antibiotics and tonsillectomy

Clinical observations suggesting precipitation, exacerbation, and maintenance of guttate and other forms of psoriasis by pharyngeal and perianal streptococcal infections [20,202,203] are supported by laboratory evidence of proliferation of skin-homing T-cell lines in response to specific streptococcal antigens functioning as superantigens [16,17,20]. Some reports estimate up to 70% of initial presentations of psoriasis in children are associated with a recent infection [204]. Because of the frequency of this association, dermatologists often prescribe empiric systemic antibiotics for recurrence or flares of guttate psoriasis, and occasionally recommend tonsillectomy in patients with refractory psoriasis and recurrent tonsillitis. Two recent exhaustive reviews assessed the evidence for such interventions in the management of childhood psoriasis and concluded that available evidence does not support the efficacy of oral antibiotics or tonsillectomy [204,205]. Well-designed, randomized, placebo-controlled trials are necessary to accurately assess the effectiveness of these interventions. In practice, the relative safety of these interventions compared with the other therapeutic options for severe psoriasis lends support to their judicious use in select patients with documented recurrent streptococcal disease.

EMERGING THERAPIES AND TECHNOLOGY

Many effective therapies for psoriasis exist as detailed above. Precise dosing strategies and laboratory monitoring for toxicity remain areas of investigation for systemic and biologic agents. As experience and evidence of safety expand, the biologic agents may take a primary position in the treatment of children as they have in adults. The advantages of less frequent dosing, monitoring, tolerance, and short-term safety must be weighed against the unknown long-term toxicities. There is increasing evidence of the importance of a novel T-cell population, Th17 cells, in autoimmune disease including psoriasis. Th17 cells are stimulated by IL-23 (which shares the p40 subunit with IL-12) to produce IL-17 and IL-22, the latter of which has been recently shown to mediate IL-23-induced dermal inflammation and acanthosis in psoriasis [206]. A new monoclonal antibody directed against the p40 subunit of IL-12 looks promising in preliminary studies in adults [206,207]. Further, as the field of pharmacogenetics expands, it may be possible to predict which patients will respond to therapy or be susceptible to toxicity of various treatments [208,209].

SUMMARY

Treating children with psoriasis represents one of the most rewarding yet constantly challenging endeavors in dermatology. These patients require time, energy, enthusiasm, empathy, and current, comprehensive knowledge of the unique clinical presentations in children and available therapies, including clinical action spectrum, mechanism of action, potential toxicity, and monitoring. Longitudinal trials examining the epidemiology and natural history of psoriasis, as well as the safety and efficacy of current and emerging treatments, are desperately needed in the pediatric population.

Partner with the patient, family, and other multidisciplinary providers to form an educational and therapeutic alliance. Early in the course of disease, schedule frequent visits for reinforcement of the therapeutic plan, education, clinical and treatment monitoring, and support. As the disease and the patient's physical, psychosocial and emotional level of functioning evolve, so too will the requirement for follow-up and monitoring. Patient advocacy and education groups, such as the National Psoriasis Foundation (www.psoriasis.org; 800-723-9166) are excellent resources and can serve as an extension of your comprehensive care.

Acknowledgments
Special thanks to Patricia B. McClelland, RN, for her time, expertise and thoughtful contributions to the phototherapy section of this article.

References
[1] Beattie PE, Lewis-Jones MS. A comparative study of impairment of quality of life in children with skin disease and children with other chronic childhood diseases. Br J Dermatol 2006;155(1):145–51.
[2] Benoit S, Hamm H. Childhood psoriasis. Clin Dermatol 2007;25(6):555–62.
[3] Farber EM, Nall L. Childhood psoriasis. Cutis 1999;64(5):309–14.
[4] Farber EM, Nall ML. The natural history of psoriasis in 5,600 patients. Dermatologica 1974;148(1):1–18.
[5] Kumar B, Jain R, Sandhu K, et al. Epidemiology of childhood psoriasis: a study of 419 patients from northern India. Int J Dermatol 2004;43(9):654–8.
[6] Lewkowicz D, Gottlieb AB. Pediatric psoriasis and psoriatic arthritis. Dermatol Ther 2004;17(5):364–75.
[7] Morris A, Rogers M, Fischer G, et al. Childhood psoriasis: a clinical review of 1262 cases. Pediatr Dermatol 2001;18(3):188–98.
[8] Rogers M. Childhood psoriasis. Curr Opin Pediatr 2002;14(4):404–9.
[9] Raychaudhuri SP, Gross J. A comparative study of pediatric onset psoriasis with adult onset psoriasis. Pediatr Dermatol 2000;17(3):174–8.
[10] Burden AD. Management of psoriasis in childhood. Clin Exp Dermatol 1999;24(5):341–5.
[11] Neville EA, Finn OA. Psoriasiform napkin dermatitis—a follow-up study. Br J Dermatol 1975;92(3):279–85.
[12] Boje Rasmussen H, Hagdrup H, Schmidt H. Psoriasiform napkin dermatitis. Acta Derm Venereol 1986;66(6):534–6.
[13] Farber EM, Mullen RH, Jacobs AH, et al. Infantile psoriasis: a follow-up study. Pediatr Dermatol 1986;3(3):237–43.
[14] Darley CR, Cunliffe WJ, Green CM, et al. Safety and efficacy of calcipotriol ointment (Dovonex) in treating children with psoriasis vulgaris. Br J Dermatol 1996;135(3):390–3.
[15] Baadsgaard O, Fisher G, Voorhees JJ, et al. The role of immune system in the pathogenesis of psoriasis. J Invest Dermatol 1990;95(5 Suppl):32S–4S.
[16] Baker BS, Brown DW, Fischetti VA, et al. Skin T cell proliferative response to M protein and other cell wall and membrane proteins of group A streptococci in chronic plaque psoriasis. Clin Exp Immunol 2001;124(3):516–21.

[17] Brown DW, Baker BS, Ovigne JM, et al. Non-M protein(s) on the cell wall and membrane of group A streptococci induce(s) IFN-gamma production by dermal CD4+ T cells in psoriasis. Arch Dermatol Res 2001;293(4):165–70.

[18] Eberhard BA, Sundel RP, Newburger JW, et al. Psoriatic eruption in Kawasaki disease. J Pediatr 2000;137(4):578–80.

[19] Han MH, Jang KA, Sung KJ, et al. A case of guttate psoriasis following Kawasaki disease. Br J Dermatol 2000;142(3):548–50.

[20] Rasmussen JE. The relationship between infection with group A beta hemolytic streptococci and the development of psoriasis. Pediatr Infect Dis J 2000;19(2):153–4.

[21] Farber EM, Nall ML, Watson W. Natural history of psoriasis in 61 twin pairs. Arch Dermatol 1974;109(2):207–11.

[22] Burden AD. Identifying a gene for psoriasis on chromosome 6 (Psors1). Br J Dermatol 2000;143(2):238–41.

[23] Enerback C, Martinsson T, Inerot A, et al. Evidence that HLA-Cw6 determines early onset of psoriasis, obtained using sequence-specific primers (PCR-SSP). Acta Derm Venereol 1997;77(4):273–6.

[24] Ikaheimo I, Tiilikainen A, Karvonen J, et al. HLA risk haplotype Cw6,DR7,DQA1*0201 and HLA-Cw6 with reference to the clinical picture of psoriasis vulgaris. Arch Dermatol Res 1996;288(7):363–5.

[25] Nair RP, Stuart PE, Nistor I, et al. Sequence and haplotype analysis supports HLA-C as the psoriasis susceptibility 1 gene. Am J Hum Genet 2006;78(5):827–51.

[26] Tiilikainen A, Lassus A, Karvonen J, et al. Psoriasis and HLA-Cw6. Br J Dermatol 1980;102(2):179–84.

[27] Carroll JM, Romero MR, Watt FM. Suprabasal integrin expression in the epidermis of transgenic mice results in developmental defects and a phenotype resembling psoriasis. Cell 1995;83(6):957–68.

[28] Wrone-Smith T, Mitra RS, Thompson CB, et al. Keratinocytes derived from psoriatic plaques are resistant to apoptosis compared with normal skin. Am J Pathol 1997;151(5):1321–9.

[29] Bhushan M, McLaughlin B, Weiss JB, et al. Levels of endothelial cell stimulating angiogenesis factor and vascular endothelial growth factor are elevated in psoriasis. Br J Dermatol 1999;141(6):1054–60.

[30] Menssen A, Trommler P, Vollmer S, et al. Evidence for an antigen-specific cellular immune response in skin lesions of patients with psoriasis vulgaris. J Immunol 1995;155(8): 4078–83.

[31] Leung DY, Travers JB, Giorno R, et al. Evidence for a streptococcal superantigen-driven process in acute guttate psoriasis. J Clin Invest 1995;96(5):2106–12.

[32] MacDonald A, Burden AD. Psoriasis: advances in pathophysiology and management. Postgrad Med J 2007;83(985):690–7.

[33] Gottlieb A, Korman NJ, Gordon KB, et al. Guidelines of care for the management of psoriasis and psoriatic arthritis: Section 2. Psoriatic arthritis: overview and guidelines of care for treatment with an emphasis on the biologics. J Am Acad Dermatol 2008;58(5):851–64.

[34] Stoll ML, Lio P, Sundel RP, et al. Comparison of Vancouver and International League of Associations for Rheumatology classification criteria for juvenile psoriatic arthritis. Arthritis Rheum 2008;59(1):51–8.

[35] Ferrandiz C, Pujol RM, Garcia-Patos V, et al. Psoriasis of early and late onset: a clinical and epidemiologic study from Spain. J Am Acad Dermatol 2002;46(6):867–73.

[36] Gelfand JM, Berlin J, Van Voorhees A, et al. Lymphoma rates are low but increased in patients with psoriasis: results from a population-based cohort study in the United Kingdom. Arch Dermatol 2003;139(11):1425–9.

[37] Cohen AD, Gilutz H, Henkin Y, et al. Psoriasis and the metabolic syndrome. Acta Derm Venereol 2007;87(6):506–9.

[38] Cohen AD, Sherf M, Vidavsky L, et al. Association between psoriasis and the metabolic syndrome. A cross-sectional study. Dermatology 2008;216(2):152–5.

[39] Yates VM, Watkinson G, Kelman A. Further evidence for an association between psoriasis, Crohn's disease and ulcerative colitis. Br J Dermatol 1982;106(3):323–30.

[40] Beretta-Piccoli BC, Sauvain MJ, Gal I, et al. Synovitis, acne, pustulosis, hyperostosis, osteitis (SAPHO) syndrome in childhood: a report of ten cases and review of the literature. Eur J Pediatr 2000;159(8):594–601.

[41] Abel EA, DiCicco LM, Orenberg EK, et al. Drugs in exacerbation of psoriasis. J Am Acad Dermatol 1986;15(5 Pt 1):1007–22.

[42] Mallon E, Bunce M, Savoie H, et al. HLA-C and guttate psoriasis. Br J Dermatol 2000;143(6):1177–82.

[43] Martin BA, Chalmers RJ, Telfer NR. How great is the risk of further psoriasis following a single episode of acute guttate psoriasis? Arch Dermatol 1996;132(6):717–8.

[44] Johnson TM, Duvic M, Rapini RP, et al. AIDS exacerbates psoriasis. N Engl J Med 1985;313(22):1415.

[45] Lazar AP, Roenigk HH Jr. Acquired immunodeficiency syndrome (AIDS) can exacerbate psoriasis. J Am Acad Dermatol 1988;18(1 Pt 1):144.

[46] Warino L, Balkrishnan R, Feldman SR. Clobetasol propionate for psoriasis: are ointments really more potent? J Drugs Dermatol 2006;5(6):527–32.

[47] Lebwohl M. Combination, rotational and sequential therapy. In: Weinstein G, Gottlieb A, editors. Therapy of moderate to severe psoriasis. 2nd edition. New York: Marcel Dekker; 2003. p. 179–95.

[48] Leman J, Burden D. Psoriasis in children: a guide to its diagnosis and management. Paediatr Drugs 2001;3(9):673–80.

[49] Cornell RC, Stoughton RB. Correlation of the vasoconstriction assay and clinical activity in psoriasis. Arch Dermatol 1985;121(1):63–7.

[50] Maibach HI, Wester RC. Issues in measuring percutaneous absorption of topical corticosteroids. Int J Dermatol. 1992;31(Suppl 1):21–5.

[51] Lebwohl M. A clinician's paradigm in the treatment of psoriasis. J Am Acad Dermatol 2005;53 1(Suppl 1):S59–69.

[52] Feldman SR. Tachyphylaxis to topical corticosteroids: the more you use them, the less they work? Clin Dermatol 2006;24(3):229–30 [discussion: 230].

[53] Comaish JS. Tar and related compounds in the therapy of psoriasis. Clin Exp Dermatol 1981;6(6):639–45.

[54] Lin AN, Moses K. Tar revisited. Int J Dermatol 1985;24(4):216–8.

[55] Cram DL. Psoriasis: treatment with a tar gel. Cutis 1976;17(6):1197–203.

[56] Farber EM, Psoriasis Nall L. A review of recent advances in treatment. Drugs 1984;28(4):324–46.

[57] Lowe NJ, Breeding JH, Wortzman MS. New coal tar extract and coal tar shampoos. Evaluation by epidermal cell DNA synthesis suppression assay. Arch Dermatol 1982;118(7):487–9.

[58] Borska L, Fiala Z, Krejsek J, et al. Immunologic changes in TNF-alpha, sE-selectin, sP-selectin, sICAM-1, and IL-8 in pediatric patients treated for psoriasis with the Goeckerman regimen. Pediatr Dermatol 2007;24(6):607–12.

[59] Stoughton RB, DeQuoy P, Walter JF. Crude coal tar plus near ultraviolet light suppresses DNA synthesis in epidermis. Arch Dermatol 1978;114(1):43–5.

[60] Sharma V, Kaur I, Kumar B. Calcipotriol versus coal tar: a prospective randomized study in stable plaque psoriasis. Int J Dermatol 2003;42(10):834–8.

[61] van Schooten FJ, Godschalk R. Coal tar therapy. Is it carcinogenic? Drug Saf 1996;15(6):374–7.

[62] Pion IA, Koenig KL, Lim HW. Is dermatologic usage of coal tar carcinogenic? A review of the literature. Dermatol Surg 1995;21(3):227–31.

[63] Pittelkow MR, Perry HO, Muller SA, et al. Skin cancer in patients with psoriasis treated with coal tar. A 25-year follow-up study. Arch Dermatol 1981;117(8):465–8.

[64] Ashton RE, Andre P, Lowe NJ, et al. Anthralin: historical and current perspectives. J Am Acad Dermatol 1983;9(2):173–92.

[65] Ingram JT. The approach to psoriasis. Br Med J 1953;2(4836):591–4.

[66] Reichert U, Jacques Y, Grangeret M, et al. Antirespiratory and antiproliferative activity of anthralin in cultured human keratinocytes. J Invest Dermatol 1985;84(2):130–4.

[67] Peus D, Beyerle A, Rittner HL, et al. Anti-psoriatic drug anthralin activates JNK via lipid per-oxidation: mononuclear cells are more sensitive than keratinocytes. J Invest Dermatol 2000;114(4):688–92.

[68] Zvulunov A, Anisfeld A, Metzker A. Efficacy of short-contact therapy with dithranol in child-hood psoriasis. Int J Dermatol 1994;33(11):808–10.

[69] Runne U, Kunze J. Short-duration ('minutes') therapy with dithranol for psoriasis: a new out-patient regimen. Br J Dermatol 1982;106(2):135–9.

[70] Guerrier CJ, Porter DI. An open assessment of 0.1% dithranol in a 17% urea base ('Psora-drate' 0.1%) in the treatment of psoriasis of children. Curr Med Res Opin 1983;8(6):446–50.

[71] Koo JY. New developments in topical sequential therapy for psoriasis. Skin Therapy Lett 2005;10(9):1–4.

[72] Lebwohl M, Ali S. Treatment of psoriasis. Part 1. Topical therapy and phototherapy. J Am Acad Dermatol 2001;45(4):487–98 [quiz: 499–502].

[73] Reichrath J, Muller SM, Kerber A, et al. Biologic effects of topical calcipotriol (MC 903) treatment in psoriatic skin. J Am Acad Dermatol 1997;36(1):19–28.

[74] Reichrath J, Perez A, Muller SM, et al. Topical calcitriol (1,25-dihydroxyvitamin D3) treat-ment of psoriasis: an immunohistological evaluation. Acta Derm Venereol 1997;77(4): 268–72.

[75] Lebwohl M, Siskin SB, Epinette W, et al. A multicenter trial of calcipotriene ointment and halobetasol ointment compared with either agent alone for the treatment of psoriasis. J Am Acad Dermatol 1996;35(2 Pt 1):268–9.

[76] Koo J, Blum RR, Lebwohl M. A randomized, multicenter study of calcipotriene ointment and clobetasol propionate foam in the sequential treatment of localized plaque-type psoriasis: short- and long-term outcomes. J Am Acad Dermatol 2006;55(4):637–41.

[77] White S, Vender R, Thaci D, et al. Use of calcipotriene cream (Dovonex cream) following acute treatment of psoriasis vulgaris with the calcipotriene/betamethasone dipropionate two-compound product (Taclonex): a randomized, parallel-group clinical trial. Am J Clin Dermatol 2006;7(3):177–84.

[78] Oranje AP, Marcoux D, Svensson A, et al. Topical calcipotriol in childhood psoriasis. J Am Acad Dermatol 1997;36(2 Pt 1):203–8.

[79] Choi YJ, Hann SK, Chang SN, et al. Infantile psoriasis: successful treatment with topical calcipotriol. Pediatr Dermatol 2000;17(3):242–4.

[80] Travis LB, Silverberg NB. Psoriasis in infancy: therapy with calcipotriene ointment. Cutis 2001;68(5):341–4.

[81] Bourke JF, Mumford R, Whittaker P, et al. The effects of topical calcipotriol on systemic cal-cium homeostasis in patients with chronic plaque psoriasis. J Am Acad Dermatol 1997;37(6):929–34.

[82] Esgleyes-Ribot T, Chandraratna RA, Lew-Kaya DA, et al. Response of psoriasis to a new topical retinoid, AGN 190168. J Am Acad Dermatol Apr 1994;30(4):581–90.

[83] Marks R. Early clinical development of tazarotene. Br J Dermatol 1996;135(Suppl 49): 26–31.

[84] Lebwohl MG, Breneman DL, Goffe BS, et al. Tazarotene 0.1% gel plus corticosteroid cream in the treatment of plaque psoriasis. J Am Acad Dermatol 1998;39(4 Pt 1):590–6.

[85] Bianchi L, Soda R, Diluvio L, et al. Tazarotene 0.1% gel for psoriasis of the fingernails and toenails: an open, prospective study. Br J Dermatol 2003;149(1):207–9.

[86] Diluvio L, Campione E, Paterno EJ, et al. Childhood nail psoriasis: a useful treatment with tazarotene 0.05%. Pediatr Dermatol 2007;24(3):332–3.

[87] Nghiem P, Pearson G, Langley RG. Tacrolimus and pimecrolimus: from clever prokaryotes to inhibiting calcineurin and treating atopic dermatitis. J Am Acad Dermatol 2002;46(2): 228–41.

[88] Bigby M. Pimecrolimus and tacrolimus for the treatment of intertriginous and facial psoriasis: are they effective? Arch Dermatol 2005;141(9):1152–3.

[89] Clayton TH, Harrison PV, Nicholls R, et al. Topical tacrolimus for facial psoriasis. Br J Dermatol 2003;149(2):419–20.

[90] Freeman AK, Linowski GJ, Brady C, et al. Tacrolimus ointment for the treatment of psoriasis on the face and intertriginous areas. J Am Acad Dermatol 2003;48(4):564–8.

[91] Gribetz C, Ling M, Lebwohl M, et al. Pimecrolimus cream 1% in the treatment of intertriginous psoriasis: a double-blind, randomized study. J Am Acad Dermatol 2004;51(5): 731–8.

[92] Kreuter A, Sommer A, Hyun J, et al. 1% pimecrolimus, 0.005% calcipotriol, and 0.1% betamethasone in the treatment of intertriginous psoriasis: a double-blind, randomized controlled study. Arch Dermatol 2006;142(9):1138–43.

[93] Lebwohl M, Freeman AK, Chapman MS, et al. Tacrolimus ointment is effective for facial and intertriginous psoriasis. J Am Acad Dermatol 2004;51(5):723–30.

[94] Yamamoto T, Nishioka K. Topical tacrolimus is effective for facial lesions of psoriasis. Acta Derm Venereol 2000;80(6):451.

[95] Yamamoto T, Nishioka K. Topical tacrolimus: an effective therapy for facial psoriasis. Eur J Dermatol 2003;13(5):471–3.

[96] Yamamoto T, Nishioka K. Successful treatment with topical tacrolimus for oral psoriasis. J Eur Acad Dermatol Venereol 2006;20(9):1137–8.

[97] Ahn SJ, Oh SH, Chang SE, et al. A case of infantile psoriasis with pseudoainhum successfully treated with topical pimecrolimus and low-dose narrowband UVB phototherapy. J Eur Acad Dermatol Venereol 2006;20(10):1332–4.

[98] Amichai B. Psoriasis of the glans penis in a child successfully treated with Elidel (pimecrolimus) cream. J Eur Acad Dermatol Venereol 2004;18(6):742–3.

[99] Brune A, Miller DW, Lin P, et al. Tacrolimus ointment is effective for psoriasis on the face and intertriginous areas in pediatric patients. Pediatr Dermatol 2007;24(1):76–80.

[100] Mansouri P, Farshi S. Pimecrolimus 1 percent cream in the treatment of psoriasis in a child. Dermatol Online J 2006;12(2):7.

[101] Steele JA, Choi C, Kwong PC. Topical tacrolimus in the treatment of inverse psoriasis in children. J Am Acad Dermatol 2005;53(4):713–6.

[102] Krochmal L, Wang JC, Patel B, et al. Topical corticosteroid compounding: effects on physicochemical stability and skin penetration rate. J Am Acad Dermatol 1989;21(5 Pt 1): 979–84.

[103] Taylor JR, Halprin KM. Percutaneous absorption of salicylic acid. Arch Dermatol 1975;111(6):740–3.

[104] Lebwohl M, Ali S. Treatment of psoriasis. Part 2. Systemic therapies. J Am Acad Dermatol 2001;45(5):649–61 [quiz: 644–62].

[105] Koo J. Systemic sequential therapy of psoriasis: a new paradigm for improved therapeutic results. J Am Acad Dermatol 1999;41(3 Pt 2):S25–8.

[106] Koo JY. Using topical multimodal strategies for patients with psoriasis. Cutis 2007;79 (1 Suppl 2):11–7.

[107] Patton TJ, Zirwas MJ, Wolverton SE. Systemic retinoids. In: Wolverton SE, editor. Comprehensive dermatologic drug therapy. 2nd edition. Philadelphia: Saunders (Elsevier); 2007. p. 275–300.

[108] Kopp T, Karlhofer F, Szepfalusi Z, et al. Successful use of acitretin in conjunction with narrowband ultraviolet B phototherapy in a child with severe pustular psoriasis, von Zumbusch type. Br J Dermatol 2004;151(4):912–6.

[109] Lee CS, Koo J. A review of acitretin, a systemic retinoid for the treatment of psoriasis. Expert Opin Pharmacother 2005;6(10):1725–34.

[110] Rosinska D, Wolska H, Jablonska S, et al. Etretinate in severe psoriasis of children. Pediatr Dermatol 1988;5(4):266–72.

[111] Shelnitz LS, Esterly NB, Honig PJ. Etretinate therapy for generalized pustular psoriasis in children. Arch Dermatol 1987;123(2):230–3.

[112] Al-Shobaili H, Al-Khenaizan S. Childhood generalized pustular psoriasis: successful treatment with isotretinoin. Pediatr Dermatol 2007;24(5):563–4.

[113] Lacour M, Mehta-Nikhar B, Atherton DJ, et al. An appraisal of acitretin therapy in children with inherited disorders of keratinization. Br J Dermatol 1996;134(6):1023–9.

[114] Brecher AR, Orlow SJ. Oral retinoid therapy for dermatologic conditions in children and adolescents. J Am Acad Dermatol 2003;49(2):171–82 [quiz: 176–83].

[115] Gold JA, Shupack JL, Nemec MA. Ocular side effects of the retinoids. Int J Dermatol 1989;28(4):218–25.

[116] Zech LA, Gross EG, Peck GL, et al. Changes in plasma cholesterol and triglyceride levels after treatment with oral isotretinoin. A prospective study. Arch Dermatol 1983;119(12):987–93.

[117] Lestringant GG, Frossard PM, Agarwal M, et al. Variations in lipid and lipoprotein levels during isotretinoin treatment for acne vulgaris with special emphasis on HDL-cholesterol. Int J Dermatol 1997;36(11):859–62.

[118] Nesher G, Zuckner J. Rheumatologic complications of vitamin A and retinoids. Semin Arthritis Rheum 1995;24(4):291–6.

[119] Halverstam CP, Zeichner J, Lebwohl M. Lack of significant skeletal changes after long-term, low-dose retinoid therapy: case report and review of the literature. J Cutan Med Surg 2006;10(6):291–9.

[120] Ruiz-Maldonado R, Tamayo-Sanchez L, Orozco-Covarrubias ML. The use of retinoids in the pediatric patient. Dermatol Clin 1998;16(3):553–69.

[121] Van Zander J, Orlow SJ. Efficacy and safety of oral retinoids in psoriasis. Expert Opin Drug Saf 2005;4(1):129–38.

[122] Milstone LM, McGuire J, Ablow RC. Premature epiphyseal closure in a child receiving oral 13-cis-retinoic acid. J Am Acad Dermatol 1982;7(5):663–6.

[123] Prendiville J, Bingham EA, Burrows D. Premature epiphyseal closure—a complication of etretinate therapy in children. J Am Acad Dermatol 1986;15(6):1259–62.

[124] Katugampola RP, Finlay AY. Oral retinoid therapy for disorders of keratinization: single-centre retrospective 25 years' experience on 23 patients. Br J Dermatol 2006;154(2): 267–76.

[125] Jones MD, Pais MJ, Omiya B. Bony overgrowths and abnormal calcifications about the spine. Radiol Clin North Am 1988;26(6):1213–34.

[126] MacDonald A, Burden AD. Noninvasive monitoring for methotrexate hepatotoxicity. Br J Dermatol 2005;152(3):405–8.

[127] Cronstein BN. The mechanism of action of methotrexate. Rheum Dis Clin North Am 1997;23(4):739–55.

[128] Callen JP, Wolverton SE. Methotrexate. In: Wolverton SE, editor. Comprehensive dermatologic drug therapy. 2nd edition. Philadelphia: Saunders Elsevier; 2007. p. 163–81.

[129] Kumar B, Dhar S, Handa S, et al. Methotrexate in childhood psoriasis. Pediatr Dermatol 1994;11(3):271–3.

[130] Paller AS. Dermatologic uses of methotrexate in children: indications and guidelines. Pediatr Dermatol 1985;2(3):238–43.

[131] Swords S, Lauer SJ, Nopper AJ. Principles of treatment in pediatric dermatology: systemic treatment. In: Schachner LA, Hansen RC, editors. Pediatric dermatology. 3rd edition. Philadelphia: Elsevier; 2003. p. 133–43.

[132] Dupuis LL, Koren G, Silverman ED, et al. Influence of food on the bioavailability of oral methotrexate in children. J Rheumatol 1995;22(8):1570–3.

[133] Hendel L, Hendel J, Johnsen A, et al. Intestinal function and methotrexate absorption in psoriatic patients. Clin Exp Dermatol 1982;7(5):491–7.

[134] Dogra S, Handa S, Kanwar AJ. Methotrexate in severe childhood psoriasis. Pediatr Dermatol 2004;21(3):283–4.

[135] Scott RB, Surana R. Erythrodermic psoriasis in childhood. A young Negro child treated with methotrexate. Am J Dis Child 1968;116(2):218–21.

[136] Graham LD, Myones BL, Rivas-Chacon RF, et al. Morbidity associated with long-term methotrexate therapy in juvenile rheumatoid arthritis. J Pediatr 1992;120(3):468–73.

[137] Kremer JM, Hamilton RA. The effects of nonsteroidal antiinflammatory drugs on methotrexate (MTX) pharmacokinetics: impairment of renal clearance of MTX at weekly maintenance doses but not at 7.5 mg. J Rheumatol 1995;22(11):2072–7.

[138] Wallace CA, Smith AL, Sherry DD. Pilot investigation of naproxen/methotrexate interaction in patients with juvenile rheumatoid arthritis. J Rheumatol 1993;20(10):1764–8.

[139] Thomas DR, Dover JS, Camp RD. Pancytopenia induced by the interaction between methotrexate and trimethoprim-sulfamethoxazole. J Am Acad Dermatol 1987;17(6):1055–6.

[140] Gutierrez-Urena S, Molina JF, Garcia CO, et al. Pancytopenia secondary to methotrexate therapy in rheumatoid arthritis. Arthritis Rheum 1996;39(2):272–6.

[141] Gisondi P, Fantuzzi F, Malerba M, et al. Folic acid in general medicine and dermatology. J Dermatolog Treat 2007;18(3):138–46.

[142] Morgan S, Alarcon GS, Krumdieck CL. Folic acid supplementation during methotrexate therapy: it makes sense. J Rheumatol 1993;20(6):929–30.

[143] Morgan SL, Baggott JE, Lee JY, et al. Folic acid supplementation prevents deficient blood folate levels and hyperhomocysteinemia during longterm, low dose methotrexate therapy for rheumatoid arthritis: implications for cardiovascular disease prevention. J Rheumatol 1998;25(3):441–6.

[144] Morgan SL, Baggott JE, Vaughn WH, et al. Supplementation with folic acid during methotrexate therapy for rheumatoid arthritis. A double-blind, placebo-controlled trial. Ann Intern Med 1994;121(11):833–41.

[145] Morgan SL, Baggott JE, Vaughn WH, et al. The effect of folic acid supplementation on the toxicity of low-dose methotrexate in patients with rheumatoid arthritis. Arthritis Rheum 1990;33(1):9–18.

[146] van Ede AE, Laan RF, Rood MJ, et al. Effect of folic or folinic acid supplementation on the toxicity and efficacy of methotrexate in rheumatoid arthritis: a forty-eight week, multicenter, randomized, double-blind, placebo-controlled study. Arthritis Rheum 2001;44(7):1515–24.

[147] Roenigk HH Jr, Auerbach R, Maibach H, et al. Methotrexate in psoriasis: consensus conference. J Am Acad Dermatol 1998;38(3):478–85.

[148] Pereira GM, Miller JF, Shevach EM. Mechanism of action of cyclosporine A in vivo. II. T cell priming in vivo to alloantigen can be mediated by an IL-2-independent cyclosporine A-resistant pathway. J Immunol 1990;144(6):2109–16.

[149] Harper JI, Ahmed I, Barclay G, et al. Cyclosporin for severe childhood atopic dermatitis: short course versus continuous therapy. Br J Dermatol 2000;142(1):52–8.

[150] Leonardi S, Marchese G, Rotolo N, et al. Cyclosporin is safe and effective in severe atopic dermatitis of childhood. Report of three cases. Minerva Pediatr 2004;56(2):231–7.

[151] Zaki I, Emerson R, Allen BR. Treatment of severe atopic dermatitis in childhood with cyclosporin. Br J Dermatol 1996;135(Suppl 48):21–4.

[152] Berth-Jones J, Voorhees JJ. Consensus conference on cyclosporin A microemulsion for psoriasis, June 1996. Br J Dermatol 1996;135(5):775–7.

[153] Pereira TM, Vieira AP, Fernandes JC, et al. Cyclosporin A treatment in severe childhood psoriasis. J Eur Acad Dermatol Venereol 2006;20(6):651–6.

[154] Perrett CM, Ilchyshyn A, Berth-Jones J. Cyclosporin in childhood psoriasis. J Dermatolog Treat 2003;14(2):113–8.

[155] Heydendael VM, Spuls PI, Ten Berge IJ, et al. Cyclosporin trough levels: is monitoring necessary during short-term treatment in psoriasis? A systematic review and clinical data on trough levels. Br J Dermatol 2002;147(1):122–9.

[156] Mockli G, Kabra PM, Kurtz TW. Laboratory monitoring of cyclosporine levels: guidelines for the dermatologist. J Am Acad Dermatol 1990;23(6 Pt 2):1275–8 [discussion: 1278–79].

[157] Alli N, Gungor E, Karakayali G, et al. The use of cyclosporin in a child with generalized pustular psoriasis. Br J Dermatol 1998;139(4):754–5.
[158] Kilic SS, Hacimustafaoglu M, Celebi S, et al. Low dose cyclosporin A treatment in generalized pustular psoriasis. Pediatr Dermatol 2001;18(3):246–8.
[159] Mahe E, Bodemer C, Pruszkowski A, et al. Cyclosporine in childhood psoriasis. Arch Dermatol 2001;137(11):1532–3.
[160] Ellis CN. Safety issues with cyclosporine. Int J Dermatol 1997;36(Suppl 1):7–10.
[161] Goeckerman WH. The treatment of psoriasis. Northwest Med 1925;24:229–31.
[162] Ibbotson SH, Bilsland D, Cox NH, et al. An update and guidance on narrowband ultraviolet B phototherapy: a British photodermatology group workshop report. Br J Dermatol 2004;151(2):283–97.
[163] Kist JM, Van Voorhees AS. Narrowband ultraviolet B therapy for psoriasis and other skin disorders. Adv Dermatol 2005;21:235–50.
[164] Jain VK, Aggarwal K, Jain K, et al. Narrow-band UV-B phototherapy in childhood psoriasis. Int J Dermatol 2007;46(3):320–2.
[165] Koo J, Bandow G, Feldman SR. The art and practice of UVB phototherapy for the treatment of psoriasis. In: Weinstein GD, Gottlieb AB, editors. Therapy of moderate to severe psoriasis. 2nd edition. New York: Marcel Dekker; 2003. p. 53–90.
[166] Tay YK, Morelli JG, Weston WL. Experience with UVB phototherapy in children. Pediatr Dermatol 1996;13(5):406–9.
[167] McClelland PB. Fundamentals of phototherapy. In: National Psoriasis Foundation Guide to Phototherapy. San Francisco (CA): National Psoriasis Foundation; 2008.
[168] al-Fouzan AS, Nanda A. UVB phototherapy in childhood psoriasis. Pediatr Dermatol 1995;12(1):66.
[169] Pasic A, Ceovic R, Lipozencic J, et al. Phototherapy in pediatric patients. Pediatr Dermatol 2003;20(1):71–7.
[170] Dawe RS, Cameron H, Yule S, et al. A randomized controlled trial of narrowband ultraviolet B vs bath-psoralen plus ultraviolet A photochemotherapy for psoriasis. Br J Dermatol 2003;148(6):1194–204.
[171] Parrish JA, Jaenicke KF. Action spectrum for phototherapy of psoriasis. J Invest Dermatol 1981;76(5):359–62.
[172] Van Weelden H, Baart de la Faille H, Young E, et al. Comparison of narrow-band UV-B phototherapy and PUVA photochemotherapy in the treatment of psoriasis. Acta Derm Venereol 1990;70(3):212–5.
[173] Walters IB, Burack LH, Coven TR, et al. Suberythemogenic narrow-band UVB is markedly more effective than conventional UVB in treatment of psoriasis vulgaris. J Am Acad Dermatol 1999;40(6 Pt 1):893–900.
[174] Dawe RS, Wainwright NJ, Cameron H, et al. Narrow-band (TL-01) ultraviolet B phototherapy for chronic plaque psoriasis: three times or five times weekly treatment? Br J Dermatol 1998;138(5):833–9.
[175] Leenutaphong V, Nimkulrat P, Sudtim S. Comparison of phototherapy two times and four times a week with low doses of narrow-band ultraviolet B in Asian patients with psoriasis. Photodermatol Photoimmunol Photomed 2000;16(5):202–6.
[176] Zanolli MD, Feldman SR. Phototherapy treatment protocols: for psoriasis and other phototherapy responsive dermatoses. 2nd edition. Abingdon (UK): Taylor & Francis; 2005.
[177] Green C, Ferguson J, Lakshmipathi T, et al. 311 nm UVB phototherapy—an effective treatment for psoriasis. Br J Dermatol 1988;119(6):691–6.
[178] Dawe RS, Ferguson J. History of psoriasis response to sunlight does not predict outcome of UVB phototherapy. Clin Exp Dermatol 2004;29(4):413–4.
[179] Boer J. A positive correlation between history of psoriasis response to sunlight and the response to UVB phototherapy. What are the consequences? Clin Exp Dermatol 2005;30(4):453–4 [author reply: 454].

[180] Woo WK, McKenna KE. Combination TL01 ultraviolet B phototherapy and topical calcipotriol for psoriasis: a prospective randomized placebo-controlled clinical trial. Br J Dermatol 2003;149(1):146–50.

[181] Behrens S, Grundmann-Kollmann M, Schiener R, et al. Combination phototherapy of psoriasis with narrow-band UVB irradiation and topical tazarotene gel. J Am Acad Dermatol 2000;42(3):493–5.

[182] Carrozza P, Hausermann P, Nestle FO, et al. Clinical efficacy of narrow-band UVB (311 nm) combined with dithranol in psoriasis. An open pilot study. Dermatology 2000;200(1):35–9.

[183] Lebwohl M, Hecker D, Martinez J, et al. Interactions between calcipotriene and ultraviolet light. J Am Acad Dermatol 1997;37(1):93–5.

[184] Spuls PI, Rozenblit M, Lebwohl M. Retrospective study of the efficacy of narrowband UVB and acitretin. J Dermatolog Treat. 2003;14(Suppl 2):17–20.

[185] Kim HS, Kim GM, Kim SY. Two-stage therapy for childhood generalized pustular psoriasis: low-dose cyclosporin for induction and maintenance with acitretin/narrowband ultraviolet B phototherapy. Pediatr Dermatol 2006;23(3):306–8.

[186] Calzavara-Pinton PG, Zane C, Candiago E, et al. Blisters on psoriatic lesions treated with TL-01 lamps. Dermatology 2000;200(2):115–9.

[187] George SA, Ferguson J. Lesional blistering following narrow-band (TL-01) UVB phototherapy for psoriasis: a report of four cases. Br J Dermatol 1992;127(4):445–6.

[188] Diffey BL, Farr PM. The challenge of follow-up in narrowband ultraviolet B phototherapy. Br J Dermatol 2007;157(2):344–9.

[189] Schiener R, Brockow T, Franke A, et al. Bath PUVA and saltwater baths followed by UV-B phototherapy as treatments for psoriasis: a randomized controlled trial. Arch Dermatol 2007;143(5):586–96.

[190] Wolff K. Side-effects of psoralen photochemotherapy (PUVA). Br J Dermatol 1990;122(Suppl 36):117–25.

[191] Delrosso G, Bornacina C, Farinelli P, et al. Bath PUVA and psoriasis: Is a milder treatment a worse treatment? Dermatology 2008;216(3):191–3.

[192] Tahir R, Mujtaba G. Comparative efficacy of psoralen-UVA photochemotherapy versus narrow band UVB phototherapy in the treatment of psoriasis. J Coll Physicians Surg Pak 2004;14(10):593–5.

[193] Spuls PI, Hadi S, Rivera L, et al. Retrospective analysis of the treatment of psoriasis of the palms and soles. J Dermatolog Treat. 2003;14(Suppl 2):21–5.

[194] Esposito M, Mazzotta A, de Felice C, et al. Treatment of erythrodermic psoriasis with etanercept. Br J Dermatol 2006;155(1):156–9.

[195] Hawrot AC, Metry DW, Theos AJ, et al. Etanercept for psoriasis in the pediatric population: experience in nine patients. Pediatr Dermatol 2006;23(1):67–71.

[196] Paller AS, Siegfried EC, Langley RG, et al. Etanercept treatment for children and adolescents with plaque psoriasis. N Engl J Med 2008;358(3):241–51.

[197] Papoutsaki M, Costanzo A, Massotta A, et al. Etanercept for the treatment of severe childhood psoriasis. Br J Dermatol 2006;154(1):181–3.

[198] Farnsworth NN, George SJ, Hsu S. Successful use of infliximab following a failed course of etanercept in a pediatric patient. Dermatol Online J 2005;11(3):11.

[199] Menter MA, Cush JM. Successful treatment of pediatric psoriasis with infliximab. Pediatr Dermatol 2004;21(1):87–8.

[200] Pereira TM, Vieira AP, Fernandes JC, et al. Anti-TNF-alpha therapy in childhood pustular psoriasis. Dermatology 2006;213(4):350–2.

[201] Cordoro KM, Feldman SR. TNF-alpha inhibitors in dermatology. Skin Therapy Lett 2007;12(7):4–6.

[202] Honig PJ. Guttate psoriasis associated with perianal streptococcal disease. J Pediatr 1988;113(6):1037–9.

[203] Rasmussen JE. Psoriasis in children. Dermatol Clin 1986;4(1):99–106.

[204] Wilson JK, Al-Suwaidan SN, Krowchuk D, et al. Treatment of psoriasis in children: is there a role for antibiotic therapy and tonsillectomy? Pediatr Dermatol 2003;20(1):11–5.

[205] Owen CM, Chalmers RJ, O'Sullivan T, et al. A systematic review of antistreptococcal interventions for guttate and chronic plaque psoriasis. Br J Dermatol 2001;145(6):886–90.

[206] Zheng Y, Danilenko DM, Valdez P, et al. Interleukin-22, a T(H)17 cytokine, mediates IL-23-induced dermal inflammation and acanthosis. Nature 2007;445(7128):648–51.

[207] Kauffman CL, Aria N, Toichi E, et al. A phase I study evaluating the safety, pharmacokinetics, and clinical response of a human IL-12 p40 antibody in subjects with plaque psoriasis. J Invest Dermatol 2004;123(6):1037–44.

[208] Berkun Y, Levartovsky D, Rubinow A, et al. Methotrexate related adverse effects in patients with rheumatoid arthritis are associated with the A1298C polymorphism of the MTHFR gene. Ann Rheum Dis 2004;63(10):1227–31.

[209] Young HS, Summers AM, Read IR, et al. Interaction between genetic control of vascular endothelial growth factor production and retinoid responsiveness in psoriasis. J Invest Dermatol 2006;126(2):453–9.

[210] Hutton KP, Orenberg EK, Jacobs AH. Childhood psoriasis. Cutis 1987;39(1):26–7.

[211] Burden AD, Stapleton M, Beck MH. Dithranol allergy: fact or fiction? Contact Derm 1992;27(5):291–3.

[212] Kumar B, Kumar R, Kaur I. Coal tar therapy in palmoplantar psoriasis: old wine in an old bottle? Int J Dermatol 1997;36(4):309–12.

[213] Kono H, Inokuma S, Matsuzaki Y, et al. Two cases of methotrexate induced lymphomas in rheumatoid arthritis: an association with increased serum IgE. J Rheumatol 1999;26(10):2249–53.

[214] Lee CS, Koo JYM. Cyclosporine. In: Wolverton S, editor. Comprehensive dermatologic drug therapy. 2nd edition. Philadelphia: Saunders (Elsevier); 2007. p. 219–37.

Update on the Natural History and Systemic Treatment of Psoriasis

Stephen K. Richardson, MD[a], Joel M. Gelfand, MD, MSCE[b],*

[a]Florida State University College of Medicine/Dermatology Associates of Tallahassee, 1714 Mahan Center Boulevard, Tallahassee, FL 32308, USA
[b]Department of Dermatology, Center for Clinical Epidemiology and Biostatistics, University of Pennsylvania, 3600 Spruce Street, 2 Maloney Building, Philadelphia, PA 19104, USA

EDITORIAL COMMENTS

Dr. Richardson and Dr. Gelfand deliver a scientific overview of the fast-moving advances in our understanding and treatment of psoriasis. Scaling, red, itchy, burning, and fissured skin are all visually disturbing components of the "heartbreak of psoriasis." In a series of studies, Dr. Gelfand and his collaborators have redefined psoriasis as a systemic disease with adverse impacts on the heart, brain, endocrine system, and, indeed, life itself. Recognition that it is an independent risk factor for myocardial infarction, stroke, diabetes, lymphoma, and mortality will assist physicians in educating and promoting preventative care for affected patients. At the same time, a revolution in our ability to treat severe disease with an ever-increasing array of innovative agents has occurred. Whether these targeted drugs modify the risks while providing relief of the skin signs is a story waiting to unfold. I think you will enjoy this outstanding article!

William D. James, MD

P soriasis is a common inflammatory disease of the skin and joints. Its cause remains unknown; however, it has been linked to complex interactions between predisposing genes and the environment. The pathophysiology of psoriasis is characterized by epidermal hyperproliferation, enhanced antigen presentation, helper T-cell (Th)1 and Th17 cytokine production, T-cell expansion, and angiogenesis. Tremendous advances in our understanding of this disorder has led to the development of novel therapeutics and the Food and Drug Administration (FDA) approval of more systemic agents for its treatment in the last 5 years than in the previous 50 years combined. Our improved

---

This work was supported in part by grant no. K23-AR051125 (JMG).

Dr. Gelfand is an investigator or receives grant funding from Amgen, Centocor, and Abbott. He is a consultant for Amgen, Centocor, and Genetech. Dr. Richardson is an advisor (Speaker's Bureau) for Abbott.

Corresponding author. E-mail address: joel.gelfand@uphs.upenn.edu (J.M. Gelfand).

0882-0880/08/$ – see front matter
doi:10.1016/j.yadr.2008.09.006

understanding of the pathogenesis of psoriasis has led to epidemiologic studies that have contributed to further characterization of its natural history. In this article, the authors focus on specific advances in our understanding of the pathogenesis, natural history, and systemic treatment of psoriasis, which are of major clinical relevance to the clinician.

KEY ADVANCES IN THE PATHOGENESIS OF PSORIASIS

The biologic basis of psoriasis informs its natural history and treatment options. Here, the authors briefly review key discoveries in the pathogenesis of psoriasis relevant to the clinician and refer the reader to several comprehensive reviews for a more detailed discussion [1–4]. Psoriasis was initially believed to be a primary disorder of keratinocytes; however, advances in molecular biology and immunology proved its cause to be much more complex. In 1995, Gottleib and colleagues [5–7] demonstrated that psoriasis could be treated successfully with the lymphocyte-selective toxin DAB389-IL-2, a discovery that heralded a new era in our approach to treating psoriasis, one focused on developing therapeutics to inhibit immunologic targets. It is now believed that the clinical phenotype of psoriatic skin arises from the interplay between inflammatory cytokines and cells that make up the cutaneous microenvironment (ie, lymphocytes, antigen-presenting cells [APCs], endothelial cells, and keratinocytes).

Lymphocytes are believed to play a central role in the pathogenesis of psoriasis; recent work has demonstrated how various lymphocyte subsets contribute to this disorder. In particular, Th1 lymphocytes have been identified as a primary source of inflammatory cytokine production in psoriatic skin; regulatory T cells, which normally suppress effector T-cell activity, are dysfunctional in the blood and skin of patients who have psoriasis; and recently identified Th17 cells produce the cytokine interleukin (IL)-17, which is critical to the establishment and maintenance of autoimmunity, and IL-22, which is primarily involved in the process of epidermal differentiation and hyperproliferation. APCs (ie, plasmacytoid and myeloid dendritic cells) and endothelial cells lining the dermal microvasculature have also been shown to play a role in psoriatic disease. In particular, dermal dendritic cells have been shown to contribute to the production of Th1 cytokines and the recruitment of inflammatory cells into psoriatic plaques. The production of IL-20 and IL-23 by myeloid dendritic cells has been reported to promote keratinocyte proliferation, up-regulate inflammatory gene products, and stimulate T-cell activation, all of which contribute to psoriatic lesions [8,9]. Endothelial cells play a critical role in recruiting inflammatory cells through their expression of E-selectin, which enhances the homing of cutaneous lymphocyte-associated antigen-positive T cells into the skin. Angiogenesis is stimulated by the inflammatory process and studies demonstrate that circulating levels of vascular endothelial growth factor correlate with psoriasis activity [10].

Whether psoriasis reflects an abnormal response to an unidentified antigen or a reaction to the aberrant production of endogenous/exogenous immune cell activators remains uncertain. However, it is clear that the response of keratinocytes to locally produced cytokines underlies the formation of cutaneous lesions. In addition, keratinocytes have been shown to produce their own cytokines, such as IL-6 and transforming growth factor-alpha, which may act in concert to promote their own proliferation in an autocrine fashion [11].

Underlying its immunopathogenesis is a complex role for genetics in promoting psoriasis disease susceptibility. More than 20 genetic loci containing varying numbers of genes, many of which have no known function, have been associated with psoriasis susceptibility. The strongest association was identified on a locus within the class I major histocompatibility complex on chromosome 6p21, known as PSORS1. This region is believed to account for 35% to 50% of psoriasis heritability. The PSORS1 locus contains fewer than 10 genes, 3 of which have been strongly implicated in psoriatic disease: human leukocyte antigen-C, CCHCR1, and CDSN. The HLA-Cw6 allele is present in up to 85% of individuals who develop psoriasis under the age of 40; these patients typically have more severe disease than individuals who develop psoriasis at a later time in life. Only 15% of individuals who develop psoriasis over the age of 40 express the HLA-Cw6 allele. Although much progress has been made toward dissecting the genetic components of this disease, few genes have been definitively implicated in its pathogenesis, and genetic testing is not clinically useful. For example, only 10% of individuals who express the HLA-Cw6 allele go on to develop psoriasis [12].

KEY ADVANCES IN THE NATURAL HISTORY OF PSORIASIS

Recent studies have broadened our knowledge of how genetics and environmental factors may lead to psoriasis and how the pathophysiology of psoriasis or its associated psychosocial behaviors and treatments may lead to adverse health outcomes (Fig. 1).

What are the risk factors for developing psoriasis?

Genetics are believed to play a key role in the development of psoriasis. It is estimated that approximately 40% of individuals suffering from psoriasis or psoriatic arthritis (PsA) have a first-degree relative who has the disease [13]. In addition, concordance rates as high as 70% have been reported among identical twins [14]. Given the strong genetic component of psoriasis, patients who have psoriasis are often concerned about the heritability of the disease. Family studies indicate that if both parents have psoriasis then the offspring have a 50% chance of developing the disease; if only one parent has psoriasis then the risk for a child to develop psoriasis is 16%. If neither parent is affected but a child develops psoriasis then his/her siblings have an 8% risk for developing the disease. Men have a higher risk for transmitting psoriasis to offspring than women, likely because of genomic imprinting, which is an epigenetic effect that causes differential expression of a gene depending on the gender of the transmitting parent [15].

Because genetics are immutable, modifiable environmental risk factors for psoriasis are of special interest. Data from analytic epidemiologic studies (eg, case-control and nested cohort studies) with appropriate control for

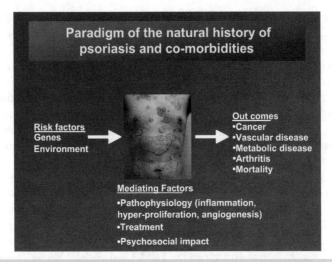

Fig. 1. The relationship among risk factors for developing psoriasis, mediating factors associated with the disease, and the risk for various health outcomes is complex. Obesity and smoking have recently been demonstrated to increase the risk for developing psoriasis. Increasingly, epidemiologic studies are controlling for these factors to determine which outcomes are directly related to having psoriasis, as opposed to being mediated by confounding factors such as smoking and obesity.

confounding variables have recently identified smoking and obesity as risk factors for the development of psoriasis. A large cohort study of more than 78,000 nurses from the United States demonstrated a "dose–response" relationship for obesity and smoking on the risk for developing incident psoriasis [16,17]. Similarly, a cohort study from the General Practice Research Database in the United Kingdom of almost 4000 incident cases of psoriasis confirmed that current smoking and obesity are independent risk factors for developing psoriasis. Finally, in a case-control study of 560 psoriasis patients seen by dermatologists, smoking and obesity were also found to be independent risk factors for the development of psoriasis [18]. The consistency of the findings across different study populations and study designs, and the dose–response relationships observed, strongly support the validity of these associations. Both smoking and obesity trigger Th1–mediated immunologic pathways, suggesting a plausible biologic explanation for these associations [19].

Clinical implications of risk factors for psoriasis

The importance of family history in the risk for developing psoriasis necessitates that clinicians be knowledgeable on counseling patients regarding the risk for their offspring to develop the disease. Furthermore, the identification of obesity and smoking as consistent and reproducible risk factors for the development of psoriasis may provide an opportunity for prevention of this chronic disease through behavior modification. For example, in the nurses' cohort study, it was estimated that 30% of new psoriasis cases were due to being overweight (body mass index >25) [16]. Future studies are necessary to determine if maintenance of ideal body weight and avoidance of smoking will truly lower one's risk for developing psoriasis. Until such data are available, it is prudent to recommend weight management and smoking avoidance to individuals at greatest risk for developing the disease (eg, those who have a positive family history).

Which major comorbidities are patients who have psoriasis at increased risk for developing?

Patients who have psoriasis may be at increased risk for developing other diseases because of shared genetic pathways, common immune mechanisms, treatment-related toxicities, psoriasis-associated behaviors such as smoking and excess alcohol use, and the associated psychosocial burden of the disease (see Fig. 1). For example, psoriasis patients have an increased prevalence of Crohn's disease, which may be because of shared genetic loci; the psoriasis susceptibility loci, PSORS8, has been shown to overlap with a Crohn's disease locus on chromosome 16q [20,21]. Moreover, chronic Th1 inflammation, central to the pathophysiology of psoriasis, can also lead to seemingly diverse conditions such as insulin resistance, atherosclerosis, and thrombosis [22]. Therapies for psoriasis frequently are immunosuppressive, which could lead to a higher risk for infections and cancer. Similarly, psoriasis is associated with smoking, excess alcohol use, mood disorders, and decrements in income, all of which could lead to adverse health outcomes [23,24]. More recent epidemiologic research has focused on determining which health outcomes in patients who have psoriasis may be direct consequences of the disease itself.

Psoriatic arthritis

Patients who have psoriasis are at significant risk for developing PsA. The frequency of PsA appears to be strongly related to the degree of skin severity. For example, a population-based study indicated that the prevalence of PsA in patients who have less than 1% body surface area (BSA), 1% to 2% BSA, 3% to 10% BSA, and more than 10% BSA was 6%, 14%, 18%, and 56%, respectively [25]. Similarly, nail involvement is another clinical predictor of PsA. For example, nail lesions are seen in 80% to 90% of patients who have concomitant PsA compared with 46% among those who have psoriasis uncomplicated by arthritis [26]. Skin disease occurs concurrently or before the development of PsA in more than 80% of cases. Studies of PsA from rheumatology referral centers indicate that the disease can be progressive and can be associated with permanent disability and excess mortality [27,28]. Studies of PsA in the general population and in the dermatology setting indicate that the disease may be less disabling and require fewer treatments of symptom management [29,30]. Having multiple joints involved at baseline and having elevated markers of systemic inflammation (eg, erythrocyte sedimentation rate, C-reactive protein) predict a more aggressive course for PsA, whereas severity of skin disease is a poor predictor of the severity of joint disease or its progression [25,30].

Cardiovascular and metabolic disease
Studies from the early 1970s first identified that patients who have psoriasis have higher frequencies of atherosclerotic disease and thrombotic complications [31]. More recently, studies have indicated that patients who have severe psoriasis have excess rates of cardiovascular disease that is not accounted for by traditional cardiovascular risk factors (obesity, hypertension, diabetes, hyperlipidemia, and smoking). For example, Gelfand and colleagues [32] demonstrated in a large observational cohort study that patients who have mild and severe psoriasis (identified by treatment patterns) have an increased risk for myocardial infarction and that the adjusted relative risk for myocardial infarction is greatest in younger patients who have severe disease. Similarly, Ludwig and colleagues [33] demonstrated that the prevalence and severity of coronary artery disease in 32 well-characterized patients who had severe psoriasis was greater than matched controls, even when controlling for major cardiovascular risk factors.

The prevalence of obesity, diabetes, and metabolic syndrome has been shown to be increased in psoriasis patients in the general population and in referral centers [34]. At least one study has demonstrated a higher prevalence of diabetes in patients who have psoriasis independent of traditional diabetes risk factors such as age, gender, obesity, hypertension, and hyperlipidemia, indicating that the disease itself, or possibly its chronic treatments, may predispose to the development of diabetes [19].

Cancer
The immunologic nature of psoriasis, and therapies that are immunosuppressive or mutagenic, may predispose patients who have psoriasis to an increased risk for cancer. A higher incidence of nonmelanoma skin cancer has been reported in psoriasis patients and findings regarding internal cancers such as lung, breast, colon, and prostate are conflicting [35–41]. Lymphoma has been of special interest because inflammatory conditions may be associated with a higher risk for lymphoproliferative disease. Studies of the risk for internal lymphoma in psoriasis patients have yielded inconsistent results. The largest study to date found no increased risk for non-Hodgkin's lymphoma, but did observe an increased risk for Hodgkin's lymphoma and a markedly increased relative risk for cutaneous T-cell lymphoma (CTCL) [42]. This association of psoriasis with CTCL may be due to misdiagnosis of early CTCL as psoriasis or may be related to chronic lymphoproliferation leading to CTCL [42]. Recently, the results of 30 years of follow-up of psoriasis patients treated with psoralen-UV-A (PUVA) found that patients who received PUVA and were exposed to high levels of methotrexate (≥36 months) had an increased incidence of lymphoma compared with the general population (incidence rate ratio 4.39, 95% CI 1.59–12.06) [43]. Increased rates of lymphoma were also observed in other patient categories created by the investigator (eg, PUVA patients who received >300 UV-B treatments, patients who had skin types 1 or 2, patients who received >200 PUVA treatments), but these were

not statistically significant, possibly because of limitations of statistical power or incomplete capture of outcomes.

Psychiatric disease
Multiple studies, most of which are descriptive, have examined psychologic characteristics of patients who have psoriasis [44–46]. A wide range of problems have been described, such as depression, anxiety, obsessive behavior, sexual dysfunction, and suicidal ideation [47–52]. A study comparing 50 patients who had psoriasis in outpatient clinics to 50 healthy controls found that patients who had psoriasis had a higher average Beck Depression Inventory score (16.96 versus 5.48, respectively, $P < .01$) [53]. Suicidal ideation was found to be present in 7.2% of patients hospitalized for psoriasis, in 2.5% of psoriasis outpatients, and in 2.4% to 3.3% of general medical patients, suggesting that patients who have more severe disease may suffer greater emotional impairment [44]. Psychologic distress may also impair response to psoriasis therapies. For example, in a cohort of psoriasis patients treated with PUVA, pathologic or high-level worry was a significant predictor of time taken for PUVA to clear psoriasis, whereas clinical severity of psoriasis, skin phenotype, alcohol intake, anxiety, and depression were not [54].

Clinical implications of comorbidities in psoriasis
The emerging data on comorbidities in psoriasis have important clinical implications for the care of these patients. First, the dermatologist must play a central role in the initial diagnosis of PsA, given that the skin disease typically precedes the onset of joint disease. Early diagnosis of PsA may lead to improved joint function and a decreased risk for future disability. Second, given the high prevalence of concomitant PsA in patients who have extensive psoriasis, dermatologists should consider joint symptoms when selecting a therapy to treat the skin disease. For example, methotrexate and tumor necrosis factor (TNF) inhibitors are considered disease-modifying antirheumatic drugs that may prevent joint destruction in patients who have PsA. Data from controlled clinical trials indicate that etanercept decreases fatigue symptoms in psoriasis patients who have concomitant PsA and also may improve symptoms suggestive of depression [55]. Furthermore, the broad evidence of elevated cardiovascular risk associated with psoriasis has resulted in new consensus statements suggesting that dermatologists play a role by either screening for cardiovascular risk factors in patients who have psoriasis or by encouraging the patient to follow up with his/her primary care physician for appropriate screenings and interventions aimed at lowering cardiovascular risk [56]. The importance of optimizing medical care for patients who have psoriasis is emphasized by recent studies indicating that severe psoriasis patients die 3 to 4 years earlier than patients who do not have psoriasis, a finding similar to estimates of years of life lost because of severe hypertension [57]. Finally, the mental health status of patients who have psoriasis should be assessed because mood disorders such as depression and anxiety are highly prevalent in this patient population and also may impair response to treatment.

KEY ADVANCES IN THE TREATMENT OF PSORIASIS

What are the current food and drug administration–approved systemic biologics available for the treatment of moderate/severe plaque psoriasis? What are their associated risks and benefits?

The therapeutic paradigm for treating psoriasis with systemic agents continues to evolve. Recent consensus statements suggest that indications for systemic psoriasis treatment or phototherapy are psoriasis affecting greater than or equal to 5% BSA, psoriasis affecting vulnerable areas (eg, palmar-plantar), psoriasis with concomitant PsA, pustular, erythrodermic, and guttate psoriasis variants, and psoriasis unresponsive to topical medications in which significant physical, social, or emotional impairments are involved [58]. Traditional therapies include methotrexate, acitretin, cyclosporine, phototherapy (including laser devices), and PUVA. In this article, the authors focus on recently approved biologic therapies for psoriasis. A biologic therapy is a compound engineered from living organisms. Biologics for psoriasis vary in structure (eg, humanized versus chimeric, antibody versus fusion protein), target (eg, cytokines versus T cells), route of administration, safety, efficacy, and monitoring requirements. TNF inhibitors were first approved for use in 1998 and have been studied extensively in clinical trials across multiple diseases and in long-term cohort studies in multiple populations involving tens of thousands of patients. By comparison, T-cell inhibitors for psoriasis have been studied predominantly in psoriasis patients, and no large, long-term, cohort studies of these drugs have been published. A summary of relevant characteristics of biologics is shown in Tables 1 and 2.

The tumor necrosis factor inhibitors

TNF-α is a 17-kD polypeptide that plays a central role in the regulation of innate immune responses. It is involved in stimulating the production of inflammatory cytokines, inducing the expression of cell surface adhesion molecules, enhancing the phagocytic/bactericidal properties of macrophages, and activating apoptotic pathways on association with membrane-bound forms of its receptors, TNF-R1 (p55) and TNF-R2 (p75). These receptors also exist in soluble forms, which regulate TNF-α bioavailability in the circulation.

TNF-α is produced by various cells, ranging from lymphocytes and monocytes, to keratinocytes, mast cells, and APCs in the skin. It is believed to contribute to the pathogenesis of psoriasis through its ability to promote immune cell trafficking to the skin and induce keratinocyte proliferation [59–61]. At present, three anti-TNF therapeutics are available for the treatment of autoimmune conditions: the fusion protein, etanercept, and two recombinant monoclonal antibodies (infliximab and adalimumab). Specific characteristics and safety issues of special interest with regard to these agents are now discussed.

Adalimumab. Adalimumab is a recombinant human monoclonal antibody that blocks the interaction between TNF-α and its p55/p75 cell surface receptor. It differs from infliximab in that it is fully human, which theoretically may decrease the risk for autoantibody formation against it. Nevertheless, neutralizing antibodies

Table 1
Overview of biologic dosing and efficacy

Biologic	Structure	Target	Dosing	Pharmacokinetics	PASI 75[a]
Adalimumab	Human monoclonal antibody	Soluble and membrane-bound TNF-α	80 mg SC followed by 40 mg SC 1wk later, then 40 mg SC qow	Half-life: 10–20 d	68% at wk 12 [95,134]
Alefacept	Fusion protein	LFA-3	15 mg IM qwk for 12 wk	Half-life: 11.25 d	33% during 14-wk study period
Efalizumab	Humanized monoclonal antibody	LFA-1	0.7 mg/kg SC followed by 1 mg/kg qwk	Half-life: 6.21 d	27% at wk 12
Etanercept	Fusion protein	Soluble TNF-α, lymphotoxin-α	50 mg SC biw for 12wk, then 50 mg SC qwk	Half-life: 4–12.5 d	34% at wk 12 (based on 25-mg SC biw dosing); 49% at wk 12 (based on 50-mg biw dosing)
Infliximab	Chimeric monoclonal antibody	Soluble and membrane-bound TNF-α	5 mg/kg IV at wk 0, 2, and 6, then q8wk	Half-life: 8–9.5 d	80% at wk 10

Data from Thomson PDR. Physician's Desk Reference. 61st edition. Montvale, New Jersey; 2007.
Abbreviations: biw, 2 times per week; IV, intravenous; IM, intramuscular; LFA, leukocyte function–associated antigen; PASI, psoriasis area and severity index; q8wk, every 8 weeks; qow, every other week; qwk, every week; SC, subcutaneous; TB, tuberculosis.
[a] Data from Kurd SK, et al. Update on the epidemiology and systemic treatment of psoriasis. Expert Rev Clin Immunol 2007;3(2):171–85.

Table 2
Overview of biologic monitoring and safety

Biologic	FDA-required screening and monitoring[a]	Common adverse effects (>5%)	Uncommon adverse effects (0.1%–5%)	Rare adverse effects (<0.1%)	Black box warnings
Adalimumab	Screen for latent TB Evaluate patients at risk for HBV or who had prior HBV infection	Injection site reaction; +ANA; upper respiratory infection; headache; nausea; elevated alk phos, cholesterol	Neutralizing antibodies; serious infection	TB; malignancy; lupus-like syndrome; hypersensitivity; hepatitis B reactivation; demyelination; congestive heart failure; pancytopenia	Infection (TB, sepsis, fungal, and opportunistic)
Alefacept	Measure CD4 count before and during treatment Evaluate for signs/symptoms of liver injury	Lymphopenia	LFT elevation; serious infection	Malignancy; hypersensitivity	None
Efalizumab	Measure platelet count before and during treatment (monthly with treatment initiation, then q 3 mo with ongoing treatment) Follow for worsening psoriasis during or on discontinuation of treatment	Flu-like symptoms; mild psoriasis flare; lymphocytosis	Severe psoriasis flare; serious infection; thrombocytopenia; arthritis; hypersensitivity; LFT elevation	Malignancies; hemolytic anemia; pancytopenia; interstitial pneumonia; toxic epidermal necrolysis; aseptic meningitis	Risk of serious infections leading to hospitalizations or death, including bacterial sepsis, viral meningitis, invasive fungal disease, opportunistic infections, and progressive multifocal leukoencephalopathy resulting from JC virus infection. Warning issued October, 2008.

Etanercept	Evaluate patients at risk for HBV or who had prior HBV infection Screen for latent TB	Injection site reaction; +ANA	Serious infection	TB; malignancy; lupus-like syndrome; hypersensitivity; hepatitis B reactivation; demyelination; congestive heart failure; pancytopenia	Infection (bacterial, sepsis, and TB)
Infliximab	Screen for latent TB Evaluate patients at risk for HBV or who had prior HBV infection Evaluate for signs/symptoms of liver injury	Infusion reaction; +ANA; elevated liver function tests; neutralizing antibodies	Hypersensitivity; serious infection	Severe hepatic injury; TB; malignancy; lupus-like syndrome; hypersensitivity; hepatitis B reactivation; demyelination; congestive heart failure; pancytopenia	Infection (TB, sepsis, fungal, and opportunistic) Hepatosplenic T-cell lymphoma

Abbreviations: alk phos, alkaline phosphatase; +ANA, antinuclear antibodies; FDA, Food and Drug Administration; HBV, hepatitis B virus; LFTs, liver function tests; q, every; TB, tuberculosis.

^a Note that published guidelines suggest that latent TB be screened for before initiating therapy with all TNF inhibitors; many practitioners screen for latent TB before starting any biologic and then annually if the patient continues on the drug. Practitioners vary in their monitoring practices for biologics, but most monitor complete blood count and liver function tests periodically during treatment.

may develop to adalimumab in patients treated with this biologic [62]. In January 2008, adalimumab received FDA approval for the treatment of adult patients who have moderate-to-severe plaque psoriasis and are candidates for systemic therapy or phototherapy, or among whom other systemic therapies may not be appropriate. It is also approved for the treatment of PsA, rheumatoid arthritis (RA) juvenile idiopathic arthritis, ankylosing spondylitis, and Crohn's disease. The half-life of adalimumab ranges from 10 to 20 days, and it achieves a peak concentration approximately 130 hours after administration, with an absolute bioavailability of 64%. For the treatment of psoriasis, adalimumab is administered as a subcutaneous injection with an initial 80-mg dose, followed by a 40-mg dose 1 week later. Subsequent maintenance doses of 40 mg should be administered every other week thereafter [63].

Infliximab. Infliximab is a chimeric recombinant monoclonal antibody consisting of a human immunoglobulin (Ig)G1 constant region fused to a murine variable region that recognizes and binds to human TNF-α. It is FDA approved for the treatment of PsA, RA, ankylosing spondylitis, Crohn's disease, ulcerative colitis, and chronic severe plaque psoriasis. Serum concentrations vary and are directly related to the administered dose. Infliximab concentrations of greater than 0.1 mg/kg are detected in most patients up to 14 weeks after treatment [60]. The serum half-life of infliximab ranges from 8 to 9.5 days. It is administered intravenously over a 2- to 3-hour period at an infusion dose of 5 mg/kg. Treatments are recommended at 2 weeks, 6 weeks, and 8 weeks after the initial dose. It may then be dosed every 8 weeks thereafter. Among the biologics, infliximab provides the most rapid onset of clinical improvement among patients who have moderate-to-severe psoriasis, with approximately 80% of patients achieving a psoriasis area and severity index (PASI) 75 by treatment week 10 [64]. When used as a monotherapy, however, treatment efficacy has been observed to decrease over time [65]. This loss of efficacy has been attributed to increased metabolism of the drug, possibly secondary to the generation of neutralizing autoantibodies. The development of neutralizing antibodies is associated with an increased risk for infusion reactions [65]. Such reactions may be serious; thus, strategies to reduce the incidence of neutralizing antibodies should be considered. It has been suggested that combining infliximab therapy with methotrexate may decrease the development of neutralizing antibodies and loss of efficacy, as was reported among patients who had Crohn's disease [65]. Furthermore, intermittent dosing of infliximab for psoriasis is similarly associated with an increased risk for neutralizing antibody formation and loss of efficacy over time; thus, intermittent dosing is discouraged [66]. Although infliximab acts quickly, it requires intravenous administration in a medical setting, and thus is not as convenient as self-administered medications.

Etanercept. Etanercept is a recombinant dimer of human soluble TNF-R2 (p75), consisting of the extracellular ligand-binding portion of p75 fused to a human IgG1Fc region; it exhibits a higher affinity (~50 fold) for TNF-α than its endogenous soluble counterpart. Unique among the TNF inhibitors, etanercept also binds lymphotoxin-α (TNF-β), a member of the TNF family of cytokines. Etanercept reversibly binds to TNF-α in the circulation, thus competitively inhibiting its ability to associate with its endogenous receptors. Etanercept is FDA approved for the treatment of PsA, RA, ankylosing spondylitis, and moderate-to-severe plaque psoriasis. It has a serum half-life of between 4 and 25 days, achieving peak plasma concentrations approximately 48 hours after dosing [67]. The bioavailability of subcutaneous etanercept is approximately 58% [68]. Etanercept is self-administered by the patient as a 50-mg subcutaneous injection, typically twice weekly for the first 12 weeks, then weekly thereafter. Etanercept efficacy may be affected by patient weight, particularly in those who are extremely obese (body mass index >40) [69].

Tumor necrosis factor inhibitors: comparisons
Although etanercept effectively neutralizes soluble forms of TNF-α, it exhibits minimal affinity for membrane-bound forms and is incapable of inducing complement fixation and the apoptosis of cells. In contrast, the antibody-based therapeutics (infliximab and adalimumab) inhibit soluble and membrane-bound forms of TNF-α. Their association with membrane-bound forms accounts for their ability to induce apoptosis of targeted cells by way of complement fixation and antibody-dependent cell-mediated cytotoxicity [70,71]. Etanercept also differs from antibody-based therapies with regard to its affinity for TNF. Unlike infliximab and adalimumab, etanercept sheds approximately 50% of soluble TNF within 10 minutes of binding [71], whereas the antibody-based therapeutics exhibit irreversible high affinity binding to both soluble and membrane-bound TNF. With regard to pharmacokinetics, the subcutaneous dosing of etanercept and adalimumab allows for more uniform serum concentration-time profiles at steady state, whereas the intravenous infusion of infliximab accounts for elevated peak-to-trough ratios [72].

Aside from their shared ability to inhibit TNF function, differences between etanercept and the antibody-based therapeutics with regard to their effects on cytokine production by Th cells have been revealed by recent laboratory studies. More specifically, results from cell culture experiments found that TNF inhibition by infliximab led to strong suppression of genes mediating Th1 cytokine production (eg, interferon [IFN]-g), whereas a similar effect was not appreciated among etanercept-treated cells [73].

Given the importance of Th1 cytokines such as IFN-γ in promoting cell-mediated immune responses, their suppression by infliximab may account for the increased reactivation of *Mycobacterium tuberculosis* reported among patients [73]. This characteristic, however, may prove beneficial in the setting of certain autoimmune disorders characterized by enhanced Th1 cytokine production, such as inflammatory bowel disease. In particular, antibody-based TNF inhibitors have proved efficacious in the management of Crohn's disease, a Th1-mediated disorder, whereas etanercept has not proved effective in this setting [74–76]. Differences in the pharmacokinetic and pharmacodynamic profiles of the TNF inhibitors may also contribute to differences in their clinical efficacy and safety in the management of specific disease states.

Tumor necrosis factor inhibitors: adverse effects/safety

Given their immunosuppressive properties, patients should be screened for signs of infection or malignancy before the initiation of therapy and during the course of treatment. The TNF inhibitors are contraindicated among patients who have active, chronic, or localized infections. In addition, they should not be administered to patients receiving the IL-1 receptor antagonist anakinra because this substantially increases the risk for infection.

Relative contraindications to treatment include a personal history of congestive heart failure or a family history of demyelinating disease (eg, multiple sclerosis). Injection site and infusion reactions are the most common side effects reported among patients receiving anti–TNF-α therapy. Other adverse effects include a potentially increased risk for infection, lymphoma, demyelinating disease, congestive heart failure, and autoantibody formation. In particular, infliximab at doses greater than 5 mg/kg is contraindicated in patients who have moderate-to-severe congestive heart failure because studies suggest that it may increase the risk for mortality in this patient population [77,78]. Adalimumab, infliximab, and etanercept are all pregnancy category B medications and are metabolized by proteolysis.

Consideration should be given to vaccination against common serious infections such as pneumonia and influenza before the initiation of therapy whenever possible because treatment during therapy, although likely efficacious, may result in decreased antibody titer responses against vaccination antigens [79,80]. Live vaccines are generally contraindicated during treatment with TNF inhibitors. The authors now discuss additional safety issues related to the use of these medications, which are of special interest.

Safety issues related to malignancy

Theoretic concern exists that TNF inhibitors may increase the risk for malignancy, such as lymphoma. Observational cohort studies of TNF inhibitors for the treatment of RA have reported an increased risk for lymphoma among treated patients [81,82]. Whether this finding represents a disease-associated predisposition for lymphoma or a drug/treatment-associated phenomenon remains to be determined. Studies that have controlled for the severity of RA have not found an increased risk for lymphoma in RA patients treated with TNF inhibitors [83]. A meta-analysis of randomized, controlled trials involving the use of infliximab and adalimumab for the treatment of RA reported an increased risk for solid organ malignancies, of which 35% were skin cancers, among patients [84]. Observational studies in patients who have RA have also found a modest increased risk for nonmelanoma skin cancer in patients treated with TNF inhibitors [85]. An increased risk for solid organ cancer was also reported among patients receiving etancercept and cyclophosphamide concurrently for the treatment of Wegener's granulomatosis in a randomized, controlled trial [86]. Thus, one should consider avoiding the concurrent use of TNF inhibitors with cyclophosphamide [86]. The applicability of malignancy risk associated with TNF inhibitors in the psoriasis population is not clear because psoriasis patients are generally treated with monotherapy, whereas the patients treated with TNF inhibitors for RA are commonly treated with concomitant immunosuppressives, which could alter the safety profile of these drugs.

Safety issues related to viral hepatitis and tuberculosis

Among psoriasis and RA patients who have concomitant hepatitis C virus (HCV) infection, no exacerbation of liver disease was reported in the setting of anti–TNF-α therapy (ie, etanercept, adalimumab, infliximab) [87–89]. In fact, TNF-α inhibition may be beneficial in the management of HCV infection because excess TNF is believed to contribute to the hepatic inflammation and fibrosis characteristic of this condition. A recent retrospective survey and prospective trial reported no substantial change in liver transaminases or HCV load among RA patients who underwent treatment with etanercept or infliximab for their arthritis [90]. Furthermore, a randomized controlled trial demonstrated that etanercept may be useful as adjuvant therapy (eg, in addition to IFN-α-2b and ribavirin) for HCV infection [91].

Patients who are chronically infected with hepatitis B virus (HBV) require special attention when being treated with anti–TNF-α therapy. More specifically, HBV reactivation and associated fatalities have been reported among patients treated with TNF-α inhibitors (ie, infliximab) [92]. Thus, consideration should be given to screening prospective treatment subjects for HBV if they are at risk for chronic HBV infection (see www.cdc.gov/ncidod/diseases/hepatitis/b/Bserology.htm). If the patient is chronically infected with HBV, then therapies that are not immunosuppressive or hepatotoxic are preferred. In situations in which TNF inhibitors must be used in a patient who has chronic HBV infection, close monitoring should occur. Additionally, concomitant treatment of HBV may be considered. For example, a small case series reported no changes in serum transaminases or viral load among chronic HBV patients receiving concomitant TNF inhibitor therapy and lamivudine [93].

The risk for tuberculosis (TB) among patients on TNF inhibitor therapy appears to be greatest among those receiving antibody-based therapeutics (ie, infliximab and adalimumab), as opposed to receptor-based therapy (ie, etanercept). Infliximab has been associated with a 4- to 20-fold increased risk for TB infection [94]. Checking a purified protein derivative (tuberculin) (PPD) is recommended, based on consensus guidelines, before initiation of treatment with all TNF inhibitors because all three may increase the risk for reactivation of latent TB [95]. Patients should also be monitored for signs/symptoms of active TB during treatment. If active disease is detected, further anti-TNF therapy should be withheld until the infection is effectively treated or resolved. If a patient tests positive for latent disease, treatment of latent TB should be initiated according to standard guidelines and TNF-inhibitor therapy may be considered [96,97]. Patients who have had the BCG vaccine may have a positive PPD even in the absence of infection; thus, alternative screening methods would be appropriate in this setting, such as QuantiFERON-TB Gold (www.quantiferon. com) or T-SPOT.TB assays. These whole blood tests have higher specificity than the traditional tuberculin skin test, ranging from 96% to 100% among BCG-vaccinated subjects, while having comparable sensitivity [94]. A PPD should not be performed before QuantiFERON-TB Gold or T-SPOT.TB assays because theoretically it can result in a higher risk for false-positive results [98].

It has been estimated that screening for latent TB (risk assessment, tuberculin skin testing, and chest radiograph) before anti-TNF therapy may decrease the rate of TB infection by as much as 90% [99]. Although TB screening, and subsequent treatment in positive cases, reduces the incidence of disease reactivation among patients who then receive TNF inhibitor therapy, one study reported the development of TB among 19% of patients who received adequate chemoprophylaxis before anti-TNF therapy [100].

Safety issues related to demyelinating diseases
Occasional reports have been made of new-onset demyelinating events among patients treated with TNF inhibitor therapy. Furthermore, a randomized controlled trial of the TNF inhibitor lenercept for treatment of multiple sclerosis demonstrated that TNF inhibition may lead to a higher rate of disease exacerbations compared with placebo [101]. A definitive link between TNF inhibitor treatment and new-onset demyelinating disease has been raised but remains uncertain. Whether TNF inhibitor therapy unmasks an underlying predisposition for autoimmune neurologic disease, promotes it, or has no direct association with it remains unclear. A recommendation to cease TNF inhibitor use on development of neurologic symptoms, and to avoid use among patients who have pre-existing demyelinating disease, has been made, given rare reports of new-onset demyelinating events among treated patients. It has also been recommended that TNF inhibitor therapy be avoided in patients who have a first-degree relative affected by demyelinating disease [102]. The impact of the T-cell inhibitors used for psoriasis on the risk for demyelination events has not been well characterized; however, such events have been reported to occur in individuals treated with efalizumab [103].

Inhibitors of T-cell activation
Alefacept
Alefacept is a human recombinant dimeric fusion protein consisting of the terminal end of leukocyte function–associated antigen-3 (LFA-3) bound to the Fc portion of human IgG1. Under normal circumstances, endogenous LFA-3, which is expressed on the surface of APCs, is recognized by CD2, which is preferentially expressed at high levels by natural killer cells and effector/memory CD4 and CD8 T cells. The interaction of APC LFA-3 with CD2 on the T-cell surface plays an essential costimulatory role in T-cell activation. By binding to CD2, alefacept inhibits T-cell costimulation and activation [104]. In addition, alefacept may induce the selective apoptosis of effector/memory T cells through its simultaneous binding of CD2 on the T-cell surface and the FcγRIII receptor expressed by natural killer cells, which recognizes the Fc portion of

alefacept [105]. Recent data suggest that alefacept may exhibit both agonistic and antagonistic properties with regard to the expression of specific cytokines (ie, the suppression of inflammatory cytokines and induction of IL-8, STAT1, and Mig) [106]. Gene expression patterns specific to responders and nonresponders to alefacept have also been identified [106].

Alefacept is FDA approved for the treatment of adults who have chronic moderate-to-severe plaque psoriasis. After drug administration, peak plasma concentrations of alefacept are achieved between 24 and 192 hours; its elimination half-life is approximately 12 days [107]. Alefacept is administered as a weekly intramuscular injection of 15 mg for 12 consecutive weeks. In a recent international phase 3 trial, a PASI 75 was achieved by 33% of patients receiving alefacept 15 mg intramuscularly weekly and by 13% of placebo-treated patients during the 14-week study period [108]. Recent studies suggest that longer courses of treatment (16 weeks) or repeated courses may lead to enhanced efficacy [109–111]. Although not FDA approved for PsA, recent trials indicate that alefacept may also improve PsA symptoms [112]. It has been used as monotherapy, and in combination with methotrexate, in this setting with promising results [112,113].

In comparison to the TNF inhibitors, alefacept appears to exhibit lower treatment efficacy with a delayed onset of action. Clinical improvement usually occurs late during the treatment course, with maximal responses often noted weeks after the final dose. The potential for long periods of disease remission on cessation of therapy exists; however, this occurs in only a few patients [114]. It is recommended that a CD4+ T-cell count be established at baseline, with subsequent re-evaluation every 2 weeks throughout the 12-week treatment course (therapy should be discontinued if the count falls below 250/uL). Approximately 10% of patients require temporary discontinuation of therapy secondary to dose-dependent lymphopenia [115].

The most common side effects associated with alefacept therapy include injection site reactions, headaches, chills, nausea, and upper respiratory symptoms. Few patients experience lymphopenia, serious infections, malignancies, and elevated serum transaminases. The FDA recommends that alefacept not be administered to patients who have HIV or CD4+ T-cell counts below normal, given the risk for lymphopenia [115]. Alefacept should be used with caution among patients who have a history of systemic malignancy or are at increased risk for infection. Studies addressing the efficacy of influenza and pneumococcal vaccines among treated patients have not been published at this time; however, a study of psoriasis patients exposed to ΦX174 neoantigen and recall antigen tetanus toxoid immunization, after a 12-week treatment course with alefacept, revealed intact CD4+ T-cell–mediated antibody titer responses that were comparable to controls [116]. Large, long-term follow-up studies of alefacept treatment of psoriasis will be necessary to define its safety profile further.

Efalizumab
Efalizumab is a humanized, recombinant, IgG1 monoclonal antibody against the CD11a subunit of leukocyte function–associated antigen-1 (LFA-1).

LFA-1 is endogenously expressed on the surface of T cells. Its ligand, intercellular adhesion molecule-1 (ICAM-1), is expressed on the surface of dermal endothelial cells and APCs. The interaction of LFA-1 with ICAM-1 on the surface of APCs promotes T-cell activation and cytotoxicity [117]. In addition, its recognition of ICAM-1 expressed on the dermal microvasculature promotes the firm adhesion and subsequent migration of lymphocytes into the cutaneous microenvironment. Thus, inhibition of LFA-1 decreases lymphocyte migration to the skin and activation by APCs.

Efalizumab is FDA approved for the treatment of moderate-to-severe plaque psoriasis. Peak plasma concentrations are achieved approximately 2 to 3 days after subcutaneous injection of the drug, with an elimination half-life of approximately 6 days [118]. Treatment is initiated with a 0.7 mg/kg subcutaneous conditioning dose, followed by weekly 1.0 mg/kg subcutaneous injections for an indefinite period of time depending on patient response to therapy.

In a 2003 phase 3 study, 27% of patients who had moderate-to-severe plaque psoriasis achieved a PASI 75 after 12 weeks of treatment with efalizumab at a weekly subcutaneous dose of 1 mg/kg, whereas only 4% of the placebo group achieved a similar result [117]. The most common side effects associated with treatment include flu-like symptoms (on initial dosing), leukocytosis/lymphocytosis, and nonserious infections.

Treated patients have a small risk for hemolytic anemia and thrombocytopenia that is not well understood. It is therefore recommended that treated patients undergo monthly evaluation of their platelet count for the first 3 months, and every 3 months thereafter.

A few patients treated with efalizumab have experienced a flare of their disease or a change in the nature of their psoriasis during treatment [119]. Additionally, some patients may experience worsening of their disease on discontinuation of therapy [103]. It has been estimated that approximately 5% of patients will experience a rebound flare on cessation of therapy [120]. In clinical trials, serious disease flares characterized by inflammatory, pustular, and erythrodermic psoriasis affected 0.7% of patients [121]. Based on a small trial, inflammatory flares associated with efalizumab appear to respond best to cyclosporine or methotrexate, as compared with oral steroids or retinoids [122].

Efalizumab must be used with caution among patients who have a history of systemic malignancy or are at increased risk for infection. The package insert recommends against the administration of acellular, live, and live attenuated vaccines during treatment. Although a decreased response to tetanus booster has been reported among treated patients (with titers still in the protective range), no studies addressing the safety or efficacy of the pneumococcal and influenza vaccine in this setting have been reported to date [123]. Large, long-term follow-up studies of efalizumab treatment of psoriasis will be necessary to define its safety profile further.

What novel biologic agents are currently under investigation?

The discovery of the proinflammatory cytokines, IL-12 and IL-23, in the past 2 decades has led to increasing interest in their potential roles as mediators of psoriatic disease. Both are involved in the regulation of cell-mediated immune responses. IL-12 is involved in the activation of natural killer cells and has been shown to promote the differentiation of naïve CD4 T-cells into effector/memory cells that secrete Th1 cytokines [124]. IL-23 stimulates the production of TNF, IL-6, IL-17, and IL-22 by a unique subset of Th cells called Th17 cells [125]. The production of IL-17 has been shown to induce the production of inflammatory cytokines by multiple cell types [126] (including macrophages, fibroblasts, and endothelial cells) and is believed to play a pivotal role in sustaining inflammatory responses in multiple autoimmune disorders [127]. IL-22 has been shown to play a role in cutaneous inflammatory processes and may promote psoriatic lesions through its inhibitory effects on keratinocyte differentiation [127].

IL-12 and IL-23 share structural similarity in that both possess an IL-12p40 subunit. Their receptors are also similar in that they share the IL-12Rβ1 subunit, which recognizes IL-12p40. Elevated levels of IL-12p40 mRNA have been reported in the skin lesions of psoriasis patients [128]. Several studies have correlated clinical improvement in psoriasis lesions with marked reductions in IL-12 and IL-23 expression levels in affected skin [128], further supporting a pathogenic role for these cytokines in psoriasis. To evaluate the therapeutic efficacy of IL-12/23 blockade on psoriasis, a recombinant human monoclonal antibody against IL-12p40 (CNTO 1275) was recently developed (Centocor Corp., Malvern, PA).

A phase 2 study ustekinumab (CNTO 1275) among patients who had moderate-to-severe plaque psoriasis reported a PASI 75 by week 12 in 52% of patients who received one 45-mg intravenous dose, in 59% of patients who received one 90-mg dose, and in 81% of patients who received four weekly 90-mg doses; compared with 2% who received placebo [129]. Twenty-three percent to 52% of patients achieved a PASI 90, depending on the dose.

In a recently conducted phase 3 study, 67% to 76% of patients receiving ustekinumab achieved a PASI 75 at 12 weeks depending upon the administered dose (45mg versus 90mg at week 0, week 4, then every 12 weeks) [130]. Among partial responders receiving the higher dose, an increase in dosing frequency from every 12 to every 8 weeks was associated with a significant improvement in clinical response. Adverse events among treatment groups were similar. Clinical responses were best sustained among patients receiving maintenance dosing [131].

Another monoclonal antibody against IL-12/23 has been developed (ABT-874; Abbot Laboratories, Abbott Park, IL) and studied in the setting of Crohn's disease and, more recently, psoriasis. A phase 2 trial among Crohn's disease patients receiving subcutaneous ABT-784 for 7 weeks resulted in marked improvements in patient symptom scores, with no serious adverse effects [132]. A phase 2 trial to assess its safety and efficacy in the treatment of moderate-to-severe chronic plaque psoriasis was recently conducted [133]. More than 90% of patients receiving repeated doses of this agent, in varying amounts and duration, achieved a PASI 75 after 12 weeks.

These studies provide early evidence that IL-12/23 monoclonal antibody therapy may offer a safe and efficacious treatment alternative for patients who have moderate-to-severe plaque psoriasis.

SUMMARY

The onset of psoriatic disease and its associated comorbidities involves the interplay among a myriad of genetic and environmental risk factors. As we gain further insight into the immunopathogenesis of psoriasis, we hope it will provide the basis for the development of safer, more efficacious, and more durable therapeutics in the future. Given its enormous toll on patient health and quality of life, steps should be taken to prevent or decrease the risk for psoriasis-associated comorbidities through behavior modification and use of preventative health screenings and treatments. Future studies will need to be performed to determine if successful treatment of psoriasis will lead to a decreased risk for developing psoriasis-associated comorbidities over time.

References

[1] Liu Y, Bowcock KJ. Psoriasis: genetic associations and immune system changes. Genes Immun 2007;8:1–12.

[2] Lowes MA, Bowcock AM, Krueger JG. Pathogenesis and therapy of psoriasis. Nature 2007;445:866–73.

[3] Griffiths CE, Barker JN. Pathogenesis and clinical features of psoriasis. Lancet 2007;370: 263–71.

[4] Elder JT, Nair RP, Henseler T, et al. The genetics of psoriasis 2001: the odyssey continues. Arch Dermatol 2001;137:1447–54.

[5] Gottlieb SL, Gilleaudeau P, Johnson R, et al. Response of psoriasis to a lymphocyte-selective toxin (DAB389IL-2) suggests a primary immune, but not keratinocyte, pathogenic basis. Nat Med 1995;1(5):442–7.

[6] Abrams LM Jr, Guzzo CA, Jegasothy BV, et al. CTLA4Ig-mediated blockade of T-cell costimulation in patients with psoriasis vulgaris. J Clin Invest 1999;103(9):1243–52.

[7] Wrone-Smith T, Nickoloff BJ. Dermal injection of immunocytes induces psoriasis. J Clin Invest 1996;98(1878–87).

[8] Wang F LE, Lowes MA, Haider AS, et al. Prominent production of IL-20 by CD68+/CD11c+ myeloid-derived cells in psoriasis: gene regulation and cellular effect. J Invest Dermatol 2006;2006(7):1590–9.

[9] Lee E, TW, Oestreicher JL, et al. Increased expression of interleukin 23 p19 and p40 in lesional skin of patients with psoriasis vulgaris. J Exp Med 2004;199(1):125–30.

[10] Creamer D, Allen M, Jaggar R, et al. Mediation of systemic vascular hyperpermeability in severe psoriasis by circulating vascular endothelial growth factor. Arch Dermatol 2002;138:791–6.

[11] Krueger JG, Krane JF, Carter DM, et al. Role of growth factors, cytokines, and their receptors in the pathogenesis of psoriasis. J Invest Dermatol 1990;94:135s–40s.

[12] Trembath RC, Clough RL, Rosbotham JL, et al. Identification of a major susceptibility locus on chromosome 6p and evidence for further disease loci revealed by a two stage genome-wide search in psoriasis. Hum Mol Genet 1997;6:813–20.

[13] Gladman DD, Anhorn KA, Schachter RK, et al. HLA antigens in psoriatic arthritis. J Rheumatol 1986;13(3):586–92.

[14] Valdimarsson H. The genetic basis of psoriasis. Clin Dermatol 2007;25(6):563–7.

[15] Rahman P, Elder JT. Genetic epidemiology of psoriasis and psoriatic arthritis. Ann Rheum Dis 2005;64(Suppl 2):37–9.

[16] Setty AR, Curhan G, Choi HK. Obesity, waist circumference, weight change, and the risk of psoriasis in women: Nurses' Health Study II. Arch Intern Med 2007;167(15):1670–5.

[17] Setty AR, Curhan G, Choi HK. Smoking and the risk of psoriasis in women: Nurses' Health Study II. Am J Med 2007;120:953–9.

[18] Naldi L, Chatenoud L, Linder D, et al. Shin DB Cigarette smoking, body mass index, and stressful life events as risk factors for psoriasis: results from an Italian case-control study. J Invest Dermatol 2005;125:61–7.

[19] Neimann AL, Shin DB, Wang X, et al. Prevalence of cardiovascular risk factors in patients with psoriasis. J Am Acad Dermatol 2006;55(5):829–35.

[20] Karason A, Gudjonsson JE, Upmanyu R, et al. A susceptibility gene for psoriatic arthritis maps to chromosome 16q: evidence for imprinting. Am J Hum Genet 2003;72(1): 125–31.

[21] Lee FI, Bellary SV, Francis C. Increased occurrence of psoriasis in patients with Crohn's disease and their relatives. Am J Gastroenterol 1990;85:962–3.

[22] Gottlieb AB, Chao C, Dann F. Psoriasis comorbidities. J Dermatolog Treat 2008;19:5–21.

[23] Kurd SK, Richardson SK, Gelfand JM. Update on the epidemiology and systemic treatment of psoriasis. Expert Review of Clinical Immunology 2007;3:171–85.

[24] Horn EJ, Fox KM, Patel V, et al. Association of patient-reported psoriasis severity with income and employment. J Am Acad Dermatol 2007;57:963–71.

[25] Gelfand JM, Gladmann DD, Mease PJ, et al. Epidemiology of psoriatic arthritis in the population of the United States. J Am Acad Dermatol 2005;53:573–7.

[26] Cohen MR, Reda DJ, Clegg DO. Baseline relationships between psoriasis and psoriatic arthritis: analysis of 221 patients with active psoriatic arthritis. Department of Veterans Affairs Cooperative Study Group on Seronegative Spondyloarthropathies. J Rheumatol 1999;26(1752–1756).

[27] Gladman DD, Shuckett R, Russell ML, et al. Psoriatic arthritis (PSA) – an analysis of 220 patients. QJM 1987;62:127–41.

[28] Wong K, Gladman DD, Husted J, et al. Mortality studies in psoriatic arthritis: results from a single outpatient clinic. Causes and risk of death. Arthritis Rheum 1997;40:1868–72.

[29] Shbeeb M, Uramoto KM, Gibson LE, et al. The epidemiology of psoriatic arthritis in Olmsted County, Minnesota, USA, 1982–1991. J Rheumatol 2000;27:1247–50.

[30] Gladman DD, Farewell VT, Nadeau C. Clinical indicators of progression in psoriatic arthritis: multivariate relative risk model. J Rheumatol 1995;4:675–9.

[31] McDonald CJ, Calabresi P. Occlusive vascular disease in psoriatic patients. N Engl J Med 1973;288:912.

[32] Gelfand JM, Niemann A, Shin DB, et al. Risk of myocardial infarction in patients with psoriasis. JAMA 2006;296(14):1735–41.

[33] Ludwig R, Herzog C, Rostock A, et al. Psoriasis: a possible risk factor for development of coronary artery calcification. Br J Dermatol 2006;156(2):271–6.

[34] Cohen AD, Sherf M, Vidavsky L, et al. Association between psoriasis and the metabolic syndrome. A cross-sectional study. Dermatology 2008;216:152–5.

[35] Paul CF, Ho VC, McGeown C, et al. Risk of malignancies in psoriasis patients treated with cyclosporine: a 5 y cohort study. J Invest Dermatol 2003;120(2):211–6.

[36] Stern RS, Vakeva LH. Noncutaneous malignant tumors in the PUVA follow-up study: 1975–1996. J Invest Dermatol 1997;108(6):897–900.

[37] Hannuksela-Svahn A, Sigurgeirsson B, Pukkala E, et al. Trioxsalen bath PUVA did not increase the risk of squamous cell skin carcinoma and cutaneous malignant melanoma in a joint analysis of 944 Swedish and Finnish patients with psoriasis. Br J Dermatol 1999;141(3):497–501.

[38] Frentz G, Olsen JH, Avrach WW. Malignant tumours and psoriasis: climatotherapy at the dead sea. Br J Dermatol 1999;141(6):1088–91.

[39] Boffetta P, Gridley G, Lindelof B. Cancer risk in a population-based cohort of patients hospitalized for psoriasis in Sweden. J Invest Dermatol 2001;117(6):1531–7.

[40] Hannuksela-Svahn A, Pukkala E, Laara E, et al. Psoriasis, its treatment, and cancer in a cohort of Finnish patients. J Invest Dermatol 2000;114(3):587–90.

[41] Frentz G, Olsen JH. Malignant tumours and psoriasis: a follow-up study. Br J Dermatol 1999;140(2):237–42.

[42] Gelfand JM, Shin DB, Neimann AL, et al. The risk of lymphoma in patients with psoriasis. J Invest Dermatol 2006;126(10):2194–201.

[43] Stern RS. Lymphoma risk in psoriasis: results of the PUVA follow-up study. Arch Dermatol 2006;142(9):1132–5.

[44] Gupta MA, Gupta AK. Depression and suicidal ideation in dermatology patients with acne, alopecia areata, atopic dermatitis and psoriasis. Br J Dermatol 1998;139(5):846–50.

[45] Gupta MA, Schork NJ, Gupta AK, et al. Suicidal ideation in psoriasis. Int J Dermatol 1993;32(3):188–90.

[46] Polenghi MM, Molinari E, Gala C, et al. Experience with psoriasis in a psychosomatic dermatology clinic. Acta Derm Venereol Suppl (Stockh) 1994;186:65–6.

[47] Gupta MA, Gupta AK, Haberman HF. Psoriasis and psychiatry: an update. Gen Hosp Psychiatry 1987;9(3):157–66.

[48] Rubino IA, Sonnino A, Pezzarossa B, et al. Personality disorders and psychiatric symptoms in psoriasis. Psychol Rep 1995;77(2):547–53.

[49] Vidoni D, Campiutti E, D'Aronco R, et al. Psoriasis and alexithymia. Acta Derm Venereol Suppl (Stockh) 1989;146:91–2.

[50] Gupta MA, Gupta AK, Watteel GN. Early onset (< 40 years age) psoriasis is comorbid with greater psychopathology than late onset psoriasis: a study of 137 patients. Acta Derm Venereol 1996;76(6):464–6.

[51] Richards HL, Fortune DG, Weidmann A, et al. Detection of psychological distress in patients with psoriasis: low consensus between dermatologist and patient. Br J Dermatol 2004;151(6):1227–33.

[52] Ginsburg IH, Link BG. Feelings of stigmatization in patients with psoriasis. J Am Acad Dermatol 1989;20(1):53–63.

[53] Devrimci-Ozguven H, Kundakci TN, Kumbasar H, et al. The depression, anxiety, life satisfaction and affective expression levels in psoriasis patients. J Eur Acad Dermatol Venereol 2000;14(4):267–71.

[54] Fortune DG, Richards HL, Kirby B, et al. Psychological distress impairs clearance of psoriasis in patients treated with photochemotherapy. Arch Dermatol 2003;139(6):752–6.

[55] Tyring S, Gottlieb A, Papp K, et al. Etanercept and clinical outcomes, fatigue, and depression in psoriasis: double-blind placebo-controlled randomised phase III trial. Lancet 2006;367:29–35.

[56] Kimball AB, Gladman D, Gelfand JM, et al. Psoriasis foundation clinical consensus on psoriasis comorbidities and recommendations for screening. J Am Acad Dermatol 2008;58(6):1031–42.

[57] Gelfand JM, Troxel AB, Lewis JD, et al. The risk of mortality in patients with psoriasis: results from a population-based study. Arch Dermatol 2007;143(12):1493–9.

[58] Pariser DM, Bagel J, Gelfand JM, et al. National Psoriasis Foundation clinical consensus on disease severity. Arch Dermatol 2007;143:239–42.

[59] Springer TA. Adhesion receptors of the immune system. Nature 1990;346(6283):425–34.

[60] Gottlieb AB, Masud S, Ramamurthi R, et al. Pharmacodynamic and pharmacokinetic response to anti-tumor necrosis factor-alpha monoclonal antibody (infliximab) treatment of moderate to severe psoriasis vulgaris. J Am Acad Dermatol 2003;48(1):68–75.

[61] Hancock GE, Kaplan G, Cohn ZA. Keratinocyte growth regulation by the products of immune cells. J Exp Med 1988;168(4):1395–402.

[62] (adalimumab) Humira. Package insert. North Chicago: Abbott Laboraties; 2008.

[63] Gordon KB, Langley RG, Leonardi C, et al. Clinical response to adalimumab treatment in patients with moderate to severe psoriasis: double-blind, randomized controlled trial and open-label extension study. J Am Acad Dermatol 2006;55(4):598–606.

[64] Reich K, Nestle FO, Papp K, et al. Infliximab induction and maintenance therapy for moderate-to-severe psoriasis: a phase III, multicentre, double-blind trial. Lancet 2005;366(9494):1367–74.

[65] Baert F, Norman M, Vermeire S, et al. Influence of immunogenicity on the long-term efficacy of infliximab in Crohn's disease. NEJM 2003;348:601–8.

[66] Menter A, Feldman SR, Weinstein GD, et al. A randomized comparison of continuous vs. intermittent infliximab maintenance regimens over 1 year in the treatment of moderate-to-severe plaque psoriasis. J Am Acad Dermatol 2006;56:31.e1–31.e15.

[67] Moreland LW, Schiff MH, Baumgartner SW, et al. Etancercept therapy in rheumatoid arthritis: a randomized, controlled trial. Ann Intern Med 1999;130(6):478–86.

[68] Zhou H, Mayer PR, Wajdula J, et al. Unaltered etanercept pharmacokinetics with concurrent methotrexate in patients with rheumatoid arthritis. J Clin Pharmacol 2004;44(11):1235–43.

[69] Clark L, Lebwohl M. The effect of weight on the efficacy of biologic therapy in patients with psoriasis. J Am Acad Dermatol 2008;58:443–6.

[70] Shen C, Assche GV, Colpaert S, et al. Adalimumab induces apoptosis of human monocytes: a comparative study with infliximab and etanercept. Aliment Pharmacol Ther 2005;21:251–8.

[71] Wallis RS, Ehlers S. Tumor necrosis factor and granuloma biology: explaining the differential infection risk of etanercept and infliximab. Semin Arthritis Rheum 2005;34(5 Suppl 1):34–8.

[72] Nestorov I. Clinical pharmacokinetics of TNF antagonists: how do they differ? Semin Arthritis Rheum 2005;34(5 Suppl. 1):12–8.

[73] Haider AS, Cardinale IR, Whynot JA, et al. Effects of etanercept are distinct from infliximab in modulating proinflammatory genes in activated human leukocytes. J Investig Dermatol Symp Proc 2007;12:9–15.

[74] Rutgeerts P, D'Haens G, Targan S, et al. Efficacy and safety of retreatment with anti-tumor necrosis factor antibody (infliximab) to maintain remission in Crohn's disease. Gastroenterology 1999;117:761–9.

[75] Sandborn WJ, Hanauer SB, Katz S, et al. Etanercept for active Crohn's disease: a randomized, double-blind, placebo-controlled trial. Gastroenterology 2001;121:1088–94.

[76] Hanauer SB, Sandborn WJ, Rutgeerts P, et al. Human anti-tumor necrosis factor monoclonal antibody (adalimumab) in Crohn's disease: the CLASSIC-I trial. Gastroenterology 2006;130:323–33.

[77] Chung ES, Packer M, Lo KH, et al. Randomized, double-blind, placebo-controlled, pilot trial of infliximab, a chimeric monoclonal antibody to tumor necrosis factor-α in patients with moderate-to-severe heart failure: results of the anti-TNF Therapy Against Congestive Heart Failure (ATTACH) trial. Circulation 2003;107:3133–40.

[78] Centocor. Remicade (Inflximab) prescribing information. Malvern PU 2006.

[79] Mease PJ, Ritchlin CT, Martin RW, et al. Pneumococcal vaccine response in psoriatic arthritis patients during treatment with etanercept. J Rheumatol 2004;31:1356–61.

[80] Fomin I, Caspi D, Levy V, et al. Vaccination against influenza in rheumatoid arthritis: the effect of disease modifying drugs, including TNF alpha blocker. Ann Rheum Dis 2006;65:191–4.

[81] Geborek P, Bladstrom A, Turesson C, et al. Tumour necrosis factor blockers do not increase overall tumour risk in patients with rheumatoid arthritis, but may be associated with an increased risk of lymphomas. Ann Rheum Dis;64:699–703.

[82] Wolfe F, Michaud K. Lymphoma in rheumatoid arthritis: the effect of methotrexate and anti-tumor necrosis factor therapy in 18,572 patients. Arthritis Rheum 2004;50:1741–51.

[83] Wolfe F, Michaud K. The effect of methotrexate and anti-tumor necrosis factor therapy on the risk of lymphoma in rheumatoid arthritis in 19,562 patients during 89,710 person-years of observation. Arthritis Rheum 2007;56:1433–9.

[84] Bongartz T, Sutton AJ, Sweeting MJ, et al. Anti-TNF antibody therapy in rheumatoid arthritis and the risk of serious infections and malignancies: systematic review and meta-analysis of rare harmful effects in randomized controlled trials. JAMA 2006;295:2275–85.

[85] Wolfe F, Michaud K. Biologic treatment of rheumatoid arthritis and the risk of malignancy: analyses from a large US observational study. Arthritis Rheum 2007;56:2886–95.

[86] Stone JH, Holbrook JT, Marriott MA, et al. Wegener's Granulomatosis Etanercept Trial Research Group. Solid malignancies among patients in the Wegener's Granulomatosis Etanercept Trial. Arthritis Rheum 2006;54:1608–18.

[87] Magliocco MA, Gottlieb AB. Etanercept therapy for patients with psoriatic arthritis and concurrent hepatitis C virus infection: report of 3 cases. J Am Acad Dermatol 2004;51(4):580–4.

[88] Aslanidis S, Vassiliadis T, Pyrpasopoulou A, et al. Inhibition of TNFalpha does not induce viral reactivation in patients with chronic hepatitis C infection: two cases. Clin Rheumatol 2007;26(2):61–264.

[89] Bellisai F, Giannitti C, Donvito A, et al. Combination therapy with cyclosporine A and anti-TNF-alpha agents in the treatment of rheumatoid arthritis and concomitant hepatitis C virus infection. Clin Rheumatol 2007;26(7):1127–9.

[90] Parke FA, Reveille JD. Anti-tumor necrosis factor agents for rheumatoid arthritis in the setting of chronic hepatitis C infection. Arthritis Rheum 2004;51:800–4.

[91] Zein NN, Etanercept Study Group. Etanercept as an adjuvant to interferon and ribavirin in treatment-naive patients with chronic hepatitis C virus infection: a phase 2 randomized, double-blind, placebo-controlled study. J Hepatol 2005;42:315–22.

[92] Nathan DM, Angus PW, Gibson PR. Hepatitis B and C virus infections and anti-tumor necrosis factor-alpha therapy: guidelines for clinical approach. J Gastroenterol Hepatol 2006;21(9):1366–71.

[93] Roux CH, Brocq O, Breuil V, et al. Safety of anti-TNF-alpha therapy in rheumatoid arthritis and spondylarthropathies with concurrent B or C chronic hepatitis. Rheumatology 2006;45:1294–7.

[94] Theis VS, Rhodes JM. Review article: minimizing tuberculosis during anti-tumor necrosis factor-alpha treatment of inflammatory bowel disease. Ailment Pharmacol Ther 2008;27:19–30.

[95] Lebwohl M, Bagel J, Gelfand JM, et al. From the medical board of the National Psoriasis Foundation: monitoring and vaccinations in patients treated with biologics for psoriasis. J Am Acad Dermatol 2008;58:94–105.

[96] Hochberg MC, Lebwohl MG, Plevy SE, et al. The benefit/risk profile of TNF-blocking agents: findings of a consensus panel. Semin Arthritis Rheum 2005;34:819–36.

[97] CDC Morbidity and Mortality Week Report. Targeted tuberculin testing and treatment of latent tuberculosis infection 2000;49(RR06):1–54.

[98] CDC Morbidity and Mortality Week Report. Guidelines for using the QuantiFERON-TB Test for diagnosing latent mycobacterial tuberculosis infection 2003;52(RR02):15–8.

[99] Perez JL, Kupper H, Spencer-Green GT. Impact of screening for latent TB prior to initiation of anti-TNF therapy in North America and Europe. Ann Rheum Dis 2006;64(Suppl. III):86A.

[100] Sichletidis L, Settas L, Spyratos D, et al. Tuberculosis in patients receiving anti-TNF agents despite chemoprophylaxis. Int J Tuberc Lung Dis 2006;10:1127–32.

[101] The Lenercept Multiple Sclerosis Study Group and the University of British Columbia MS/MRI Analysis Group. TNF neutralization in MS: results of a randomized, placebo-controlled multicenter study. Neurology 1999;53:457–65.

[102] Codoro KM, Feldman SR. TNF-α inhibitors in dermatology. Skin Therapy Lett 2007;12.

[103] (efalizumab) Raptiva. Package insert. South San Francisco (CA): Genentech, Inc.; 2007.

[104] Ellis CN, Krueger GG. Treatment of chronic plaque psoriasis by selective targeting of memory effector T lymphocytes. N Engl J Med 2001;345(4):248–55.

[105] Cooper JC, Morgan G, Harding S, et al. Alefacept selectively promotes NK cell-mediated deletion of CD45RO+ human T cells. Eur J Immunol 2003;33(3):666–75.

[106] Haider AS, Lowes MA, Gardner H, et al. Novel insight into the agonistic mechanism of alefacept in vivo: differentially expressed genes may serve as biomarkers of response in psoriasis patients. J Immunol 2007;178(11):7442–9.

[107] Vaishnaw AK, TenHoor CN. Pharmacokinetics, biologic activity, and tolerability of alefacept by intravenous and intramuscular administration. J Pharmacokinet Pharmacodyn 2002;29:415–26.

[108] Lebwohl M, Christophers E, Langley R, et al. For the Alefacept clinical study group. An international, randomized, double-blind, placebo-controlled phase 3 trial of intramuscular alefacept in patients with chronic plaque psoriasis. Arch Dermatol 2003;139(6):719–27.

[109] Gribetz CH, Blum R, Brady C, et al. An extended 16-week course of alefacept in the treatment of chronic plaque psoriasis. J Am Acad Dermatol 2005;53:73–5.

[110] Menter A, Cather JC, Baker D, et al. The efficacy of multiple courses of alefacept in patients with moderate to severe chronic plaque psoriasis. J Am Acad Dermatol 2006;54:61–3.

[111] Goffe B, Papp K, Gratton D, et al. An integrated analysis of thirteen trials summarizing the long-term safety of alefacept in psoriasis patients who have received up to nine courses of therapy. Clin Ther 2005;27:1912–21.

[112] Mease PJ, Gladman DD, Keystone EC. Alefacept in Psoriatic Arthritis Study Group. Alefacept in combination with methotrexate for the treatment of psoriatic arthritis: results of a randomized, double-blind, placebo-controlled study. Arthritis Rheum 2006;54:1638–45.

[113] Kraan MC, van Kuijk AW, Dinant HJ, et al. Alefacept treatment in psoriatic arthritis: reduction of the effector T cell population in peripheral blood and synovial tissue is associated with improvement of clinical signs of arthritis. Arthritis Rheum 2002;46:2776–84.

[114] Gordon KB, Langley RG. Remittive effects of intramuscular alefacept in psoriasis. J Drugs Dermatol 2003;2(6):624–8.

[115] Amevive (alefacept) prescribing information. Biogen Inc. (Cambridge, MA) 2005.

[116] Gottlieb AB, Casale T, Frankel E, et al. CD4+ T-cell-directed antibody responses are maintained in patients with psoriasis receiving alefacept: results of a randomized study. J Am Acad Dermatol 2003;49:816–25.

[117] Gordon KB, Papp KA, Hamilton TK, et al. Efalizumab Study Group. Efalizumab for patients with moderate to severe plaque psoriasis: a randomized controlled trial. JAMA 2003;290(23):3073–80.

[118] Raptiva (efalizumab) package insert. South San Francisco (CA): Genentech, Inc.; 2003.

[119] Hamilton TK. Clinical considerations of efalizumab therapy in patients with psoriasis. Semin Cutan Med Surg 2005;24:19–27.

[120] Cather JC, Menter A. Modulating T cell responses for the treatment of psoriasis: a focus on efalizumab. Expert Opin Biol Ther 2003;3:361–70.

[121] Carey W, Glazer S, Gottlieb AB, et al. Relapse, rebound, and psoriasis adverse events: an advisory group report. J Am Acad Dermatol 2006;54(4 Suppl. 1):S171–81.

[122] Papp KA, Toth D, Rosoph L. Approaches to discontinuing efalizumab: an open-label study of therapies for managing inflammatory recurrence. BMC Dermatol 2006;6:9.

[123] Krueger J, Ochs H, Patel P, et al. Impact of efalizumab T cell modulation on immune response in psoriasis patients. J Investig Dermatol 2005;124(Suppl. 4):264.

[124] Robertson MJ, Ritz J. Interleukin 12: basic biology and potential application in cancer treatment. Oncologist 1996;1:88–97.

[125] Aggarwal S, Ghilardi N, Xie MH, et al. Interleukin-23 promotes a distinct CD4 T cell activation state characterized by the production of interleukin-17. J Biol Chem 2003;278:1910.

[126] Kuligowska M, Odrowaz-Sypniewska G. Role of interleukin-17 in cartilage and bone destruction in rheumatoid arthritis. Ortop Traumatol Rehabil 2004;6(2):235–41.

[127] Nograles KE, Zaba LC, Guttman-Yassky E, et al. Th17 cytokines interleukin (IL)-17 and IL-22 modulate distinct inflammatory and keratinocyte-response pathways. Br J Dermatol 2008 Aug 5 [Epub ahead of print].

[128] Torti DC, Feldman SR. Interleukin-12, interleukin-23 and psoriasis: current prospects. J Am Acad Dermatol 2007;57(6):1059–68.

[129] Krueger JG, Langley RG, Leonardi C, et al. Psoriasis Study Group. A human interleukin-12/23 monoclonal antibody for the treatment of psoriasis. N Engl J Med 2007;356(6): 580–92.

[130] Papp KA, Langley RG, Lebwohl M, et al. Efficacy and safety of ustekinumab, a human interleukin-12/23 monoclonal antibody, in patients with psoriasis: 52-week results from a randomised, double-blind, placebo-controlled trial (PHOENIX 2). Lancet 2008;371(9625):1675–84.

[131] Leonardi CL, Kimball AB, Papp KA, et al. Efficacy and safety of ustekinumab, a human interleukin-12/23 monoclonal antibody, in patients with psoriasis: 76-week results from a randomised, double-blind, placebo-controlled trial (PHOENIX 1). Lancet 2008;371(9625):1665–74.

[132] Sandborn WJ. How future tumor necrosis factor antagonists and other compounds will meet the remaining challenges in Crohn's disease. Rev Gastroenterol Disord 2004;4(Suppl):S25–33.

[133] Kimball AB, Gordon KB, Langley RG, et al. Safety and efficacy of ABT-874, a fully human interleukin 12/23 monoclonal antibody, in the treatment of moderate to severe chronic plaque psoriasis: results of a randomized, placebo-controlled, phase 2 trial. Arch Dermatol 2008;144:200–7.

[134] Menter A, Tyring SK, Gordon K, et al. Adalimumab therapy for moderate to severe psoriasis: a randomized, controlled phase III trial. J Am Acad Dermatol 2007;58:106–15.

Recent Advances in Acne Vulgaris Research: Insights and Clinical Implications

Kevin C. Wang, MD, PhD[a], Lee T. Zane, MD, MAS[a,b,*]

[a]Department of Dermatology, University of California at San Francisco School of Medicine, 1701 Divisadero Street, 3rd Floor, San Francisco, CA 94115, USA

[b]Anacor Pharmaceuticals, 1020 East Meadow Circle, Palo Alto, CA 94303, USA

EDITORIAL COMMENT

Acne is dermatology's signature disease. We are the physicians who have described, discovered and led the way to all important advances in the understanding of this common malady. Drs. Wang and Zane review for us the most recent advances in acne and place these into appropriate perspective. The areas covered range from the most basic science findings to the psychosocial implication of this highly visible disease. Our patients always want to know how diet influences their condition. The authors review the recent investigations and guide us through the strengths and weaknesses of the methods used in the research specified. Get up-to-date on acne; read this!

William James, MD

Acne vulgaris is a common disorder that affects many adolescents and adults, and is one of the leading cutaneous disorders seen in consultation by dermatologists worldwide. Despite its high prevalence, the understanding of acne, its treatment, and its effect on patients continues to expand. This article discusses some recent advances in acne research, highlighting a few key studies in both the basic science and clinical realms.

DIETARY INFLUENCES ON ACNE

Dermatologists' beliefs about the role of diet in acne were profoundly shaped by the results of an experiment conducted by Fulton and coworkers in 1969 [1]. In this oft-cited single-blind, crossover study, 65 subjects were assigned to consume either an enriched chocolate bar or a control bar lacking cocoa

This work was not supported by any specific funding source.

*Corresponding author. Anacor Pharmaceuticals, 1020 East Meadow Circle, Palo Alto, CA 94303. *E-mail address:* lzane@anacor.com (L.T. Zane).

0882-0880/08/$ – see front matter
doi:10.1016/j.yadr.2008.09.002

butter and chocolate liquor. Changes in lesion count during each ingestion period were categorized as worse (increased by 30% or more); improved (decreased by 30% or more); or same (less than 30% change in either direction). Because no statistically significant differences were found between the chocolate and control bars across the three ordinal categories or in sebum characteristics, it was concluded that ingestion of high amounts of chocolate "did not materially affect the course of acne vulgaris or the output or composition of sebum."

Unfortunately, however, the results of this study were widely overinterpreted, dismissing the potential effect of dietary ingestions on acne and the study has been criticized on a number of methodologic grounds. A small study in 1971 subsequently found no differences in count or grade of acne among medical students who were asked to consume the one food they thought would worsen their acne for 7 days [2]. Since then, although a few important observational studies have been recently published examining the role of diet in acne [3,4], no other dietary interventional studies exploring this association were published for another 35 years.

In 2007, Smith and colleagues [5] published the results of a randomized, single-blind, dietary intervention trial examining the effect of 12 weeks of a high-protein, low-glycemic-load (LGL) diet versus a conventional high-glycemic-load diet on total acne lesion counts and select endocrinologic parameters in young male patients with mild-to-moderate facial acne vulgaris. In this study, 50 male patients, age 15 to 25 years, with mild-to-moderate facial acne taking no medications known to affect acne or glucose metabolism were randomized to receive one of two interventions. The LGL intervention group received dietary education on how to substitute higher glycemic index foods with higher-protein, lower glycemic index alternatives along with some sample staple foods. They were encouraged to consume a recommended diet consisting of 25% protein, 45% low glycemic index carbohydrates, and 30% fats on a daily basis for 12 weeks. The control group received samples of carbohydrate-rich staples and were encouraged to eat these or similar foods daily. A standardized noncomedogenic topical cleanser was also provided and patients were instructed to use it during a 2-week run-in period before the dietary intervention period and throughout the study.

Forty-three subjects completed the study per protocol (23 in the LGL group, 20 in the control group). Although both groups experienced substantial reductions in total acne lesion count at 12 weeks compared with baseline, the LGL group was found to have statistically significantly greater reductions (mean, −54%) compared with the control group (mean, −40%). In addition, compared with controls, the LGL group also experienced statistically significant reductions in body weight, body mass index, percentage body fat, and waist circumference, and favorable changes in multiple biochemical parameters.

These results suggest that following an LGL diet may enhance improvement of facial acne when combined with a standardized noncomedogenic cleanser. Additionally, the changes in physical and endocrinologic parameters suggest that decreases in total energy intake, body weight, and indices of androgenicity and insulin resistance may also be associated with observed improvements in acne. It may be difficult to dissect out the individual contributions each of these factors has on the overall improvement of facial acne. Indeed, these factors are quite likely interrelated: LGL diets are known to improve insulin resistance [6]; mild insulin resistance has been observed in women with acne [7]; androgen and insulin-like growth factor levels have been correlated with sebaceous gland size and activity [8,9] and acne lesion counts in adult women [10]; and weight loss has been associated with improved indices of androgenicity in women with hyperandrogenic conditions, such as polycystic ovary syndrome (PCOS) [11]. The effect of change in body mass index as an effect modifier in this relationship deserves further exploration, as does the substantial improvement in acne lesion counts observed in the control diet group, particularly in the setting of "unfavorable" changes in weight and some key biochemical parameters. The use of the standardized cleanser may help to explain the improvement among controls, as may such factors as regression to the mean of acne severity and subjects' increased attention to their acne in this study. In the face of these limitations, however, this study promises to figure as another important chapter in the story of dietary influences on acne vulgaris.

ACNE PATHOGENESIS

Traditionally, acne has been thought of as a multifactorial disease of the folliculosebaceous unit, involving excess sebum production, abnormal follicular hyperkeratinization, overgrowth of *Propionibacterium acnes*, and inflammation. Recent laboratory and clinical investigations into the roles of the innate immune system and extracellular matrix remodeling proteins have shed additional light on this pathogenetic process.

Further defining the role of the sex hormones

The prominent role of hormones in the pathophysiology of acne has long been recognized and corroborated by clinical and experimental observations and therapeutic experience [12,13]. Although acne is not considered a primary endocrine disorder, androgens, such as dihydrotestosterone, dehydroepiandrosterone sulfate, and testosterone, and growth hormone and insulin-like growth factors, have all been implicated in the pathogenesis of acne [13]. The precise mechanism by which these hormones exert their influence on sebaceous glands has not been fully elucidated.

Androgens exert their effects by binding to the nuclear androgen receptor [14] and changes in isoenzyme or androgen receptor levels have been implicated in the development of hyperandrogenism and associated skin diseases, such as acne, seborrhea, hirsutism, and androgenetic alopecia. Both in vitro and in vivo studies have demonstrated that the folliculo-sebaceous unit possesses the necessary enzymes for local synthesis and metabolism of androgens [15–17]. Interestingly, stress factors, such as the corticotropin-releasing hormone, have been found to increase expression of some of these key enzymes of androgenesis in sebocytes, suggesting a biochemical link between the stress response and sebaceous gland activity [18].

Although ethinylestradiol-containing oral contraceptives have been shown to be effective in acne treatment, little is known about the role of estrogens in the pathogenesis of acne. Estrogens exert their actions through intracellular receptors or by cell surface receptors, which activate specific second messenger signaling pathways [19]. Estrogens may counteract the effects of androgens locally within the sebaceous gland, inhibit systemic production of androgens by gonadal tissues through negative feedback inhibition, or down-regulate expression of genes important in sebaceous gland proliferation or lipid production. Interestingly, significant differences in the expression of estrogen receptors ERα and ERβ have been found between normal and acne-bearing skin [20,21].

Toll-like receptors and immune system

Toll-like receptors (TLRs) are "pathogen-associated pattern recognition receptors" that recognize particular pathogen-associated molecular patterns conserved among microorganisms and elicit specific immune responses (reviewed in [22]). Expressed on many immune cells and at sites of host-pathogen interaction, such as the skin [23], TLRs are instrumental in launching innate immune responses and influencing adaptive immunity.

Recent results suggest that keratinocytes and sebocytes may be activated by *P acnes* by TLRs and CD14 leading to the production of inflammatory cytokines, such as interleukin (IL)-12 and IL-8 [23]. This cytokine response is a T helper-1–type immune response [24], and is mediated through increased expression of TLR-2 and TLR-4 by *P acnes*. Furthermore, because TLRs are vital players in infectious and inflammatory diseases, they have been identified as potential therapeutic targets.

Role of matrix metalloproteinases

Although the precise inflammatory mediators activated in acne have not been fully described, advances in gene array expression profiling have helped to identify individual candidate genes [25]. Significant up-regulation of genes involved in mediating inflammation and extracellular matrix remodeling, such as the matrix metalloproteinases (MMPs), has been recently identified from acne lesional tissue [26,27]. MMPs are a group of zinc-dependent endopeptidases that selectively degrade various components of extracellular matrix and nonmatrix proteins [28]. MMP-1 and MMP-3 are up-regulated in skin lesions from acne patients [27], and down-regulation of some MMPs is seen in the setting of improving acne during isotretinoin treatment.

ASSOCIATED CLINICAL CONDITIONS

Several clinical syndromes characteristically include acne vulgaris as a component. Greater mechanistic understanding of some of these syndromes may provide insight into acne pathogenesis.

Polycystic ovary syndrome

PCOS affects approximately 5% to 10% of reproductive-aged women and is commonly characterized by elevated androgen levels or clinical hyperandrogenism [29,30]. The most recent clinical definition of PCOS has as one of its three cardinal criteria the dermatologic manifestations of hyperandrogenism, including hirsutism, acne vulgaris, and androgenetic alopecia [29].

Past studies have estimated the prevalence of acne vulgaris in PCOS patients at between 10% and 35% [31]. In addition to biochemical data, such as elevated luteinizing hormone/follicle-stimulating hormone ratios, the critical role of androgens in the pathogenesis of acne is supported by several observed clinical phenomena including first presentations of acne during onset of adrenarche; absence of acne in androgen receptor–deficient individuals; and presence of acne in patients with hyperandrogenism states, such as adrenal or ovarian tumors. Recent evidence from studies of serum hormone levels in middle-aged women with acne [10] raises the intriguing possibility that androgen receptor sensitivity at the local follicular unit, rather than systemic serum androgen levels, plays a more significant role, and that this state of functional hyperandrogenism may be associated with clinical manifestations of insulin resistance in PCOS patients [32].

Interestingly, the effects of androgen on pilosebaceous units in the skin can vary by anatomic location, producing pathophysiologic effects on hair growth and differentiation, sebaceous gland size and activity, and follicular keratinization [33]. It is likely that local factors other than androgen plasma levels also play a part in the development of acne through regulation of local androgen synthesis; some of the newer molecular candidates implicated include insulin-like growth factor-1 [10]. Taken together, there is now strong evidence that the acne lesions are the result of a combination of effects from circulating serum androgens and the modulation of their enzymatic activity in local tissues, with significant contributions from reciprocal growth hormone production. The exact mechanisms of action and the identity of other players involved in acne pathogenesis at the molecular level will no doubt provide a springboard for novel therapeutic approaches in the future.

Pyogenic arthritis, pyoderma gangrenosum, and acne syndrome

The *P*yogenic *A*rthritis, *P*yoderma gangrenosum, and *A*cne (PAPA) syndrome is a rare autosomal-dominant genetic disorder characterized by arthritis at a young age and prominent skin changes (acne and pyoderma gangrenosum) starting around puberty [34]. Acne affects most individuals with PAPA syndrome but to a variable degree, and is usually of the nodular type. In most of the reported cases, episodes of skin and joint flares are often precipitated by mild physical trauma, which may correlate with the postulated pathogenesis involving increased inflammatory sensitivity [35]. Recently, mutations in the CD2 binding protein 1 (CD2BP1) have been found in patients with PAPA syndrome [36]. CD2BP1 is part of an inflammatory pathway associated with other autoinflammatory diseases, such as familial Mediterranean fever, hyper IgD and periodic fever syndrome, Muckle-Wells syndrome, familial cold autoinflammatory syndrome, and neonatal-onset multisystem inflammatory disease [37].

It is unclear whether the presence of inflammatory lesions of acne in PAPA syndrome represents a coincidental association or a manifestation of a shared inflammatory etiology. The increased IL-1β production seen in PAPA syndrome and the effectiveness of anakinra [38] and infliximab [39] in its treatment argue for activation of a systemic signaling cascade centered on inflammatory cytokines, such as tumor necrosis factor-α. With the new data on the involvement of MMPs (see previous discussion) in acne pathogenesis, it is not unreasonable to hypothesize that the noncutaneous clinical manifestations of PAPA syndrome result from immunologic cross-reactivity between the etiologic skin microbe *P acnes* and a component of skin and joints, analogous to group A streptococcal-induced rheumatic fever, which results in inflammatory tissue remodeling.

Synovitis, acne, pustulosis, hyperostosis, osteitis syndrome

Synovitis, acne, pustulosis, hyperostosis, osteitis (SAPHO) syndrome is a systemic osteoarticular-skin disease characterized by sterile inflammatory arthro-osteitis of the anterior chest wall and various skin conditions including palmoplantar pustulosis, acne conglobata or fulminans, and pustular psoriasis [40]. It has been described in association with inflammatory bowel disease, pulmonary lesions, and skin manifestations [41]. The skin lesions may appear many years after the onset of bone lesions, however, or may be totally absent, particularly in children [40].

Cases of *P acnes* chest wall infection have been reported in patients with palmoplantar pustulosis or chronic or multifocal osteitis, supporting a role for *P acnes* in the pathogenesis of SAPHO syndrome [42]. Although it is inviting to speculate that infection with a microorganism of low virulence, such as *P acnes*, may serve as a triggering factor for SAPHO syndrome, effective antibiotic therapy against *P acnes* has not resulted in dramatic clinical improvements in the acneiform lesions of this syndrome.

THERAPEUTIC INSIGHTS

Clinicians are observing with increased frequency decreases in the clinical efficacy of antibiotic therapy in the treatment of acne, and a correspondingly growing number of resistant *P acnes* strains, which have fueled the important debate on antibiotic overuse. Although it remains controversial whether the burden of *P acnes* is a reliable predictor of acne severity or response to treatment, it is clear that presence of resistant strains of *P acnes* is correlated with poor clinical response to antibiotic therapy [43,44]. *P acnes* represents but one component in the pathogenesis of acne, however, and antimicrobial properties may represent only one aspect of an antibiotic's mechanism of action (which may also include anti-inflammatory activity). Instead, an alternative approach to understanding antibiotic resistance in vitro is to conceptualize its laboratory definition [45]: increases in the minimum inhibitory concentrations (MICs) are often used as an indicator of decreased microbial sensitivity to antibiotics. Rather than acting as strictly microbial sensitivity guides, MICs can serve as valuable indicators of the predominant mechanism of action for a particular antibiotic. For example, in bacteria with low MICs to a particular agent, that agent's antimicrobial effects likely predominate in the clinical setting, whereas in bacteria with higher MICs the antibiotic probably exerts more of an anti-inflammatory effect. It is not unreasonable still to observe some clinical improvement of acne as a result of an antibiotic's anti-inflammatory effects, even with identification of *P acnes* with higher MICs. Continued use of the antibiotic, however, may exert prolonged selection pressure favoring survival of resistant strains, thereby further increasing their prevalence.

Ross and colleagues [46] demonstrated that point mutations in the ribosomal RNA of resistant strains of *P acnes* had been found across four continents and that the phenotypic pattern of resistance determined by MIC levels corresponded to the genomic pattern of mutation. The mutations were all in essential chromosomal genes, and not transferable between bacteria, suggesting that the spread of resistance is not primarily caused by bacteria, but the transfer of resistant strains of bacteria between human hosts. The authors hypothesized that perhaps an individual may harbor different strains of *P acnes* with varying degrees of antibiotic resistance.

As a result of increasing antibiotic resistance, recommendations from both sides of the Atlantic regarding optimal use of antibiotics in acne management have been developed to preserve the use of these drugs [47,48] by avoiding overuse and minimizing the development of microbial resistance. Both guidelines suggest that once improvement is noted, oral antibiotics therapy should be discontinued and maintenance therapy instituted. Adjunctive benzoyl peroxide can also help to mitigate the development of resistance. Because of the lack of established efficacy and safety data in the treatment of acne, other commonly used oral antibiotics including cephalosporins, fluoroquinolones, aminoglycosides, and sulfonamides are not recommended for routine use [49].

Maintenance therapy

Once clinical improvement with more aggressive clearance therapy is achieved, a change to "maintenance therapy" has been advocated, especially in those patients in whom acne is most likely to recur with cessation of treatment (eg, teenagers and young adults). There have been two well-controlled studies [50,51] in the literature that provide support for the efficacy of this approach. These studies demonstrated that a significant proportion of patients continued to do well several months after they had discontinued their prior oral antibiotic regimens. Although not definitive, these studies provide support for the role of topical retinoids in acne maintenance therapy. Expanding the use of topical retinoids in acne maintenance therapy may help significantly to reduce antibiotic overuse [45], and stimulate research into how such therapies should be studied in the future.

Isotretinoin, sebaceous glands, and anti-inflammatory mechanisms

Isotretinoin (13-*cis* retinoic acid) exerts a potent effect on sebaceous glands, decreasing their size and sebaceous lipid secretory activity and inhibiting progression of sebocyte differentiation [52].

Recently, investigators have reported that isotretinoin induces apoptosis and cell cycle arrest in cultured human sebocytes [53] through a retinoic acid receptor (RAR) independent pathway, whereas inhibition of sebaceous lipid synthesis was shown to occur by the traditional retinoic acid receptor– and retinoid X receptor–mediated pathways. This mechanism not only provides a plausible explanation for observed decreases in size, shape, and lipid content of sebaceous glands in acne skin undergoing isotretinoin treatment, but helps explain the variety of clinical findings (dry skin, dry eye, meibomian gland dysfunction, and remission of acne and seborrhea) observed in patients on isotretinoin therapy.

In addition to inhibiting migration of polymorphonuclear leukocytes into the skin [54], isotretinoin has also been shown to exert an anti-inflammatory effect by reducing the up-regulation of promatrix MMP-9 and MMP-13 in the sebum of acne patients and inhibited arachidonic acid–induced secretion and mRNA expression of pro–MMP-2 and pro–MMP-9 in sebocytes in vitro [26].

Anti-inflammatory mechanisms of all-*trans* retinoic acid

TLRs may play an important role in acne pathogenesis. Indeed, activation of TLR-2 seems to mediate the host response to *P acnes*, leading to the production of a range of inflammatory cytokines [23].

Investigators have recently observed that all-*trans* retinoic acid seems to exert its anti-inflammatory effect on monocytes through a pathway involving down-regulation of TLR-2 expression and through a TLR-independent pathway [55]. It has also been observed that adapalene, a synthetic retinoid, produced decreased expression of TLR-2 and IL-10 in explants of normal and acne-involved skin and increased CD1d expression in explants from acne patients, suggesting that adapalene can modulate the epidermal immune system by increasing CD1d expression and decreasing keratinocyte IL-10 expression [56]. These immune modulations may act together to increase the interactions between dendritic cells and T lymphocytes, thereby potentially strengthening antimicrobial activity against *P acnes*. Greater elucidation of the inflammatory mechanisms of acne may aid in the design of future rational therapies not only for acne.

QUALITY OF LIFE AND HEALTH STATE UTILITIES

Health-related quality of life (QOL) represents patients' perceptions and reactions to their health [57]. Measuring acne patients' impairment in QOL, it has been argued, may aid in their management by evaluating the psychologic impact of their acne, which often may not correlate with the clinical severity of their acne; aiding in the detection of depression or need for psychologic care; and improving therapeutic outcomes [58].

Much of the work on measuring QOL in acne has been through the use of health status instruments, both global and disease-specific. Examples of global scales that have been used to evaluate acne include Skindex [59] and Dermatology Quality of Life Index [60], whereas examples of acne-specific scales include the Acne-Specific Quality of Life questionnaire [61,62] and the Acne Quality of Life scale [63]. More recently in dermatology, however, the use of patient preferences and health state utilities has received increasing attention as an important measure of QOL.

Health state utilities are quantitative measures of patient preferences for health outcomes, usually ranging from 0 (representing a health state equivalent to death) to 1 (representing perfect health). Two individuals with the same disease condition may elicit very different utility scores depending on their degree of perceived impairment (eg, a patient who is indifferent to the presence of their disease may have a utility score close to 1, whereas a patient who perceives their disease as a profoundly disabling burden may have a much lower utility score). Like health status QOL instruments, utilities can be used in clinical trials as outcome measures of treatment effect [64] and in aiding clinical decision-making "at the bedside" [65]. In addition, utilities enjoy certain advantages over disease-specific QOL instruments, including that they allow for comparison across disease states and populations (eg, utility scores for acne can be compared with those for epilepsy or asthma), and they can be used to calculate quality-adjusted life-years, which are metrics that can be used in cost-effectiveness analyses.

Several methods can be used to measure utilities, but the most common technique used in dermatology is time trade-off (TTO) [66]. In the TTO method, patients are asked how much of their remaining life expectancy they would be willing to trade for perfect health. The TTO utility is then calculated from the ratio of the shortened lifespan resulting from the trade to the original life expectancy.

Only three studies have examined acne-related health state utilities, each with important methodologic differences. Chen and colleagues [66] published a catalog of dermatology TTO utilities derived from 267 adult outpatient subjects across three hospitals including 30 patients in the "acneiform" diagnostic category. The mean TTO utility in these patients was 0.940 (median = 0.990). An earlier study using a different utility measurement methodology elicited utility scores for a multitude of medical conditions [67] and included 70 acne patients whose acne did not require treatment with medication. They were found to have a mean acne utility of 0.94. A recent, much larger, community-based study of 266 adolescent public high school students with facial acne in San Francisco conducted by Chen and colleagues [68] found a similar, although slightly higher, mean acne TTO utility score of 0.961 (median = 0.985). In addition to assessing current acne health state, these investigators also evaluated patient preferences for multiple hypothetical treatment outcomes, such as 100% clearance of acne, 50% clearance, and 100% clearance but with residual permanent scarring. Their elicited utility scores correlated well with subjects' self-rated severity scores, but not with the investigator's static global assessment.

TTO utilities for acne in the 0.94 to 0.96 range might seem surprisingly high to some readers. Utility scores depend on the characteristics of the sample and because utilities can be compared across disease states, mean utilities of other conditions in this range can provide scale: adults with epilepsy, 0.92 [69]; adolescents with myopia, 0.94 [70]; adults with skin neoplasm of uncertain behavior, 0.97 [66]. Continued research into acne health state utilities should improve understanding of the impact this condition has on the self-perception and psychologic functioning of acne patients and help to identify what features of acne predict greater disability, at the same time providing a foundation for future research into the cost-effectiveness of acne therapies.

SUMMARY

Understanding of acne vulgaris has taken major steps forward over the past few years. The renewed interest in the effect of dietary interventions on acne, the elucidation of the involvement of TLR and MMPs in acne pathogenesis, and a more detailed functional understanding of various treatment modalities at the molecular level are all promising indications that advances in therapeutics are sure to follow. Health utilities will serve not only as powerful outcome measures of treatment effects but also as clinical decision-making aids in everyday practice. It is hoped that future advances will further uncover additional molecular and cellular details of pathophysiology, leading to rational targeted design of medications, and advance clinical management through improved understanding of the psychosocial impact of acne on patients.

References

[1] Fulton JE Jr, Plewig G, Kligman AM. Effect of chocolate on acne vulgaris. JAMA 1969;210(11):2071–4.

[2] Anderson PC. Foods as the cause of acne. Am Fam Physician 1971;3(3):102–3.

[3] Cordain L, Lindeberg S, Hurtado M, et al. Acne vulgaris: a disease of western civilization. Arch Dermatol 2002;138(12):1584–90.

[4] Adebamowo CA, Spiegelman D, Berkey CS, et al. Milk consumption and acne in adolescent girls. Dermatol Online J 2006;12(4):1. Available at: http://dermatology.cdlib.org/124/original/acne/danby.html. Accessed September 22, 2008.

[5] Smith RN, Mann NJ, Braue A, et al. The effect of a high-protein, low glycemic-load diet versus a conventional, high glycemic-load diet on biochemical parameters associated with acne vulgaris: a randomized, investigator-masked, controlled trial. J Am Acad Dermatol 2007;57(2):247–56.

[6] Frost G, Keogh B, Smith D, et al. The effect of low-glycemic carbohydrate on insulin and glucose response in vivo and in vitro in patients with coronary heart disease. Metabolism 1996;45(6):669–72.

[7] Aizawa H, Niimura M. Mild insulin resistance during oral glucose tolerance test (OGTT) in women with acne. J Dermatol 1996;23(8):526–9.

[8] Strauss JS, Kligman AM, Pochi PE. The effect of androgens and estrogens on human sebaceous glands. J Invest Dermatol 1962;39:139–55.

[9] Deplewski D, Rosenfield RL. Growth hormone and insulin-like growth factors have different effects on sebaceous cell growth and differentiation. Endocrinology 1999;140(9):4089–94.

[10] Cappel M, Mauger D, Thiboutot D. Correlation between serum levels of insulin-like growth factor 1, dehydroepiandrosterone sulfate, and dihydrotestosterone and acne lesion counts in adult women. Arch Dermatol 2005;141(3):333–8.

[11] Kiddy DS, Hamilton-Fairley D, Seppala M, et al. Diet-induced changes in sex hormone binding globulin and free testosterone in women with normal or polycystic ovaries: correlation with serum insulin and insulin-like growth factor-I. Clin Endocrinol (Oxf) 1989;31(6): 757–63.

[12] Shaw JC. Acne: effect of hormones on pathogenesis and management. Am J Clin Dermatol 2002;3(8):571–8.

[13] Thiboutot D. Acne: hormonal concepts and therapy. Clin Dermatol 2004;22(5):419–28.

[14] Zouboulis CC, Degitz K. Androgen action on human skin: from basic research to clinical significance. Exp Dermatol 2004;13(Suppl 4):5–10.

[15] Fritsch M, Orfanos CE, Zouboulis CC. Sebocytes are the key regulators of androgen homeo-stasis in human skin. J Invest Dermatol 2001;116(5):793–800.

[16] Guy R, Ridden C, Kealey T. The improved organ maintenance of the human sebaceous gland: modeling in vitro the effects of epidermal growth factor, androgens, estrogens, 13-cis retinoic acid, and phenol red. J Invest Dermatol 1996;106(3):454–60.

[17] Thiboutot DM, Knaggs H, Gilliland K, et al. Activity of type 15 alpha-reductase is greater in the follicular infrainfundibulum compared with the epidermis. Br J Dermatol 1997;136(2): 166–71.

[18] Zouboulis CC, Seltmann H, Hiroi N, et al. Corticotropin-releasing hormone: an autocrine hormone that promotes lipogenesis in human sebocytes. Proc Natl Acad Sci USA 2002;99(10):7148–53.

[19] Thornton MJ. The biological actions of estrogens on skin. Exp Dermatol 2002;11(6): 487–502.

[20] Gustafsson JA. An update on estrogen receptors. Semin Perinatol 2000;24(1):66–9.

[21] Plewig G, Kligman AM. Acne and rosacea. 3rd edition. Berlin: Springer; 2003.

[22] Mempel M, Kalali BN, Ollert M, et al. Toll-like receptors in dermatology. Dermatol Clin 2007;25(4):531–40, viii.

[23] Kim J. Review of the innate immune response in acne vulgaris: activation of Toll-like recep-tor 2 in acne triggers inflammatory cytokine responses. Dermatology 2005;211(3): 193–8.

[24] Bialecka A, Mak M, Biedron R, et al. Different pro-inflammatory and immunogenic poten-tials of Propionibacterium acnes and Staphylococcus epidermidis: implications for chronic inflammatory acne. Arch Immunol Ther Exp (Warsz) 2005;53(1):79–85.

[25] Wong DJ, Chang HY. Learning more from microarrays: insights from modules and networks. J Invest Dermatol 2005;125(2):175–82.

[26] Papakonstantinou E, Aletras AJ, Glass E, et al. Matrix metalloproteinases of epithelial origin in facial sebum of patients with acne and their regulation by isotretinoin. J Invest Dermatol 2005;125(4):673–84.

[27] Trivedi NR, Gilliland KL, Zhao W, et al. Gene array expression profiling in acne lesions reveals marked upregulation of genes involved in inflammation and matrix remodeling. J Invest Dermatol 2006;126(5):1071–9.

[28] Chakraborti S, Mandal M, Das S, et al. Regulation of matrix metalloproteinases: an over-view. Mol Cell Biochem 2003;253(1–2):269–85.

[29] Lee AT, Zane LT. Dermatologic manifestations of polycystic ovary syndrome. Am J Clin Der-matol 2007;8(4):201–19.

[30] Norman RJ, Dewailly D, Legro RS, et al. Polycystic ovary syndrome. Lancet 2007;370(9588):685–97.

[31] Azziz R, Sanchez LA, Knochenhauer ES, et al. Androgen excess in women: experience with over 1000 consecutive patients. J Clin Endocrinol Metab 2004;89(2):453–62.

[32] Pugeat M, Ducluzeau PH, Mallion-Donadieu M. Association of insulin resistance with hyper-androgenia in women. Horm Res 2000;54(5-6):322–6.

[33] Deplewski D, Rosenfield RL. Role of hormones in pilosebaceous unit development. Endocr Rev 2000;21(4):363–92.

[34] Tallon B, Corkill M. Peculiarities of PAPA syndrome. Rheumatology (Oxford) 2006;45(9): 1140–3.

[35] Galeazzi M, Gasbarrini G, Ghirardello A, et al. Autoinflammatory syndromes. Clin Exp Rheumatol 2006;24(1 Suppl 40):S79–85.

[36] Wise CA, Gillum JD, Seidman CE, et al. Mutations in CD2BP1 disrupt binding to PTP PEST and are responsible for PAPA syndrome, an autoinflammatory disorder. Hum Mol Genet 2002;11(8):961–9.

[37] Inohara N, Nunez G. NODs: intracellular proteins involved in inflammation and apoptosis. Nat Rev Immunol 2003;3(5):371–82.

[38] Dierselhuis MP, Frenkel J, Wulffraat NM, et al. Anakinra for flares of pyogenic arthritis in PAPA syndrome. Rheumatology (Oxford) 2005;44(3):406–8.

[39] Stichweh DS, Punaro M, Pascual V. Dramatic improvement of pyoderma gangrenosum with infliximab in a patient with PAPA syndrome. Pediatr Dermatol 2005;22(3):262–5.

[40] Beretta-Piccoli BC, Sauvain MJ, Gal I, et al. Synovitis, acne, pustulosis, hyperostosis, osteitis (SAPHO) syndrome in childhood: a report of ten cases and review of the literature. Eur J Pediatr 2000;159(8):594–601.

[41] Hayem G, Bouchaud-Chabot A, Benali K, et al. SAPHO syndrome: a long-term follow-up study of 120 cases. Semin Arthritis Rheum 1999;29(3):159–71.

[42] Kotilainen P, Merilahti-Palo R, Lehtonen OP, et al. *Propionibacterium acnes* isolated from sternal osteitis in a patient with SAPHO syndrome. J Rheumatol 1996;23(7):1302–4.

[43] Eady EA, Cove JH, Holland KT, et al. Erythromycin resistant propionibacteria in antibiotic treated acne patients: association with therapeutic failure. Br J Dermatol 1989;121(1): 51–7.

[44] Ozolins M, Eady EA, Avery AJ, et al. Comparison of five antimicrobial regimens for treatment of mild to moderate inflammatory facial acne vulgaris in the community: randomised controlled trial. Lancet 2004;364(9452):2188–95.

[45] Zane LT. Acne maintenance therapy: expanding the role of topical retinoids? Arch Dermatol 2006;142(5):638–40.

[46] Ross JI, Snelling AM, Eady EA, et al. Phenotypic and genotypic characterization of antibiotic-resistant *Propionibacterium acnes* isolated from acne patients attending dermatology clinics in Europe, the U.S.A., Japan and Australia. Br J Dermatol 2001;144(2):339–46.

[47] Dreno B, Bettoli V, Ochsendorf F, et al. European recommendations on the use of oral antibiotics for acne. Eur J Dermatol 2004;14(6):391–9.

[48] Leyden JJ, Del Rosso JQ, Webster GF. Clinical considerations in the treatment of acne vulgaris and other inflammatory skin disorders: focus on antibiotic resistance. Cutis 2007; 79(6 Suppl):9–25.

[49] Gollnick H, Cunliffe W, Berson D, et al. Management of acne: a report from a global alliance to improve outcomes in acne. J Am Acad Dermatol 2003;49(1 Suppl):S1–S37.

[50] Thiboutot DM, Shalita AR, Yamauchi PS, et al. Adapalene gel, 0.1%, as maintenance therapy for acne vulgaris: a randomized, controlled, investigator-blind follow-up of a recent combination study. Arch Dermatol 2006;142(5):597–602.

[51] Leyden J, Thiboutot DM, Shalita AR, et al. Comparison of tazarotene and minocycline maintenance therapies in acne vulgaris: a multicenter, double-blind, randomized, parallel-group study. Arch Dermatol 2006;142(5):605–12.

[52] Harper JC, Thiboutot DM. Pathogenesis of acne: recent research advances. Adv Dermatol 2003;19:1–10.

[53] Nelson AM, Gilliland KL, Cong Z, et al. 13-cis Retinoic acid induces apoptosis and cell cycle arrest in human SEB-1 sebocytes. J Invest Dermatol 2006;126(10):2178–89.

[54] Wozel G, Chang A, Zultak M, et al. The effect of topical retinoids on the leukotriene-B4-induced migration of polymorphonuclear leukocytes into human skin. Arch Dermatol Res 1991;283(3):158–61.

[55] Liu PT, Krutzik SR, Kim J, et al. Cutting edge: all-trans retinoic acid down-regulates TLR2 expression and function. J Immunol 2005;174(5):2467–70.

[56] Tenaud I, Khammari A, Dreno B. In vitro modulation of TLR-2, CD1d and IL-10 by adapalene on normal human skin and acne inflammatory lesions. Exp Dermatol 2007;16(6):500–6.

[57] Gill TM, Feinstein AR. A critical appraisal of the quality of quality-of-life measurements. JAMA 1994;272(8):619–26.

[58] Dreno B. Assessing quality of life in patients with acne vulgaris: implications for treatment. Am J Clin Dermatol 2006;7(2):99–106.

[59] Chren MM, Lasek RJ, Quinn LM, et al. Skindex, a quality-of-life measure for patients with skin disease: reliability, validity, and responsiveness. J Invest Dermatol 1996;107(5):707–13.

[60] Finlay AY, Khan GK. Dermatology life quality index (DLQI): a simple practical measure for routine clinical use. Clin Exp Dermatol 1994;19(3):210–6.

[61] Girman CJ, Hartmaier S, Thiboutot D, et al. Evaluating health-related quality of life in patients with facial acne: development of a self-administered questionnaire for clinical trials. Qual Life Res 1996;5(5):481–90.

[62] Martin AR, Lookingbill DP, Botek A, et al. Health-related quality of life among patients with facial acne: assessment of a new acne-specific questionnaire. Clin Exp Dermatol 2001;26(5):380–5.

[63] Gupta MA, Johnson AM, Gupta AK. The development of an acne quality of life scale: reliability, validity, and relation to subjective acne severity in mild to moderate acne vulgaris. Acta Derm Venereol 1998;78(6):451–6.

[64] Nease RF Jr, Kneeland T, O'Connor GT, et al. Variation in patient utilities for outcomes of the management of chronic stable angina: implications for clinical practice guidelines. Ischemic heart disease patient outcomes research team. JAMA 1995;273(15):1185–90.

[65] Goldstein M, Tsevat J. Applying utility assessment at the bedside. In: Chapman GB, Sonnenberg FA, editors. Decision making in health care: theory, psychology, and applications. Cambridge (MA):: Cambridge University Press; 2000. p. 313–33.

[66] Chen SC, Bayoumi AM, Soon SL, et al. A catalog of dermatology utilities: a measure of the burden of skin diseases. J Investig Dermatol Symp Proc 2004;9(2):160–8.

[67] Mittmann N, Trakas K, Risebrough N, et al. Utility scores for chronic conditions in a community-dwelling population. Pharmacoeconomics 1999;15(4):369–76.

[68] Chen CL, Kuppermann M, Caughey AB, et al. A community-based study of acne-related health preferences in adolescents. Arch Dermatol 2008;144(8):988–94.

[69] Stavem K. Quality of life in epilepsy: comparison of four preference measures. Epilepsy Res 1998;29(3):201–9.

[70] Saw SM, Gazzard G, Au Eong KG, et al. Utility values and myopia in teenage school students. Br J Ophthalmol 2003;87(3):341–5.

Current Concepts: Dermatopathology of Pigmentary Alteration Disorders in the Hispanic Population

Carlos Ricotti, MD[a], Sarah A. Stechschulte, BA[b],
Clay J. Cockerell, MD[a],*

[a]University of Texas Southwestern School of Medicine, 2330 Butler Street, Suite 115,
Dallas, TX, USA
[b]University of Miami L. Miller School of Medicine, Miami, FL, USA

EDITORIAL COMMENT

For many years, textbooks of dermatology and dermatopathology were written from the standpoint of skin diseases observed in whites. Over time, it has become apparent that description of skin disease in non-white ethnic groups is equally as important. Although a number of articles and even texts have discussed skin conditions in African Americans, relatively little has been written about the clinical features of skin disorders in Hispanics, and even less has been published about the histopathology of skin diseases in this ethnic group. In this article, Dr. Carlos Ricotti presents a comprehensive overview of this subject. It is important that dermatologists and dermatopathologists understand the differences that they may encounter when evaluating these patients and the microscopic features of their skin diseases.

The Hispanic population is the fastest growing minority group in the United States and currently is 15% of the United States population [1]. The terms "Hispanic" and "Latino" tend to be used interchangeably in the United States, mainly because of an inconsistency in syntax between the English and Spanish languages. The US Census Bureau defines "Hispanic" or "Latino" as a person of Mexican, Puerto Rican, Cuban, South or Central American, or other Spanish-European culture or origin, regardless of race. As a result of its cultural, physiologic, and geographic diversity, the Hispanic population encompasses all Fitzpatrick skin phototypes. Although a broad spectrum of dermatologic diseases can be found in this patient population, several disorders are overrepresented. These disorders include but are not limited to atopic dermatitis, pigment alteration disorders, cutaneous manifestations of diabetes, and late-stage melanomas. Pigment alterations and dyschromia of the

*Corresponding author. E-mail address: ccockerell@dermpathdiagnostics.com (C.J. Cockerell).

0882-0880/08/$ – see front matter
doi:10.1016/j.yadr.2008.09.012

skin are common complaints of patients who have darker skin types. Both hyperpigmentation and hypopigmentation disorders are prevalent in the Hispanic population, may be quite noticeable, and can have negative psychosocial effects [2]. To improve medical care in this growing ethnic population, it is essential for dermatologists and dermatopathologists to become familiar with the common skin disorders encountered in Hispanic patients. This article discusses pigmentary disorders in the Hispanic population and reviews the current concepts in dermatopathology of these entities.

MELASMA

Melasma, also known as "chloasma," is one of the most prevalent pigmentation alterations of the skin and can affect a patient's quality of life significantly [3]. It is a benign, acquired hypermelanosis seen in women who have Fitzpatrick skin types II through V, characterized as hyperpigmented patches characteristically involving the malar and brow areas of the face (Fig. 1A). Although the pathogenesis is still under debate, many hypothesize that after exposure to UV irradiation, hyperfunctional melanocytes within involved skin produce increased amounts of melanin compared with uninvolved skin [4]. Interestingly, increased vascularity has been reported in melasma, and vascular endothelial growth factor is hypothesized to be a major angiogenic factor for altered vessels because it has been found to be significantly increased in this disorder [5]. The significance of this finding in regards to the pathogenesis of melasma remains to be elucidated. Sun exposure, pregnancy, estrogen, use of oral contraceptives, autoimmune thyroid disease, and certain medications such as phenytoin and phototoxic drugs are known to aggravate this condition [6]. The diagnosis of melasma can be made on clinical grounds alone, although

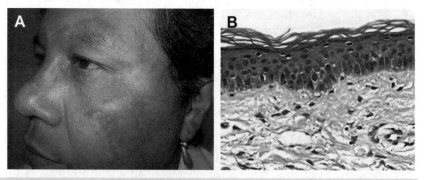

Fig. 1. (A) A woman with characteristic melasma: brown hyperpigmented patches over malar and brow areas. (B) Routine histopathology of a biopsy obtained from melasma (magnification 20×). Findings are not pathognomonic and need strict clinicopathologic correlation to make a definitive diagnosis. There is increased basal keratinocyte melanin as well as scant pigment incontinence in the papillary dermis.

the clinician may biopsy lesions that are resistant to therapy, that are suspected of being other pigmented melanocytic lesions or dermal pigmentary disorders (eg, Hori's nevus), and in cases of concomitant exogenous ochronosis. Histopathologic evaluation demonstrates increased epidermal melanin, mostly of the basal epidermal layer (Fig. 1B). Rarely, scant pigment incontinence may be observed. Melasma may worsen with the current available laser therapy, whereas other pigmentary disorders, such as nevus of Ota, may respond well to such therapy [7]. Melasma is an excellent example of a disorder in which biopsy results may assist in further therapeutic management of pigment alterations.

EXOGENOUS OCHRONOSIS

Exogenous ochronosis is an acquired hyperpigmentation disorder of the skin that is a complication of hydroquinone, phenolic compounds, antimalarial agents, benzene substances, mercury, and L-dopa [8–10]. The most frequently implicated drug is topical hydroquinone, which is used commonly alone or in combination with topical retinoids for the treatment of hyperpigmentation disorders such as postinflammatory pigmentation alteration and melasma. The most widely accepted theory for this hyperpigmentation involves the inhibition of the enzyme homogentisic oxidase by hydroquinone, leading to the accumulation of homogentisic acid [11]. The accumulated homogentisic acid then polymerizes to form ochre-colored pigment in the papillary dermis. Unlike the endogenous form, exogenous ochronosis affects the skin locally but lacks systemic manifestations such as arthralgias. The characteristic clinical findings are dark-brown hyperpigmented patches and papules located in the areas of hydroquinone application (Fig. 2A). Early diagnosis and discontinuation of topical hydroquinone cream is imperative to prevent further hyperpigmentation. The reference standard for diagnosis is skin biopsy. On histopathologic evaluation, early lesions may show only basophilic degeneration of the superficial dermal collagen (Fig. 2B). The pathognomonic islands of irregularly shaped "ochre" bodies (also referred to as "banana" bodies) observed histopathologically will be present in the superficial dermis and correspond to the "caviar" bodies (dark-brown papules) observed clinically on the skin (Fig. 2C and D). Although the clinical differential diagnosis is vast and includes melasma, the histopathologic findings are unique for exogenous ochronosis [12].

POSTINFLAMMATORY PIGMENT ALTERATION

Postinflammatory hyperpigmentation signifies an excess of melanin pigment as a consequence of cutaneous insult, such as injury or inflammation. Inflammation may result from either endogenous or exogenous insults, such as atopic dermatitis, acne, photo damage, and contact dermatitis. The hyperpigmentation becomes evident after any edema and/or erythema resolve (Fig. 3). Although postinflammatory pigment alteration may occur at any age and in either gender, darkly pigmented individuals are remarkably at risk.

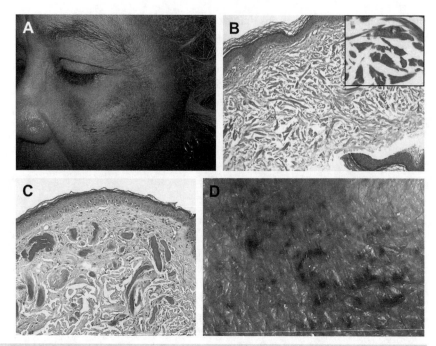

Fig. 2. (*A*) An Hispanic woman with a 2-year history of worsening pigmentation over areas on her face where she applied hydroquinone 4% cream for the treatment of melasma. A biopsy confirmed the diagnosis of exogenous ochronosis. This patient denied having any systemic manifestations of endogenous ochronosis such as arthralgias or chest pain. (*B*) Routine histopathology of early exogenous ochronosis (magnification 10×). Early on there is primarily basophilic degeneration of the collagen fibers. (*Inset*) In this specimen there were very small "ochre" bodies evident only at high-power magnification. (*C*) Pathognomonic histopathologic findings of exogenous ochronosis (magnification 10×). In the superficial dermis there are multiple "ochre" bodies with surrounding degenerated collagen fibers. (*D*) High magnification of "caviar" bodies that are noted on clinical examination of exogenous ochronosis.

Additionally, the alteration occurs earlier, more often, is of larger extent, and persists for a longer time than in individuals who have lighter skin [13].

Two forms of postinflammatory hyperpigmentation are described: epidermal and dermal. In the epidermal form, inflammatory mediators result in increased melanin synthesis and/or transfer to keratinocytes [14]. The mechanism of postinflammatory hyperpigmentation as a result of inflammation has not been elucidated completely. Several groups have shown that inflammatory mediators such as interleukin-1, endothelin-1, and/or stem cell factor directly stimulate melanocytes, resulting in an increased production of melanin with subsequent increased epidermal pigmentation. Furthermore, epidermal cell damage can lead to the release of α-melanocyte–stimulating hormone [15,16].

In the dermal form, an impaired basement membrane (as a result of inflammation) results in the descent of melanin into the dermis, where it is

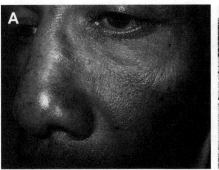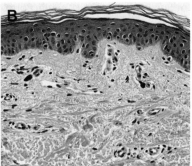

Fig. 3. (A) A dark-skinned Cuban man who had a 1-month history of brown patches with scant scale over the nasal ala and tip of nose. This patient suffered from chronic allergic rhinitis, resulting in rubbing of his nose with Kleenex. This repetitive physical assault to the skin resulted in recurring inflammation and subsequent hyperpigmentation. (B) Routine histologic examination of postinflammatory pigment alteration shows pigment incontinence (with the presence of melanophages) and increased basal keratinocytes pigmentation (magnification 20×). Sometimes these findings are subtle, but the clinical changes may be dramatic in more fair-skinned Hispanics.

phagocytosed by macrophages. An additional theory suggests epidermal migration of macrophages with concomitant melanosome phagocytosis following epidermal injury, and subsequent restoration to the dermis [17].

The epidermal form commonly resolves with time given effective treatment of the primary disorder; however, the dermal form can be permanent. Darkly pigmented individuals can require months or years for affected areas to lighten. Of note, continued inflammatory insult or exposure to UV irradiation can worsen postinflammatory hyperpigmentation.

Histologic examination of hyperpigmented areas in the epidermal form shows keratinocytes with an increased number of pigment granules. The dermal form demonstrates melanin accumulation within melanophages. These two types of hyperpigmentation are not independent of each other and usually co-exist. Concomitant histopathologic changes as a result of the primary insult, such as atopic dermatitis, may be present also. Unlike postinflammatory pigment alterations, melasma does not present with a prior inflammatory phase, and in melasma there is likely a genetic link, although the link has yet to be determined.

ERYTHEMA DYSCHROMICUM PERSTANS

Erythema dyschromicum perstans is a gradually progressive macular hyperpigmentation disorder primarily affecting Latin Americans or persons who have skin phototypes III and IV. It typically presents in the second to third decade of life, without a gender predilection. Although the etiology remains unknown, it is believed to correspond predominately with a contacted, inhaled, or ingested material causing a cell-mediated immune reaction that results in confined regions of pigmentary incontinence [18]. Some consider this disorder a variant of lichen planus. A trigger or primary etiology is never discovered in most patients, although a potential risk factor in Mexican patients is the HLA-DR4 allele [19].

The clinical differential diagnosis includes mycosis fungoides, fixed drug eruption, postinflammatory hyperpigmentation, lichen planus, and erythema multiforme. The oval shape and the ashy-gray color, characteristic of erythema dyschromicum perstans lesions, help differentiate this condition from other disorders of pigmentation in Hispanic patients (Fig. 4A). Active lesions have an elevated, slightly erythematous, raised rim.

Histologic findings differ depending on the activity of the lesion. In the active phase, interface dermatitis with melanin incontinence is the primary feature (Fig. 4B). The lymphocytic perivascular and papillary dermal infiltrate is mild in comparison with other lichenoid dermatoses such as classic lichen planus, subacute cutaneous lupus erythematosus, or dermatomyositis. There may be minimal liquefaction degeneration at the basal layer without basement membrane zone thickening. Consistent findings are dermal hemosiderin and increased dermal melanophages [20].

Inactive lesions demonstrate variable epidermal change, such as atrophy and effacement of rete ridges, have increased dermal melanophages, and illustrate a significant degree of pigment incontinence while containing nominal dermal mononuclear cell infiltrate or basal layer hydropic changes. Direct immunofluorescence microscopy has revealed nonspecific IgM, IgG, C4, and fibrinogen granular staining of colloid bodies on the active border, and immunohistochemistry results demonstrate the expression of lymphocyte activation and cell adhesion molecules [21].

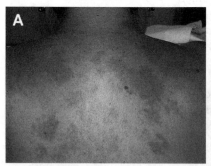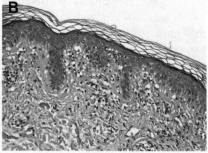

Fig. 4. (A) An Hispanic woman who has multiple gray-blue, irregular, sharply demarcated patches on her upper back. These lesions also were present on her extremities and her trunk. Based on the clinical "ashy-gray" color of the skin lesions, this disorder originally was named "dermatitis cenizientas." The English translation is "ashy dermatitis." (B) An interface dermatitis with vacuolar changes of the basal keratinocytes. Pigment incontinence is observed. Occasionally there will be scant dyskeratotic cells. The superficial lymphocytic infiltrate density varies during different stages of disorder activity.

ACANTHOSIS NIGRICANS

It has been suggested that the prevalence and health burden of diabetes is greater in older Hispanics than in older white non-Hispanics and African Americans [22]. Furthermore, the global epidemic of obesity and diabetes also has affected the younger Hispanic population and has led to an increase in the dermatologic manifestations of diabetes in Hispanic children. One common cutaneous manifestation that has predominated in the Hispanic population is acanthosis nigricans.

Acanthosis nigricans is more common in the obese Hispanic pediatric population than in white and African American children. It also has been associated with increased levels of insulin, thus suggesting that acanthosis nigricans is an associated risk factor for glucose homeostasis abnormalities including diabetes [23].

Clinically acanthosis nigricans presents as velvety, hyperpigmented plaques on intertriginous surfaces, most commonly in the axilla and the nape of the neck (Fig. 5). In the appropriate clinical setting, such as obesity, further endocrinologic work-up including glucose tolerance testing should be pursued. In patients who experience weight loss, rapid onset of acanthosis nigricans, and involvement of the areolas, dorsum of the hands, or the oral mucosa, further work-up for internal malignancy is warranted. Adenocarcinomas of the stomach and gastrointestinal tract are the most common neoplastic associations [24].

Histologically, papillomatosis with overlying hyperkeratosis is apparent. There is evident hyperpigmentation of the basal cell layer, although this hyperpigmentation may be subtle. Typically there are no deep dermal alterations, and the papillary dermis appears elongated, forming dermal projections into the overlying papillomatous epidermis. Seborrheic keratosis presents with confluent and reticulated papillomatosis, whereas epidermal nevi may have histologic features that overlap with those of acanthosis nigricans. Clinicopathologic correlation may be required to make a definitive diagnosis.

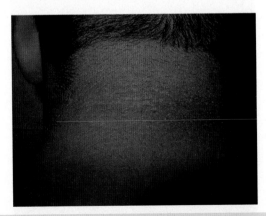

Fig. 5. Acanthosis nigricans in a 12-year-old obese Hispanic child who has glucose intolerance. There is a velvety brown, hyperpigmented plaque on the nape of the neck.

SKIN CANCER
Non-melanoma skin cancer
In general, the incidence of nonmelanoma skin cancers is lower in Hispanics than in the white non-Hispanic population [25]. The studies performed have involved Hispanic patients of all Fitzpatrick phototypes. Because a larger proportion of Hispanics than non-Hispanics have darker skin, the incidence of non-melanoma skin cancers may be underestimated in fair-skinned Hispanic patients. In darker Hispanics, basal cell carcinomas are 6.6 times more prevalent than squamous cell carcinomas [26]. Furthermore, in this patient population it has been shown that basal cell carcinomas are more commonly multiple and of the pigmented variant (Fig. 6).

Melanoma
Melanoma is the sixth most common cancer in the United States; it is predicted that 1 in 58 Americans will develop invasive melanoma [27]. Over the past 15 years, the annual rate of melanoma among Hispanics in the United States has increased to 2.9%, compared with the 3% annual increase among white non-Hispanics. Additionally, melanomas arising in minority populations have worse outcomes, are diagnosed at a later stage, and are more likely to metastasize than melanomas in white non-Hispanics. A study using California Cancer Registry data over a 15-year period found that Hispanics were twice as likely as white non-Hispanics to present with regional or distant invasive melanoma [28]. Additionally, the poorer 5-year survival rates in Hispanics compared with white non-Hispanics probably reflect diagnosis at a later stage of the disease (Fig. 7). This delay in diagnosis probably is caused by the suboptimal primary and secondary prevention in minority populations. The National Health Interview Surveys found that Hispanics are screened less frequently for

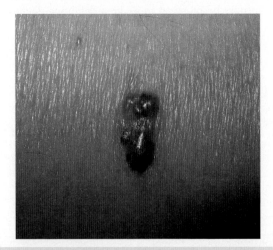

Fig. 6. Pigmented basal cell with pearly peripheral boarders and telangiectasias.

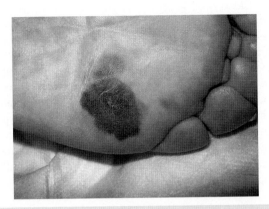

Fig. 7. Large acral melanoma in an elderly Hispanic woman.

skin cancer than white non-Hispanics [29]. Delayed diagnosis also may represent decreased awareness of skin cancer. In a study of Hispanic and white non-Hispanic high school students in Miami-Dade County in Florida, Hispanic students were less likely to wear sun-protective clothing or sunscreen with a sun protection factor greater than 15, were more likely to use tanning beds, and believed their chances of developing skin cancer were less than those of white non-Hispanics [30]. In addition to decreased public awareness, delayed diagnosis also may result from a lower index of suspicion in dark-skinned individuals by physicians and from disparities in access to medical care.

DISCUSSION

The Hispanic population is projected to reach 17% of the United States population by 2020 [31]. Unfortunately, there is a paucity of dermatologic literature geared toward Hispanic cutaneous medicine. As this population continues to grow, a thorough understanding by dermatologists and dermatopathologists of common skin disorders that afflict this subset of patients will be required to improve patient care. This succinct article discusses the most common dermatologic complaints of Hispanic patients, namely disorders of dyschromia and pigmentation alteration. It is important for the reader to understand that, like inflammatory disorders, pigmentary diseases in the Hispanic population require strict clinicopathologic correlation for definitive diagnosis. In addition, this article discusses recent data concerning skin cancer in this population.

Melasma and secondary postinflammatory pigment alteration are the most common dermatologic complaints by Hispanic patients. Although the diagnosis of these two entities is primarily clinical, dermatopathology plays a role in confirming the diagnosis and further optimizing management in patients who have recalcitrant disease. Examples include the exclusion of exogenous ochronosis in patients treated with topical hydroquinone for melasma, histopathologic evaluation of pigmented lesions, measuring disease activity in patients who have erythema dyschromicum perstans, and the evaluation of pigment in the skin for potential laser therapy.

Recently several studies have demonstrated that there are suboptimal prevention and screening efforts as well as worse skin cancer outcomes in the Hispanic population. This information has led to an attempt to increase awareness of skin cancers and skin protection in the Hispanic population.

With the increasing number of Hispanic patients, dermatologists and dermatopathologists will need to have a thorough understanding of these skin diseases to diagnose skin disorders correctly and manage them appropriately in this population.

References

[1] US Census Bureau. Hispanic population of the United States. Available at: http://www.census.gov/population/www/socdemo/hispanic/hispanic_pop_presentation.html. Accessed August 20, 2008.

[2] Pawaskar MD, Parikh P, Markowski T, et al. Melasma and its impact on health-related quality of life in Hispanic women. J Dermatolog Treat 2007;18(1):5–9.

[3] Freitag FM, Cestari TF, Leopoldo LR, et al. Effect of melasma on quality of life in a sample of women living in southern Brazil. J Eur Acad Dermatol Venereol 2008;22(6):655–62.

[4] Kang WH, Hwang JS, Lee JY, et al. Melasma: histopathological characteristics in 56 Korean patients. Br J Dermatol 2002;146(2):228–37.

[5] Kim EH, Kim YC, Lee ES, et al. The vascular characteristics of melasma. J Dermatol Sci 2007;46(2):111–6.

[6] Gupta AK, Gover MD, Nouri K, et al. The treatment of melasma: a review of clinical trials. J Am Acad Dermatol 2006;55(6):1048–65.

[7] Taylor CR, Anderson RR. Ineffective treatment of refractory melasma and postinflammatory hyperpigmentation by q-switched ruby laser. J Dermatol Surg Oncol 1994;20(9):592–7.

[8] Findlay GH, Morrison JG, Simson IW. Exogenous ochronosis and pigmented colloid milium from hydroquinone bleaching creams. Br J Dermatol 1975;93:613–22.

[9] Kaufmann D, Wegmann W. [Exogenous ochronosis after L-dopa treatment]. Pathologe 1992;13:164–6 [in German].

[10] Bruce S, Tschen JA, Chow D. Exogenous ochronosis resulting from quinine injections. J Am Acad Dermatol 1986;15(2 Pt 2):357–61.

[11] Penneys NS. Ochronosislike pigmentation from hydroquinone bleaching creams. Arch Dermatol 1985;121(10):1239–40.

[12] Phillips JI, Isaacson C, Carman H. Ochronosis in black South Africans who used skin lighteners. Am J Dermatopathol 1986;8:14–21.

[13] Cayce KA, McMichael AJ, Feldman SR. Ethnic considerations in the treatment of Hispanic and Latin-American patients with hyperpigmentation. Br J Dermatol 2004;156S:7–12.

[14] Boissy RE. Melanosome transfer to and translocation in the keratinocyte. Exp Dermatol 2003;12S:5–12.

[15] Sriwiriyanont P, Ohuchi A, Hachiya A, et al. Interaction between stem cell factor and endothelin-1: effects on melanogenesis in human skin xenografts. Lab Invest 2006;86:1115–25.

[16] Unver N, Freyschmidt-Paul P, Horster S, et al. Alterations in the epidermal–dermal melanin axis and factor XIIIa melanophages in senile lentigo and ageing skin. Br J Dermatol 2006;155:119–28.

[17] Masu S, Seiji M. Pigmentary incontinence in fixed drug eruptions. Histologic and electron microscopic findings. J Am Acad Dermatol 1983;8(4):525–32.

[18] Schwartz RA. Erythema dyschromicum perstans: the continuing enigma of Cinderella or ashy dermatosis. Int J Dermatol 2004;43(3):230–2.

[19] Correa MC, Memije EV, Vargas-Alarcón G, et al. HLA-DR association with the genetic susceptibility to develop ashy dermatosis in Mexican Mestizo patients. J Am Acad Dermatol 2007;56(4):617–20.

[20] Bolognia JL, Jorizzo JL, Rapini RP. In: Dermatology. Philadelphia: Elsevier Science; 2003. p. 195.

[21] Vasquez-Ochoa LA, Isaza-Guzmán DM, Orozco-Mora B, et al. Immunopathologic study of erythema dyschromicum perstans (ashy dermatosis). Int J Dermatol 2006;45(8):937–41.

[22] Black SA, Ray LA, Markides KS. The prevalence and health burden of self-reported diabetes in older Mexican Americans: findings from the Hispanic established populations for epidemiologic studies of the elderly. Am J Public Health 1999;89(4):546–52.

[23] Brickman WJ, Binns HJ, Jovanovic BD, et al. Acanthosis nigricans: a common finding in overweight youth. Pediatr Dermatol 2007;24(6):601–6.

[24] Muñoz Díaz F, García Carrasco C, Monge Romero MI, et al. Acanthosis nigricans as the initial paraneoplastic manifestation of gastric adenocarcinomas. Gastroenterol Hepatol 2007;30(1):14–8.

[25] Harris RB, Griffith K, Moon TE. Trends in the incidence of nonmelanoma skin cancers in southeastern Arizona, 1985–1996. J Am Acad Dermatol 2001;45(4):528–36.

[26] Halder RM, Ara CJ. Skin cancer and photoaging in ethnic skin. Dermatol Clin 2003;21(4): 725–32, x.

[27] Rouhani P, Hu S, Kirsner RS. Melanoma in Hispanic and black Americans. Cancer Control 2008;15(3):248–53.

[28] Cress RD, Holly EA. Incidence of cutaneous melanoma among non-Hispanic whites, Hispanics, Asians, and blacks: an analysis of California Cancer Registry data, 1988–93. Cancer Causes Control 1997;8(2):246–52.

[29] Saraiya M, et al. Skin cancer screening among U.S. adults from 1992, 1998, and 2000 National Health Interview Surveys. Prev Med 2003;39(2):308–14.

[30] Ma F, Collado-Mesa F, Hu S, et al. Skin cancer awareness and sun protection behaviors in white Hispanic and white non-Hispanic high school students in Miami, Florida. Arch Dermatol 2007;143(8):983–8.

[31] Ramirez RR, de la Cruz GP. The Hispanic population the United States: March 2002. Population characteristics. Current population reports. Washington (DC): US Department of Commerce, Economics and Statstics Administration. US Census Bureau; 2003.

Cutaneous Mosaicism: a Molecular and Clinical Review

Dawn H. Siegel, MD

Department of Dermatology and Pediatrics, Oregon Health & Science University,
3303 SW Bond Avenue, CH16D, Portland, OR 97239, USA

EDITORIAL COMMENT

For the past century, dermatologists have recognized the distinctive patterns of many sporadic and inherited skin conditions. These unusual, segmental, and Blaschkoid distributions have long been attributed to the concept of genetic mosaicism; however, the mechanisms by which these phenomena occur have been more recently elucidated. In this article, author Dawn Siegel, a pediatric dermatologist with experience and expertise in genodermatoses, provides an excellent cutting-edge review on the clinical presentations of cutaneous mosaicism and enlightens the reader on recent advances in our understanding of the molecular mechanisms that lead to these fascinating dermatologic disorders. Dr. Siegel reviews the cutaneous features that are suggestive of mosaicism, as well as the embryologic cell migration patterns that may result in these unique distributions of skin changes. She also discusses practical considerations for skin biopsy when investigating mosaic skin diseases. Dr. Siegel explains the concepts of gonadal, gonosomal, and segmental mosaicism, as well as functional and revertent mosaicism, and provides clinical examples of these molecular mechanisms. Some of the clinical entities reviewed in this article include: segmental neurofibromatosis, segmental Darier's disease, McCune Albright syndrome, focal dermal hypoplasia, X-linked chondrodysplasia punctata, incontinentia pigmenti, hypohidrotic ectodermal dyplasia, Proteus syndrome, and the more common segmental pigmentation disorder, which is not associated with other congenital anomalies or systemic manifestations. Dr. Siegel ends with useful clinical photographs that depict these concepts and valuable tables that define the mechanisms and summarize the clinical examples discussed in this article. Read ahead for an educational experience!

Amy Jo Nopper, MD

S ince Blaschko first reported the patterns of epidermal nevi in 1901, dermatologists have recognized that many inherited and sporadic skin conditions appear in distinct cutaneous patterns. The concept of genetic mosaicism has been used to explain these patterns. Genetic mosaicism is

E-mail address: siegeld@ohsu.edu

0882-0880/08/$ – see front matter
doi:10.1016/j.yadr.2008.09.011

defined as two or more cell populations with distinct karyotypes or genotypes in one individual. The causative genetic changes for disorders caused by mutations in a single gene have been rapidly uncovered since the publication of the results from the Human Genome Project. However, the genetic alterations in mosaic conditions have proven much more difficult to elucidate [1]. This article reviews in detail the potential mechanisms by which mosaic skin conditions may occur.

The appearance of epidermal nevi following distinct patterns on the skin was first documented by Blaschko in 1901 [2]. At the same time, Montgomery [3] proposed the theory that the patterned lines on the skin represented the dorso-ventral outgrowth, as embryonic cells follow a path of migration from the neural crest in the developing embryo. In 1976, Jackson [4] renewed interest in the subject with the publication of a review article on the lines of Blaschko. Since that time, Happle [5–7] has published many papers discussing theories related to the clinical and molecular mechanisms of cutaneous mosaicism.

PATTERNS OF CUTANEOUS MOSAICISM

The timing of the genetic alteration affects the distribution of skin changes. The location and the extent of the involvement of the mosaic changes on the skin are a reflection of the stage of development during which the genetic alteration occurred. For mutations that occur early in embryologic development, the condition may be apparent over a broader body surface area; whereas later mutations will be apparent in smaller, more confined anatomic regions.

As Blaschko noted, the nevoid changes on the skin tend to follow distinct patterns, notably an S-figure on the sides of the torso and a V-shape on the back, which he referred to as the "fountain spray" (Fig. 1A). Happle has expanded on the classification of the patterns of cutaneous mosaicism as follows: type 1, lines of Blaschko; type 2, checkerboard; type 3, phylloid; type 4, large patches without midline separation; and type 5, lateralization (Fig. 1B). Type 1a is used to define conditions following narrow lines of Blaschko (Fig. 2). In type 1b, the nevoid changes appear along broad lines of Blaschko; this is frequently seen in segmental pigmentation disorder (also referred to as patterned dyspigmentation) and in McCune-Albright syndrome. The checkerboard pattern, type 2, describes the random appearance of a flag-shaped birthmark with a sharp midline demarcation, as seen in Becker's nevus, some congenital melanocytic nevi, and some cases of segmental neurofibromatosis. Zietz [8] has proposed that vascular malformations that present in a checkerboard pattern are the result of postzygotic mutations, and that the mutations, which occur later in embryogenesis, result in more focal birthmarks, whereas the mutations that occur early in embryogenesis lead to more widespread changes. The phylloid pattern presents with leaf-like or oblong patterns. The phylloid pattern is most common, with hypopigmented patches in trisomy 13 [9]. Type 4 is defined by large patches without midline separation; the best example of this pattern is the bathing-trunk distribution of giant congenital melanocytic nevi. Finally, the lateralization pattern, type 5, is used to describe the type of nevus seen in CHILD (congenital hemidysplasia with ichthyosiform erythroderma and limb defects) syndrome, in which one half of the body is diffusely involved with a sharp cut-off at the midline and sparing of the contra-lateral side.

CELL MIGRATION

The distribution of mosaic skin changes can best be understood by reviewing the embryologic migration patterns of the affected cell type, namely the mela-nocytes, keratinocytes, and angioblasts. Melanoblasts are neural crest-derived cells that migrate via the mesenchyme as single cells during embryogenesis. Early in embryogenesis, at approximately 10-weeks gestation, the melanocytes are located diffusely in the dermis. Later, some melanocytes undergo a pre-sumed programmed cell death, while others continue the migration to the epi-dermis and basal layer of the hair matrix in the outer root sheath of the hair follicles. After arrival in the epidermis and hair follicles, the melanocytes proliferate locally. Most of what is known about melanocyte migration has been learned using mouse models and examining coat color patterns [10]. Many different patterns have been suggested as examples of the patterns of cutaneous mosaicism of melanocytes, including segmental pigmentation disor-der (also known as patterned dyspigmentation) along the lines of Blaschko (type 1a and type 1b), segmental neurofibromatosis in a checkerboard pattern (type 2), hypopigmentation in the phylloid pattern with certain mosaic chromo-somal aberrations (type 3), and congenital melanocytic nevi overlying the mid-line (type 4).

Embryonic keratinocytes undergo a dorsoventral migration pattern, later curving in lines, which likely explains the appearance of the whorls and streaks along the lines of Blaschko (type 1), such as in incontinentia pigmenti. The lines of Blaschko can also be seen in the oral mucosa, the bone, and the eye.

Angioblasts originate in the central body axis with a lateral migration. The migration is influenced by gradients of soluble factors and cell-cell interactions guiding the angioblasts through their migration [11]. Vascular birthmarks com-monly present in a segmental or dermatomal pattern, and are therefore possi-bly caused by a postzygotic mutation, leading to abnormal migration or formation of the vasculature in a localized area [8]. However, mosaicism has not yet been proven as the etiology of most vascular or melanocytic birthmarks.

Practical considerations on skin biopsies

Skin biopsy has been demonstrated to be beneficial in establishing the presence of mosaicism; however, care must be taken to select the appropriate cell type when establishing the cell lines for study. For example, Maertens and col-leagues [12] recently studied three individuals with segmental neurofibromato-sis. One had a segmental presentation of neurofibromas only, one had a segmental presentation of pigmentary changes only, and one had greater than six café-au-lait patches on the body as well as a large café-au-lait patch

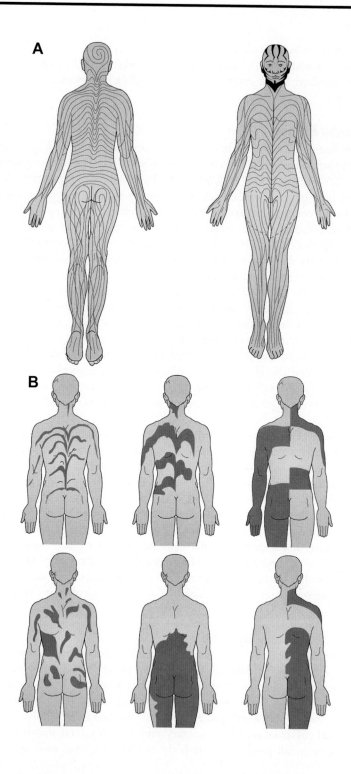

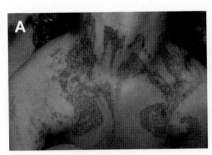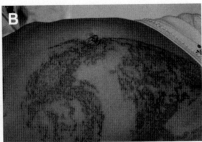

Fig. 2. Demonstration of the narrow lines of Blaschko on the neck and chest (A) and abdomen (B), showing sharp midline demarcation in a child with porokeratotic eccrine ostial and dermal duct nevus.

with underlying neurofibromas on her right hand. Several cell line cultures were established from the epidermal melanocytes and dermal fibroblasts from the café-au-lait patches and dermal fibroblasts, and Schwann cells were cultured from the neurofibromas. In the individual with segmental pigmentation defects only, mutations were found in both alleles in melanocytes, but none were identified from fibroblasts or blood. The individual with neurofibromas only had biallelic mutations in Schwann cells, but a very low positive rate in the fibroblasts. Mutations were found in both melanocytes and Schwann cells of the individual, with both café-au-lait macules and neurofibromas, but again an almost undetectable level was seen in the fibroblasts. This highlights the importance of culturing the correct cell type when performing mutational analysis on skin from segmental neurofibromatosis.

Historically, conventional cytogenetic analysis has been the most common tool for screening for chromosomal anomalies; however, this technique is time consuming, labor intensive, and requires cell culture. Array comparative genomic hybridization (CGH) is emerging as a new technique for high-resolution, genome-wide scanning in congenital anomaly syndromes [13,14]. This technique has also been referred to as chromosomal microarray analysis. Cheung and colleagues [15] reported using array CGH to detect chromosomal mosaicism from fibroblasts from patients in 12 out of 2,585 cases with birth defects and mental retardation. In the positive cases, 10 out of 12 had normal conventional blood chromosome analysis. Array CGH also has the benefit of not requiring cell culture before analysis.

Fig. 1. (A) Lines of Blaschko showing the fountain-like pattern on the back and the S-figure on the lateral trunk. (B) Patterns of mosaicism: (*top left*) type 1a, lines of Blaschko, narrow bands; (*top middle*) type 1b, lines of Blaschko, broad bands; (*top right*) type 2, checkerboard pattern; (*bottom left*) type 3, phylloid pattern; (*bottom middle*) type 4, patchy pattern without midline separation; (*bottom right*) lateralization. (*From* Itin PH, Burgdorf WHC, Happle R, et al. In Schachner LA, Hansen RC, editors. Pediatric Dermatology, 3rd edition. Figures 7.84 and 7.85. Copyright Elsevier 2003; with permission.)

MOLECULAR MECHANISMS

Gonadal mosaicism

Germ-line mosaicism, or gonadal mosaicism, occurs when there are genetically distinct cell populations in the germ-line tissues only. This has been described with transmission of an autosomal dominant condition to more than one child from unaffected parents.

Examples have included case reports of gonadal mosaic transmission of Cornelia de Lange, Pallister-Hall, and Conradi-Hünermann-Happle syndrome, as well as hereditary angioedema [16–18]. In cases of gonadal mosaicism, it is presumed that the cells containing the mutated genes are localized exclusively in the gonadal tissue. Although gonadal mosaicism is difficult to prove in females because of the challenges in accessing the gonadal tissue, gonadal mosaicism has been proven in the sperm of fathers in some of the reported cases. One example by Niu and colleagues reported two siblings born with Cornelia de Lange syndrome to unaffected parents. Cornelia de Lange syndrome is characterized by distinctive facial features, short stature, hirsutism and synophrys, long eyelashes, and subtle limb reduction defects. The disorder is caused by mutations in the Nipped-B-like (*NIPBL*) gene [19–21]. Niu and colleagues [22] reported a heterozygous missense *NIPBL* mutation in the peripheral blood sample of the affected girl, but not in the peripheral blood samples of her parents. The same mutation was identified in the sperm sample of the father, confirming gonadal mosaicism as the source of transmission of the mutation.

Gonosomal mosaicism

Gonosomal mosaicism refers to cases in which the mutations are present in both somatic tissue and in the gonadal tissue. This has been implicated in cases of segmental presentations in the parent and subsequent full-blown expression in the affected offspring. Published examples have included segmental neurofibromatosis (NF) type 1 in a parent with full expression of NF1 in the offspring. The classic example is an individual with epidermal nevi of the epidermolytic hyperkeratosis-type who has an offspring with generalized epidermolytic hyperkeratosis. Paller and colleagues [23] were able to prove that mosaic mutations in keratin 10 were present in cultured keratinocytes from the epidermal nevi in the parent, but not the normal skin or genomic DNA, and were present in the genomic DNA of the affected child.

The molecular mechanisms by which genetic mosaicism can occur include postzygotic mutations, Lyonization, chromosomal nondisjunction, revertant mosaicism, chimerism, and epigenetic mechanisms (Table 1). Key features of these mechanisms are discussed below.

Segmental mosaicism

Happle [24] has proposed two mechanisms for the segmental expression of autosomal dominant disorders. Type 1 segmental changes occur as a postzygotic mutation in a wild-type embryo; therefore, the cutaneous changes are seen only in a localized segment, while the remaining skin is unaffected.

Table 1
Mechanisms of mosaicism

Mechanism	Definition
Postzygotic (somatic) mutation	A mutation or chromosomal replication error that occurs after fertilization.
Lyonization	In females, one X-chromosome (either the maternal or the paternal X chromosome), is randomly inactivated in early embryologic development; that change is carried on in all future cell divisions
Chimerism	When an organism is composed of two or more genetically distinct cell lines with completely different genetic make-up. This may occur after bone marrow or organ transplant or maternal-fetal transfusion
Revertant mosaicism	Spontaneous correction of an inherited mutation.

Type 2 segmental mosaicism is proposed to result from loss of heterozygosity (LOH) in an otherwise heterozygous individual. Therefore, a generalized phenotype is apparent with an exaggerated expression localized to one region. There are many different theoretic explanations for how the second mutation might occur during cell division. Potential mechanisms for LOH include mitotic recombination, gene conversion, point mutation, deletion, and mitotic nondisjunction (Table 2).

Type 2 segmental mosaicism (a second-hit mutation resulting in LOH) has been proposed as the genetic etiology in an individual with typical lesions of neurofibromatosis type 1 with a superimposed "bathing-trunk" distribution café-au-lait patch, although this was not proven on a molecular level [25]. Numerous additional examples of type 2 segmental mosaicism have been reported in the literature for cases of neurofibromatosis, Hailey-Hailey disease, and Darier's disease in individuals with typical lesions and a superimposed segmental presentation [26–29].

Table 2
Mechanisms of loss of heterozygosity

Mechanism	Definition
Mitotic recombination	The formation of new combinations of alleles because of the exchange of a segment of DNA by crossing over between homologous chromosomes.
Gene conversion	One allele converts the mutated sequence of the other allele to the wild-type sequence, possibly by nonreciprocal exchange
Point mutation	A change in a single base pair
Deletion	Loss of a portion of sequence of DNA; may range from one base pair to a large portion of the chromosome.
Mitotic nondisjunction	Failure of the chromosomes to separate properly during meiosis or mitosis; the result is that one daughter cell receives both chromatids and the other receives neither chromatid

Functional mosaicism

Functional mosaicism occurs in females as a result of X-inactivation. Early in embryologic development, each cell simultaneously and selectively turns off or inactivates either the maternal or the paternal X chromosome. The inactivation is random, but once it occurs all progeny cells carry that same activated X-chromosome. This inactivation idea was originally introduced by Mary Lyon [30] in 1961, based upon her observations of striped coat color patterns in mice, and the process is now referred to as Lyonization. The mechanism for inactivation is via the X-inactivation site, located at Xq13.2 containing the *XIST* gene. There are some regions of the X-chromosome that escape this inactivation, such as the steroid sulfatase gene. Mutations in the steroid sulfatase gene result in X-linked ichthyosis. For X-linked recessive conditions, the female carriers express a variable, mild phenotype, but their male offspring will have full expression of the phenotype. X-linked dominant conditions are presumed to be lethal in males, but are fully expressed in the affected females. Females survive because many cells are present that express the unaffected X-chromosome as result of random X-inactivation. Males with XXY karyotype will survive because of the same mechanism; X-inactivation results in the presence of some cells that have an active, normal X chromosome. Males may also survive if the mutation was a postzygotic mutation resulting in somatic mosaicism, again because some cells in the body are spared and are wild type.

Revertant mosaicism

Revertant mosaicism is a mechanism that has been most often demonstrated in autosomal recessive conditions and is exemplified by the localized reversion of a severe clinical phenotype. Several examples of revertant mosaicism have been published [31–35]. On a molecular level, the reversion is based on the restoration of the wild-type amino acid sequence, which leads to a fully or partially functional protein product. One of the first descriptions in the literature of revertant mosaicism was in 1997 by Jonkman and colleagues [33], who described a patient with autosomal recessive non-Herlitz junctional epidermolysis bullosa (EB), who was a compound heterozygote for nonsense and frameshift mutations in the type XVII collagen gene, *COL17A1*. When normal, nonblistering patches of skin appeared, molecular studies revealed that normal type XVII collagen was being expressed. The mechanism of reversion hypothesized was gene conversion. In this process, it is proposed that one allele converts the mutated sequence of the other allele to the wild-type sequence, possibly by nonreciprocal exchange. Another mechanism for reversion is by mRNA rescue of a frame-shift mutation by a downstream second-site mutation. Although the original mutation is not removed, the reading frame is restored by the second mutation, leading to translation of the protein. This may either result in complete or partial correction, depending on the level of function in the restored protein. This mechanism was shown in an individual with autosomal recessive non-Herlitz junctional EB in whom studies of the keratinocytes revealed a second insertion downstream from the deletion, which restored the reading frame [32].

Recently, Pasmooij and colleagues [36] demonstrated multiple correcting second-site mutations in an individual with non-Herlitz junctional EB who showed expanding areas of normal, healthy skin. It is hypothesized that this may have been because of the expansion of clonal epidermal stem cells. It is possible that these examples of revertant mosaicism may have implications as methods for natural gene therapy for EB in the future.

Chromosomal numeric or structural abnormalities

A variety of chromosomal abnormalities can lead to mosaicism; examples include structural abnormalities, such as ring chromosomes, deletions, or duplications, and numeric abnormalities, such as in mosaic trisomy 21. Chromosomal mosaicism results from events that take place after fertilization and result in failure of the chromosomes to separate properly during cell division; this is also known as nondisjunction. After the error occurs, two different cell populations are produced: one that continues to express the normal karyotype and the other, which contains the chromosomal abnormality.

Chimerism

Chimerism occurs when an organism is made up of two cell lines from two different zygotes. It is distinguished from mosaicism because chimerism is made up of cell lines from two distinct organisms, whereas mosaicism occurs when a mitotic error mutation occurs in a single zygote. Blood chimerism can result from twin-twin transfusion in dizygotic twins [37]. Interestingly, in transplant experiments, the individuals with chimeric cells do not reject a transplant from the donor twin [38,39]. Chimerism can occur from a transfusion between a mother and her fetus as well [40]. Finally, stem cells in an organ from an allogenic donor can engraft in the host to create a chimeric individual [41].

Epigenetic mosaicism

With the publication of the results of the Human Genome Project, it became apparent that the total number of genes in the human genome was less than expected: approximately 20,000 to 25,000 genes. However, the regulation of transcription and modification was much more complex than expected. The "epigenome" is the term used to describe this regulatory network. Epigenetic regulation refers to a variety of heritable mechanisms for altering gene expression. A number of factors come into play for epigenetic regulation, and these include genetic determinants, the developmental stage of the embryo, the types of the cells in which the genes are being expressed, and the local environmental pressures on those cells [42]. The specific chemical alterations and mechanisms controlling these changes are numerous, but two examples include cytosine methylation and histone modification [43]. The epigenetic factors that control changes in gene expression can be heritable and in some cases are transmitted to the next generation. In other cases, the epigenetic controls may only be effective during embryogenesis. "Imprinting" is the term used to describe the situation in which gene expression is dependent on the sex of the transmitting parent. DNA-promoter methylation has been implicated in the silencing of numerous imprinted genes. Examples of diseases that are influenced by imprinting include Albright syndrome, Beckwith-Wiedemann syndrome, Prader-Willi syndrome, and Angelman syndrome [42–44].

Twin-spotting

Happle [5] has proposed twin-spotting as a potential mechanism for the development of coexisting birthmarks, such as nevus simplex with adjacent Mongolian spots or pigmentary nevi. His theory is based on research from plants, showing that when two different recessive mutations are located on the same chromosome, somatic recombination can lead to two daughter cells, which are each homozygous for the mutation. He initially used this concept to explain the finding of twin vascular nevi. He proposed that nevus anemicus and telangiectatic nevi (nevus simplex) occur when a gene locus carries one allele for vasodilation, while the other carries an allele for vasoconstriction. The theory is that mitotic cross-overs may give rise to two different homozygous cells. The progeny of one cell would create a nevus with dilated vasculature (nevus simplex), while the other would give rise to constricted vasculature (nevus anemicus). This theory has been further used to explain the finding of simultaneous occurrence of a vascular malformation with a neighboring pigmentary nevus.

CLINICAL EXAMPLES

Clinical examples of segmental manifestations of autosomal dominant conditions, autosomal lethal conditions, X-linked dominant, X-linked recessive, chromosomal, and sporadic conditions are discussed below (Table 3).

Autosomal dominant conditions

Segmental neurofibromatosis

Segmental neurofibromatosis can present either as type 1 segmental mosaicism in a localized area of the body in an individual who is otherwise phenotypically normal, or as type 2 segmental mosaicism with typical generalized skin lesions (such as café-au-lait macules and neurofibromas) with a superimposed segmental manifestation (such as a giant café-au-lait patch or giant plexiform neurofibroma). In type 1 segmental NF, the segmental changes may often involve one extremity or quadrant of the body. The phenotype may include a large café-au-lait patch, axillary freckling, or dermal neurofibromas (Fig. 3). Systemic complications are rare in type 1 segmental NF [45]. The proposed mechanism for the development of segmental NF1 is a postzygotic somatic mutation in the *NF1* gene. The earlier the mutation occurs, the more likely extensive skin involvement will be seen, and also the greater the likelihood gonadal tissue will be involved. Therefore, with wider segmental mosaic involvement, there is a presumed increased risk of transmission to the offspring [46].

Table 3
Selected clinical examples of mosaic conditions

X-linked-dominant mutations: lethal in the hemizygous male	Autosomal lethal mutations surviving by mosaicism (gene known)	Sporadic conditions: presumed autosomal lethal, but genetic basis not yet determined	Revertant mosaicism	Polygenic with superimposed segmental presentation
Incontinentia pigmenti (*NEMO* gene)	McCune-Albright (*GNAS* gene)	Encephalo-cerebro-cutaneous lipomatosis	Epidermolysis bullosa (*LAMB3*, *KRT14*, and *COL17A1* genes)	Linear psoriasis
Conradi-Hunermann-Happle syndrome (*EBP* gene)		Proteus syndrome		Linear lichen planus
Goltz syndrome (*PORCN* gene)				Linear systemic lupus erythematosus
CHILD syndrome (*NSDHL* gene)				Linear pemphigus vulgaris

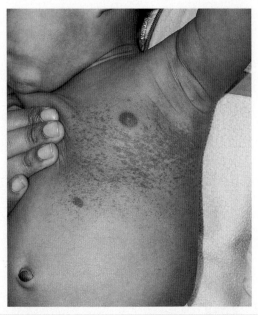

Fig. 3. Axillary freckling and café-au-lait macules in the segmental pattern on the axilla and chest of a toddler with segmental neurofibromatosis. (*Courtesy of* Alfons Krol, Portland, OR, USA).

Segmental Darier's disease

Darier-White disease (Online Mendelian Inheritance in Man gene map or OMIM #124,200) is an autosomal dominant condition characterized by warty, keratotic papules on the forehead, chest, scalp, trunk and extremities. Palmar pits, and V-shaped notching of the nails; longitudinal white or red subungual streaks on the nail beds are also noted. The hands can also display acrokeratosis verruciformis-like lesions resembling warts. The histopathologic features include acantholysis in the suprabasal layer of the epidermis. The molecular basis is a causative mutation in the ATPase, calcium dependent gene (*ATP2A2*) [47]. Several cases of segmental Darier's disease have been reported [48–50]. In segmental Darier's disease, the warty papules are localized in a Blaschko-linear pattern in one region of the body. In one example, a 41-year-old Japanese female presented with red-brown hyperkeratotic papules along the lines of Blaschko on the chest, with no additional manifestations present. A skin biopsy from the affected area revealed focal acantholytic dyskeratosis consistent with Darier's disease. Molecular analysis of the *ATP2A2* gene was performed from peripheral leukocytes, lesional skin, and normal skin. *ATP2A2* mutations were identified in the lesional skin, but not in the blood or unaffected skin, confirming a mosaic mutation [29].

Autosomal lethal mutations surviving by mosaicism

McCune-Albright syndrome

Some conditions are presumed to be lethal, with individuals only surviving when the mutated cells are present in the mosaic state. One example is

McCune-Albright syndrome, which is caused by sporadic postzygotic-activating mutations in guanine nucleotide-binding protein, alpha-stimulating activity polypeptide 1, (*GNAS1* gene) [51]. The clinical features of McCune-Albright syndrome include large, segmental, unilateral café-au-lait patches, which in some cases have been described as following the broad lines of Blaschko and in other cases have been described as having a "coast of Maine" appearance (Fig. 4). Additional features include polyostotic fibrous dysplasia and endocrine abnormalities, including precocious puberty. Transmission of McCune-Albright does not occur even if the gonadal tissue is involved because the mutation is not compatible with life when present in all cells.

X-linked conditions
X-linked dominant conditions occur predominantly in females who are presumed to survive because of the functional mosaicism created by X-inactivation. X-linked dominant conditions are generally lethal in hemizygous males, who only have one X chromosome and therefore do not have the benefit of random X-inactivation. Affected males have been reported for each of these conditions; some were shown to have Kleinfelter syndrome (XXY), while others were presumed to survive because of postzygotic mutations leading to somatic mosaicism (therefore, not all of the cells in the body harbored the mutation). X-linked recessive conditions manifest mainly in males who are hemizygous because they have only one X chromosome. Female carriers may have subtle clinical findings along the lines of Blaschko.

Focal dermal hypoplasia (Goltz syndrome)
Focal dermal hypoplasia (FDH, Goltz syndrome, OMIM #305,600) is an X-linked dominant disorder affecting both mesodermal and ectodermal structures, including the skin, eyes, teeth, and digits. The skin lesions are

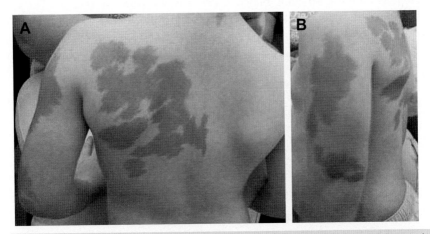

Fig. 4. Sharply demarcated café-au-lait spots along the broad lines of Blaschko on the back (A) and arm (B) in a child with McCune-Albright syndrome. (*Courtesy* of Daniel Marks, Portland, OR, USA).

characterized by atrophic, hypopigmented, linear streaks with telangiectasia and punctuate cribiform scarring, as well as subcutaneous fat herniations into the dermis along the lines of Blaschko. Raspberry-like papillomas frequently appear in the perioral and anogenital regions. The classic radiologic features are osteopathia striata (noted in the mid-portion of the lower extremities), limb reduction abnormalities, and syndactyly. Although this condition is predominantly seen in females, there have been a few males reported with FDH, likely because of Kleinfelter syndrome (47XXY) or a presumed mutation during embryologic development, making the individual mosaic for the condition and allowing for survival [52].

Recently, two separate groups reported mutations in the X-linked *PORCN* gene as the cause of Goltz syndrome [53,54]. *PORCN* encodes a putative *O*-acyltransferase, which is a regulator of the Wnt signaling pathway, which regulates cell-cell interactions during embryogenesis. Survival of the female in X-linked dominant conditions is based on the expression of functional gene products in the cells in which the X-chromosome possessing the mutation is inactivated and the normal X-chromosome is expressed. Most cases of Goltz syndrome have been sporadic. Interestingly, the familial cases have shown an imbalanced X-inactivation [53]. Whereas in most females, each X is inactivated approximately 50% of the time, in skewed X-inactivation nearly all of the X-chromosomes are normal, and there has been selection against expression of the X-chromosome carrying the mutant gene.

Conradi-Hunermann-Happle syndrome (X-linked chondrodysplasia punctata)
Conradi syndrome (OMIM #302,960) presents in the neonate with the appearance after birth of erythroderma and linear hyperkeratosis and psoriasiform scale. As the erythroderma resolves later in childhood, linear streaks with fine scale and ichthyosis along Blaschko's lines become apparent. Scarring alopecia on the scalp along Blaschko's lines is also common (Fig. 5). The extracutaneous features include limb reduction, distinctive facial features with

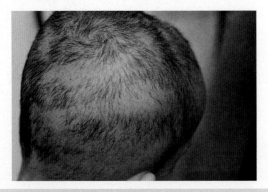

Fig. 5. Cicatricial alopecia along the lines of Blaschko on the scalp in a child with Conradi-Hunermann-Happle syndrome.

asymmetry, frontal bossing, and saddle nose. Cataracts may develop. Conradi-Hunermann-Happle syndrome is caused by mutations in the emopamil-binding protein (3b-hydroxysteroid-delta8,delta7-isomerase), which is involved in cholesterol biosynthesis [18].

Incontinentia pigmenti

Incontinentia pigmenti (IP) (OMIM #308,300) is an X-linked dominant disorder affecting the skin, teeth, hair, nails, and eyes caused by mutations in the *NEMO* (necrosis factor kappaB or NFkB essential modulator) gene [55]. The Blaschko-linear pattern of the cutaneous lesions reflects functional mosaicism because of Lyonization. *NEMO* plays a role in NFkB activation, which is protective against tumor necrosis factor-α-induced apoptosis. Cells with mutations in *NEMO* are not protected from apoptosis. Females are able to survive because of Lyonization; however, in boys the mutation is presumed to be lethal because of expression of the mutant allele in all cells. Males who survive are presumed to have had postzygotic mutations or have Kleinfelter syndrome (XXY) [56,57].

The cutaneous lesions of IP evolve through four distinct phases: the first phase is the vesiculobullous phase (Fig. 6A) and is followed by a second phase characterized by verrucous lesions (Fig. 6B). These verrucous lesions resolve, leaving prominent figurate hyperpigmented streaks and whorls along the lines of Blaschko (Fig. 6C). Finally, the lesions evolve into subtle hypopigmented atrophic streaks with absent eccrine glands and hair follicles (Fig. 6D). The teeth can be conical and peg-shaped and nail dystrophy is frequently seen in IP. The characteristic eye findings of IP include retinal vascular anomalies and optic atrophy. In some cases, neurologic changes occur including developmental delay and seizures.

Ectodermal dysplasia with immunodeficiency

Different mutations in the *NEMO* gene may result in ectodermal dysplasia with immunodeficiency in males (OMIM #300,291). These mutations are called hypomorphic mutations because they result in an altered gene product that possesses a reduced level of activity, or in which the wild-type gene product is expressed at a reduced level. Incontinentia pigmenti, on the other hand, is caused by amorphic mutations in which the altered gene product lacks the molecular function of the wild-type gene. Amorphic mutations are the same as loss-of-function mutations or null mutations. Ectodermal dysplasia with immunodeficiency (ED-ID) is an X-linked recessive disorder; the phenotype occurs in hemizygous males. Females are spared because they have one X-chromosome with the wild-type gene. The features of ED-ID are combined humoral and cell-mediated immunodeficiency and variable features of ectodermal dysplasia, including reduced sweating and dental anomalies.

X-linked recessive hypohidrotic ectodermal dysplasia

X-linked recessive hypohidrotic ectodermal dysplasia (HED/EDA1) (OMIM #305,100) also occurs in hemizygous males who have only one X

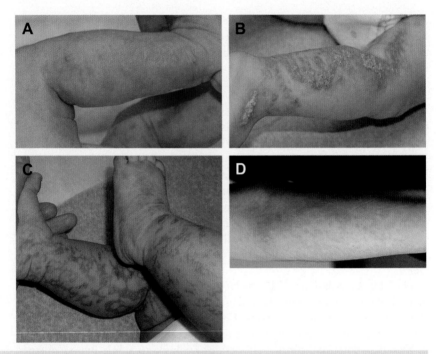

Fig. 6. (A) Linear streaks of erythema and vesicles along the lines of Blaschko on the arm of a 3-week-old girl with incontinentia pigmenti. (B) Hyperkeratotic plaques on the leg in the same patient at age 6 months. (C) Macular hyperpigmentation along the lines of Blaschko on the legs of a 10 month old with incontinentia pigmenti. (D) Hypopigmented, atrophic, hairless linear patches on the arm of the affected grandmother of the patient in (A) and (B).

chromosome. The carrier status in females may be difficult to diagnose clinically. Features in hemizygous males include a characteristic facial phenotype with full lips and periorbital ridging, thin, sparse, blond hair, lack of sweating, and abnormal teeth. The clinical features in carrier females may include patchy absence of vellus hair and stripes of hypotrichosis on the limbs and back, and mild to moderate hypotrichosis of the scalp hair. Interestingly, the functional mosaicism in these female carriers can be demonstrated using a starch iodine test, which reveals a lack of sweating along the lines of Blaschko [58]. X-linked recessive ectodermal dysplasia is caused by mutations in the ectodysplasin A gene [59].

Chromosomal mosaicism

Chromosomal mosaicism is sometimes apparent based on pigmentary alteration along the lines of Blaschko in children with developmental delay and additional congenital anomalies. Moss and colleagues [60] performed a literature search and identified 113 reports of pigmentary mosaicism associated with cytogenetic abnormalities. A wide variety of chromosomal abnormalities were reported, including structural abnormalities, balanced translocations, and polyploidy. In some cases, the chromosomal abnormalities were reported in all cells and in other cases the changes were reported as mosaic (affecting only a subset of cells). The investigators hypothesized that the pigmentary changes seen in these patients were because of disruptions of the pigmentary gene loci, which occurred because of a structural defect in the chromosome.

Other sporadic conditions

Proteus syndrome and other hemihypertrophy syndromes

Proteus syndrome was originally described by Cohen and Hayden [61] in 1979 and is named after the Greek sea-god, known for the ability to assume many different shapes. Biesecker [62] has proposed stringent diagnostic criteria for Proteus syndrome to avoid confusion with other overgrowth syndromes. The general criteria for the diagnosis of Proteus syndrome include mosaic distribution of the lesions, sporadic occurrence, and progressive course. If, in addition to these criteria, a cerebriform connective tissue nevus on the soles of the feet is present, the diagnosis of Proteus syndrome can be made. If not, then additional diagnostic criteria include asymmetric, disproportionate overgrowth of the limbs or viscera, and hyperostosis. Specific tumors can also be seen, including bilateral ovarian cystadenoma or parotid monomorphic adenoma. Finally, dysregulation of adipose tissue, vascular malformations, and lung cysts may be additional features. The overgrowth leads to severe disfigurement and functional compromise. Surgical intervention is not recommended unless "absolutely necessary," because the complication rate is high [62]. Deep vein thrombosis is one of the most common causes of death in Proteus syndrome [63]. Although there is no proven genetic basis for mosaicism, it is theorized that it is caused by mutations that would be lethal in a nonmosaic state; in other words, the embryo would not survive if the mutation was present in all cells [64].

A number of conditions are included in the differential diagnosis for Proteus syndrome, including Proteus-like syndrome, PTEN-hamartoma syndrome, Klippel-Trenaunay syndrome, and hemihyperplasia multiple lipomatosis syndrome. Recently, Biesecker's group described a new entity called "congenital lipomatosis, overgrowth, vascular malformations, and epidermal nevi" (CLOVE Syndrome). The cases described did not meet diagnostic criteria for Proteus syndrome but had the phenotype outlined above. The article pointed out that one of the distinguishing features was overgrowth of the palms and soles, with wrinkling rather than the connective tissue nevi seen in Proteus syndrome [65].

Segmental pigmentation disorder (patterned dyspigmentation)

The majority of children presenting to the pediatric dermatologist with pigmentary changes along the lines of Blaschko or large segmental café-au-lait patches do not have associated congenital anomalies or other systemic associations. This has been labeled segmental pigmentation disorder (or patterned dyspigmentation) [66]. The pigmented patches may be either solitary or multiple. They tend to measure several centimeters in diameter with a sharp midline demarcation (Fig. 7). If an individual presents with isolated pigmentary alteration, without any features suggestive of NF1, McCune-Albright syndrome, or another chromosomal abnormality, then the changes are most likely localized to the skin without systemic manifestations. The term "hypomelanosis of Ito" should be avoided in this situation, as it implies a chromosomal abnormality and association with development delay and additional congenital anomalies.

Segmental manifestations of polygenic and inflammatory skin disorders

Several inflammatory and polygenic conditions have been reported with linear or segmental presentations. Generally, these conditions present with a more severe segment overlying a milder background of generalized involvement. One possible mechanism is loss of heterozygosity in a somatic cell. Recent examples in the literature include linear psoriasis, linear lichen planus, linear systemic lupus erythematosus, linear pemphigus vulgaris, linear atopic

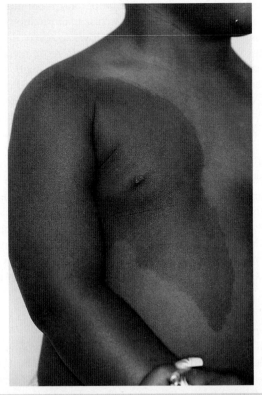

Fig. 7. Segmental pigmentation disorder demonstrated along the lines of Blaschko in an otherwise healthy young female (*Courtesy of* Amy Jo Nopper, Kansas City, MO, USA).

dermatitis, linear graft-versus-host disease, segmental granuloma annulare, and linear fixed-drug eruptions [67].

SUMMARY

Physicians have long been intrigued by the distinct patterns created by epidermal nevi and other mosaic cutaneous disorders. Although many of the molecular mechanisms underlying these disorders remain unrevealed, with the release of the results of the Human Genome Project our knowledge is rapidly increasing. The underlying genetic defects for many of the X-linked and mosaic disorders have recently been identified. Advances in technology, such as the array comparative genomic hybridization, will provide the tools for continued gene discovery and expanded understanding of the pathogenic mechanisms underlying mosaic skin conditions.

Acknowledgments

The author would like to thank Jonathon Zonana, MD for his critical review of the manuscript.

References

[1] McGrath JA. Translational benefits from research on rare genodermatoses. Australas J Dermatol 2004;45(2):89–93.

[2] Blashcko A. Die Nervenverteilung in der Haut in ihrer Beziehung zu den Erkrankungen der Haut. Vienna, Austria and Leipzig, Germany: Wilhelm Braunmuller; 1901.

[3] Mongomery D. The cause of streaks in naevus linearis. J Cutan Genito-urinary 1901;19: 455–64.

[4] Jackson R. The lines of Blashko: a review and reconsideration: observations of the cause of certain unusual linear conditions of the skin. Br J Dermatol 1976;95(4):349–60.

[5] Happle R. Mosaicism in human skin. Understanding the patterns and mechanisms. Arch Dermatol 1993;129(11):1460–70.

[6] Happle R. Dohi memorial lecture. New aspects of cutaneous mosaicism. J Dermatol 2002;29(11):681–92.

[7] Happle R. [Patterns on the skin. New aspects of their embryologic and genetic causes]. Hautarzt 2004;55(10):960–1, 964–81.

[8] Zietz S, Happle R, Hohenleutner U, et al. The venous nevus: a distinct vascular malformation suggesting mosaicism. Dermatology 2008;216(1):31–6.

[9] Happle R. Phylloid hypomelanosis is closely related to mosaic trisomy 13. Eur J Dermatol 2000;10(7):511–2.

[10] Huszar D, Sharpe A, Jaenisch R. Migration and proliferation of cultured neural crest cells in W mutant neural crest chimeras. Development 1991;112(1):131–41.

[11] Schmidt A, Brixius K, Bloch W. Endothelial precursor cell migration during vasculogenesis. Circ Res 2007;101(2):125–36.

[12] Maertens O, De Schepper S, Vandesompele J, et al. Molecular dissection of isolated disease features in mosaic neurofibromatosis type 1. Am J Hum Genet 2007;81(2):243–51.

[13] Bar-Shira A, Rosner G, Rosner S, et al. Array-based comparative genome hybridization in clinical genetics. Pediatr Res 2006;60(3):353–8.

[14] Lalani SR, Sahoo T, Sanders ME, et al. Coarctation of the aorta and mild to moderate developmental delay in a child with a de novo deletion of chromosome 15(q21.1q22.2). BMC Med Genet 2006;7:8.

[15] Cheung SW, Shaw CA, Scott DA, et al. Microarray-based CGH detects chromosomal mosaicism not revealed by conventional cytogenetics. Am J Med Genet A 2007;143A(15): 1679–86.

[16] Guarino S, Perricone C, Guarino MD, et al. Gonadal mosaicism in hereditary angioedema. Clin Genet 2006;70(1):83–5.

[17] Ng D, Johnston JJ, Turner JT, et al. Gonadal mosaicism in severe Pallister-Hall syndrome. Am J Med Genet A 2004;124A(3):296–302.

[18] Has C, Bruckner-Tuderman L, Müller D, et al. The Conradi-Hunermann-Happle syndrome (CDPX2) and emopamil binding protein: novel mutations, and somatic and gonadal mosaicism. Hum Mol Genet 2000;9(13):1951–5.

[19] Ben-Asher E, Lancet D. NIPBL gene responsible for Cornelia de Lange syndrome, a severe developmental disorder. Isr Med Assoc J 2004;6(9):571–2.

[20] Gillis LA, McCallum J, Kaur M, et al. NIPBL mutational analysis in 120 individuals with Cornelia de Lange syndrome and evaluation of genotype-phenotype correlations. Am J Hum Genet 2004;75(4):610–23.

[21] Krantz ID, McCallum J, DeScipio C, et al. Cornelia de Lange syndrome is caused by mutations in NIPBL, the human homolog of Drosophila melanogaster Nipped-B. Nat Genet 2004;36(6):631–5.

[22] Niu DM, Huang JY, Li HY, et al. Paternal gonadal mosaicism of NIPBL mutation in a father of siblings with Cornelia de Lange syndrome. Prenat Diagn 2006;26(11):1054–7.

[23] Paller AS, Syder AJ, Chan YM, et al. Genetic and clinical mosaicism in a type of epidermal nevus. N Engl J Med 1994;331(21):1408–15.

[24] Happle R. Segmental forms of autosomal dominant skin disorders: different types of severity reflect different states of zygosity. Am J Med Genet 1996;66(2):241–2.

[25] Yang CC, Happle R, Chao SC, et al. Giant cafe-au-lait macule in neurofibromatosis 1: a type 2 segmental manifestation of neurofibromatosis 1? J Am Acad Dermatol 2008;58(3):493–7.

[26] Poblete-Gutierrez P, Wiederholt T, König A, et al. Allelic loss underlies type 2 segmental Hailey-Hailey disease, providing molecular confirmation of a novel genetic concept. J Clin Invest 2004;114(10):1467–74.

[27] Ruggieri M. The different forms of neurofibromatosis. Childs Nerv Syst 1999;15(6–7):295–308.

[28] Sanderson EA, Killoran CE, Pedvis-Leftick A, et al. Localized Darier's disease in a Blaschkoid distribution: two cases of phenotypic mosaicism and a review of mosaic Darier's disease. J Dermatol 2007;34(11):761–4.

[29] Wada T, Shirakata Y, Takahashi H, et al. A Japanese case of segmental Darier's disease caused by mosaicism for the ATP2A2 mutation. Br J Dermatol 2003;149(1):185–8.

[30] Lyon MF. Gene action in the X-chromosome of the mouse (Mus musculus L.). Nature 1961;190:372–3.

[31] Darling TN, Yee C, Bauer JW, et al. Revertant mosaicism: partial correction of a germ-line mutation in COL17A1 by a frame-restoring mutation. J Clin Invest 1999;103(10):1371–7.

[32] Jonkman MF, Castellanos Nuijts M, van Essen AJ. Natural repair mechanisms in correcting pathogenic mutations in inherited skin disorders. Clin Exp Dermatol 2003;28(6):625–31.

[33] Jonkman MF, Scheffer H, Stulp R, et al. Revertant mosaicism in epidermolysis bullosa caused by mitotic gene conversion. Cell 1997;88(4):543–51.

[34] Pasmooij AM, Pas HH, Deviaene FC, et al. Multiple correcting COL17A1 mutations in patients with revertant mosaicism of epidermolysis bullosa. Am J Hum Genet 2005;77(5):727–40.

[35] Smith FJ, Morley SM, McLean WH. Novel mechanism of revertant mosaicism in Dowling-Meara epidermolysis bullosa simplex. J Invest Dermatol 2004;122(1):73–7.

[36] Pasmooij AM, Pas HH, Bolling MC, et al. Revertant mosaicism in junctional epidermolysis bullosa due to multiple correcting second-site mutations in LAMB3. J Clin Invest 2007;117(5):1240–8.

[37] Youssoufian H, Pyeritz RE. Mechanisms and consequences of somatic mosaicism in humans. Nat Rev Genet 2002;3(10):748–58.

[38] Hall JG. Twinning: mechanisms and genetic implications. Curr Opin Genet Dev 1996;6(3):343–7.

[39] van Dijk BA, Boomsma DI, de Man AJ. Blood group chimerism in human multiple births is not rare. Am J Med Genet 1996;61(3):264–8.

[40] Nguyen Huu S, et al. Feto-maternal cell trafficking: a transfer of pregnancy associated progenitor cells. Stem Cell Rev 2006;2(2):111–6.

[41] Spangrude GJ, Torok-Storb B, Little MT. Chimerism of the transplanted heart. N Engl J Med 2002;346(18):1410–2 [author reply 1410–2].

[42] Bernstein BE, Meissner A, Lander ES. The mammalian epigenome. Cell 2007;128(4): 669–81.

[43] Geiman TM, Robertson KD. Chromatin remodeling, histone modifications, and DNA methylation-how does it all fit together? J Cell Biochem 2002;87(2):117–25.

[44] Millington GW. Genomic imprinting and dermatological disease. Clin Exp Dermatol 2006;31(5):681–8.

[45] Ruggieri M, Huson SM. The clinical and diagnostic implications of mosaicism in the neurofibromatoses. Neurology 2001;56(11):1433–43.

[46] Consoli C, Moss C, Green S, et al. Gonosomal mosaicism for a nonsense mutation (R1947X) in the NF1 gene in segmental neurofibromatosis type 1. J Invest Dermatol 2005;125(3):463–6.

[47] Sakuntabhai A, Ruiz-Perez V, Carter S, et al. Mutations in *ATP2A2*, encoding a Ca2+ pump, cause Darier disease. Nat Genet 1999;21(3):271–7.

[48] Happle R, Itin PH, Brun AM. Type 2 segmental Darier disease. Eur J Dermatol 1999;9(6): 449–51.

[49] Itin PH, Buchner SA, Happle R. Segmental manifestation of Darier disease. What is the genetic background in type 1 and type 2 mosaic phenotypes? Dermatology 2000;200(3):254–7.

[50] Reese DA, Paul AY, Davis B. Unilateral segmental Darier disease following Blaschko lines: a case report and review of the literature. Cutis 2005;76(3):197–200.

[51] Diaz A, Danon M, Crawford J. McCune-Albright syndrome and disorders due to activating mutations of *GNAS1*. J Pediatr Endocrinol Metab 2007;20(8):853–80.

[52] Happle R. Cutaneous manifestation of lethal genes. Hum Genet 1986;72(3):280.

[53] Grzeschik KH, Bornholdt D, Oeffner F, et al. Deficiency of *PORCN*, a regulator of Wnt signaling, is associated with focal dermal hypoplasia. Nat Genet 2007;39(7):833–5.

[54] Wang X, Reid Sutton V, Omar Peraza-Llanes J, et al. Mutations in X-linked *PORCN*, a putative regulator of Wnt signaling, cause focal dermal hypoplasia. Nat Genet 2007;39(7):836–8.

[55] Aradhya S, Nelson DL. NF-kappaB signaling and human disease. Curr Opin Genet Dev 2001;11(3):300–6.

[56] Fusco F, Fimiani G, Tadini G, et al. Clinical diagnosis of incontinentia pigmenti in a cohort of male patients. J Am Acad Dermatol 2007;56(2):264–7.

[57] Pacheco TR, Levy M, Collyer JC, et al. Incontinentia pigmenti in male patients. J Am Acad Dermatol 2006;55(2):251–5.

[58] Clarke A, Burn J. Sweat testing to identify female carriers of X linked hypohidrotic ectodermal dysplasia. J Med Genet 1991;28(5):330–3.

[59] Schneider P, Street SL, Gaide O, et al. Mutations leading to X-linked hypohidrotic ectodermal dysplasia affect three major functional domains in the tumor necrosis factor family member ectodysplasin-A. J Biol Chem 2001;276(22):18819–27.

[60] Taibjee SM, Bennett DC, Moss C. Abnormal pigmentation in hypomelanosis of Ito and pigmentary mosaicism: the role of pigmentary genes. Br J Dermatol 2004;151(2):269–82.

[61] Cohen MM Jr, Hayden PW. A newly recognized hamartomatous syndrome. Birth Defects Orig Artic Ser 1979;15(5B):291–6.

[62] Biesecker L. The challenges of Proteus syndrome: diagnosis and management. Eur J Hum Genet 2006;14(11):1151–7.

[63] Cohen MM Jr. Causes of premature death in Proteus syndrome. Am J Med Genet 2001;101(1):1–3.

[64] Happle R. Lethal genes surviving by mosaicism: a possible explanation for sporadic birth defects involving the skin. J Am Acad Dermatol 1987;16(4):899–906.

[65] Sapp JC, Turner JT, van de Kamp JM, et al. Newly delineated syndrome of congenital lipo-matous overgrowth, vascular malformations, and epidermal nevi (CLOVE syndrome) in seven patients. Am J Med Genet A 2007;143(24):2944–58.

[66] Gibbs N, Makkar H. Neonatal dermatology. In: Eichenfield LF, Frieden IJ, Esterly NB, editors. Philadelphia: Saunders Elsevier; 2008.

[67] Happle R. Superimposed segmental manifestation of polygenic skin disorders. J Am Acad Dermatol 2007;57(4):690–9.

Advances in Hair Diseases

Maria Hordinsky, MD

Department of Dermatology, MMC 98, 420 Delaware St. SE, University of Minnesota, Minneapolis, Minnesota 55455, USA

EDITORIAL COMMENT

Hair abnormalities range from uncommon genetic conditions to some of the most common diseases we see in our clinics. Maria Hordinsky is an expert in all of them. In this comprehensive well-written review the latest information is concisely presented. A simplified classificaton of the inflammatory alopecias is now the accepted standard; treatment is recommended in ranked tiers. This practical advice is welcome. Additionally the advances in our understanding of the hair cycle and structure leads me to have hope for more rational, effective and hopefully safe, alternative therapies for androgenetic alopecia may be closer to reality.

William James, MD

THE HUMAN HAIR FOLLICLE

The hair follicle is a complicated structure that produces an equally complicated product, the hair fiber. The hair follicle also has the unique ability to completely regenerate itself. Hair grows, falls out, and then grows again. A plucked hair regrows.

Cells important to the creation of hair follicles and hair fibers include the stem cells present in the bulge region (Fig. 1) as well as dermal sheath, papilla, and cusp cells [1–3]. Unique molecules are selectively up-regulated in the human anagen hair follicle bulge region. Some of these include: KRT15, Frizzled homolog 1, Follistatin, Dickkopf Homolog 3, WNT inhibitory factor, Pleckstrin homology-like domain, family A, CD146, and endothelin receptor. The role of these unique molecules in follicle differentiation and cycling is being investigated [4].

Hair fibers originate from the hair matrix/dermal papilla region and consist of a cuticle, medulla and cortex. The follicle is surrounded by the outer root sheath, which shares many characteristics of the epidermis (Fig. 2). Advances in basic science research have established the presence of the K5/K14 keratin pair characteristic of basal epidermal cells and K6/K16 keratin pair

E-mail address: hordi001@umn.edu

0882-0880/08/$ – see front matter
doi:10.1016/j.yadr.2008.09.013

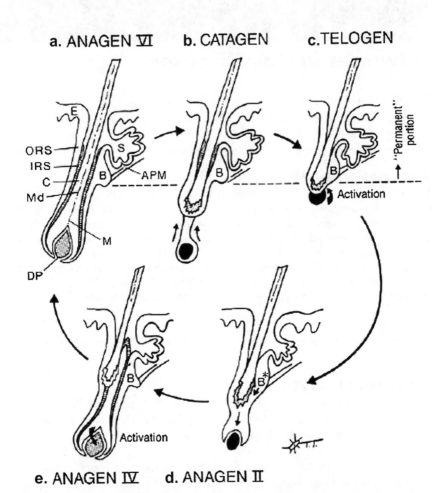

Fig. 1. Hair cycle: The bulge activation hypothesis illustrated are different phases of the hair cycle incluing (a) anagen VI, (b) catagen, (c) telogen, (d) anagen II, and (e) anagen IV. *Abbreviations:* APM, arrector pili muscle; B, bulge; C, cortex; DP, dermal papilla; E, epidermis; IRS, inner root sheath; M, matrix; Md, medulla; ORS, outer root sheath; S, sebaceous gland. B and B* denote quiescent and activated bulge cells respectively. *From* Cotsarelis G, Sun T, and Lavker R. Label Retaining Cells Reside in the Bulge Area of Pilosebaceous Unit: Implications for Follicular Stem Cells, Hair Cycle, and Skin Carcinogenesis. Cell Vol. 61, 1329–37, June 29, 1990 (Fig. 6); with permission.

characteristic of hyperproliferative keratinocytes in this outer root sheath. K19 has been found to localize to the bulge region, the site of the slow-cycling hair follicle stem cells that are capable of initiating follicular renewal at the end of the resting phase of the hair cycle [3]. The companion layer separates the outer root sheath from the inner root sheath, which consists of: Henle's layer, Huxley's layer. and the cuticle. The cuticle of the inner root sheath interdigitates with the cuticle of the hair fiber and these interdigitations are thought

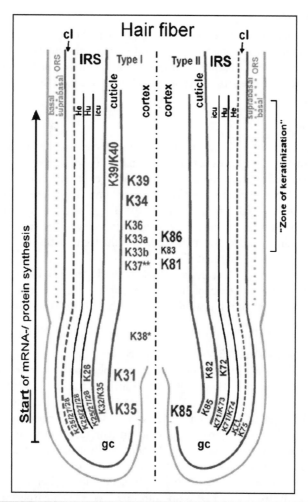

Fig. 2. Summary scheme of the expression of all hair and hair follicle-specific keratins in the human hair follicle. K37** is found in the cortex of vellus hair and medulla of sexual hairs. K38* is heterogeneously expressed in the cortex. The keratin gene designations follow the new keratin nomenclature. *From* Schweizer J, et al. Hair follicle-specific keratins and their diseases. Experimental Cell Research 313(2007):2010–20 (Fig. 3); with permission.

to be abnormal in loose anagen hair syndrome. Huxley's layer contains trichohyaline granules, which serve as a substrate for citrulline-rich proteins.

Type I and Type II keratins have been studied not only in the hair fiber, bulge region, and external root sheath, but also in the other compartments of the hair follicle as shown in Fig. 2. Of the 18 known Type I keratins, 17 are epithelial and 11 are hair keratins; of the 26 Type II keratins, 20 are epithelial and six are hair keratins. Disease-causing mutations of both hair follicle-specific and epithelial keratins have until now only been described to Type II keratins [5].

HAIR COLOR

Hair color is genetically determined and is postulated to occur with the transfer of melanosomes from melanocytes in the dermal papilla region to the developing hair fiber. Recently, a transcription factor has been described that contributes to hair color by marking which cells are to receive pigment from melanocytes [6].

HAIR CYCLE

On average, 90% of follicles are in the anagen phase of the hair cycle or the actively growing phase, postulated to last an average of 3 years. The transition phase, catagen, lasts an average of 2 weeks and represents only about 1%–2% of all scalp follicles. Telogen follicles comprise about 10% of scalp hair follicles and last an average of 3–5 months. Two other stages of the hair cycle described more recently include: exogen, the stage associated with the release of telogen fibers from follicles and kenogen, described as the lag time between exogen and new anagen fiber development [7].

Recent advances in hair follicle biology and genetics have significantly increased the understanding of human hair fiber structural abnormalities, as well as expanding the knowledge about the nonscarring and cicatricial alopecias.

STRUCTURAL HAIR ABNORMALITIES

For the clinician, hair shaft abnormalities can be broadly divided into major categories as outlined in Box 1, [8]. These include fractures of the hair shaft, irregularities and hair coiling and twisting of the hair shaft, and extraneous matter on hair shaft. Causative genes have now been described for: trichothiodystrophy, Netherton syndrome, moniliform hair found in monilethrix localized autosomal recessive hypotrichosis ,and woolly hair. Associated disorders with hair shaft abnormalities and recently described causative genes are nicely summarized in a recent review article by Cheng and Bayliss [9].

Trichothiodystrophy (TTD) is an autosomal recessive neuroectodermal disorder characterized by brittle hair and hair fibers with low sulfur content. Hair fibers characteristically show trichoschisis and, under polarized light, a "tiger tail" pattern of alternating bright and dark bands. TTD is associated with mutations in the TTDA gene, and two of seven xeroderma pigmentosum (XP) genes, XPB and XPD, both of which encode for helical subunits that unwind the double helix. Patients with TTD and defective DNA repair are not at significant risk for developing skin cancer in contrast to patients with XP. This has been related to differences in natural killer cell function, activation of apopotosis, intracellular adhesion molecule-1 expression, and mutation-induced changes in protein structure [10,11].

Multiple hair shaft abnormalities have been reported in Netherton's syndrome, including: trichorrhexis invaginata (bamboo hair), golftee hair, and torsion nodes. Other clinical features of this syndrome include ichthyosis lineraris circumflexa and an atopic diathesis. The Netherton syndrome gene

Box 1: Classification of structural hair abnormalities

Fractures of the Hair Shaft

- Longitudinal – Trichoptilosis
- Oblique – Tapered fracture
- Transverse:
  - Trichorrhexis nodosa
  - Trichoschisis
  - Trichoclasis
  - Trichorrhexis invaginata

Irregularities, Coiling and Twisting of the Hair Shaft

- Circle hairs
- Longitudinal ridging and grooving
- Monilethrix
- Pili annulati
- Pili bifurcati and pili multigemini
- Pili torti, including Corkscrew hair and Menke's disease
- Pseudopili annulati
- Pseudomonilethrix
- Tapered hairs
- Trichonodosis
- Uncombable hair or pili trianguli et canaliculi or spun glass hair
- Woolly hair

Extraneous Matter on Hair Shaft

- Bacteria – Trichomycosis axillaris
- Deposits – Lacquer, paint, glue, etc.
- Fungi – Tinea capitis, Piedra
- Pediculosis – Nits
- Peripilar Casts – Pseudonits

has been localized to chromosome 5q 32 and to a mutation in the SPINK5 gene that encodes the serine protease inhibitor LEKTI (lymphoepithelial Kazal-type-related inhibitor), which is associated with skin barrier function and immunity. LEKTI dysfunctions may cause abnormal maturation of T lymphocytes and faulty Th2 immune responses [12].

Moniliform fibers can be found in monilethrix and localized autosomal recessive hypothrichosis. Monilethrix has been associated with a mutation in Type II cortical hair keratins (hHb6 and HHB1), whereas a mutation in the lipase H (LIPH) gene underlies autosomal recessive hypotrichosis, a rare autosomal recessive disorder characterized by sparse scalp and body hair [13,14]. A mutation in the desmoglein 4 (DSG4) gene has also been reported in inherited hypotrichosis [15].

Woolly hair has been described as part of several syndromes including Naxos disease and Carvajal syndrome. Naxos disease is associated with right ventricular cardiomyopathy, diffuse nonepidermolytic palmoplantar keratoderma, and a mutation in the gene encoding plakoglobin [16]. Carvajal Syndrome is also associated with woolly hair, a palmoplantar keratoderma, and heart disease but with a mutation in the gene encoding desmoplakin [17].

HAIR CYCLE, STEM CELLS, IMMUNE PRIVILEGE

Human hair follicle stem cells are postulated to reside in the follicular bulge, the region of the follicle at the level of insertion of the arrector pili muscle. Here, the slow-cycling stem hair follicle stem cells are capable of initiating follicular renewal at the end of the resting phase of the hair cycle [3]. The region below this site is intimately involved in the hair cycle and is the part of the follicle that moves up and down during the hair cycle. It is this region that also lacks the expression of major histocompatiblity complex human leukocyte antigen (HLA) class I and class II antigens, giving it the distinction of being an immune privileged site [18]. It is this region that loses its immune privilege in alopecia areata and when injured, cicatricial or scarring alopecias occur.

CICATRICIAL ALOPECIAS

The cicatrical alopecias are an important group of disorders associated with permanent destruction of the pilosebaceous unit. Most investigators postulate that injury to the region of the insertion of the arrector pili muscle into the hair follicle and the area where follicular stem cells reside leads to permanent injury and scarring. The destruction of this region may be primary or secondary, but, in both cases, follicular orifices are lost [19]. Research and support for patients with the cicatrical alopecias is available through the Cicatrical Alopecia Research Foundation.

The current classification of the cicatricial alopecias is based on the principal inflammatory cell type: lymphocytic, neutrophilic, or mixed [20]. The lymphycytic cicatrical alopecias include: lichen plano pilaris, central centrifugal scarring alopecia, frontal fibrosing alopecia, pseudopelade, chronic cutaneous lupus erythematosus, and discoid lupus erythematosus. The neutrophilic cicatrical alopecias include: folliculitis decalvans and dissecting cellulitis and the mixed cicatrical alopecias acne keloidalis, acne necrotica and erosive pustular dermatoses of the scalp (Box 2).

Unfortunately, the histopathologic findings in scalp biopsy specimens from affected patients do not always distinguish clinical variants because clinical and histologic features may change over time. For example, predominantly neutrophilic infiltrates may change to a mixed infiltrate with many lymphocytes. Histologic features may also not necessarily correlate with clinical

Box 2: The Cicatricial Alopecias

Lymphocytic Cicatricial Alopecias
  Lichen Plano Pilaris
  Central Centrifugal Scarring Alopecia
  Frontal Fibrosing Alopecia
  Pseudopelade
  Chronic cutaneous lupus erythematosus
  Discoid Lupus Erythematosus

Neutrophilic Cicatricial Alopecias
  Folliculitis Decalvans
  Dissecting Cellulitis

Mixed Cicatrical Alopecias
  Acne Keloidalis
  Acne Necrotica
  Erosive Pustular Dermatoses of the Scalp

responses [21]. These results may leave the clinician with the challenge of figuring out whether to use immunomodulating drugs or antibiotics or both.

Treatment of the lymphocytic cicatricial alopecias can be broken into three tiers and choice of therapy stepped up based on clinical response and severity [22]. Tier 1 therapies include topical high potency ccorticosteroids or intralesional steroids, as well as topical nonsteroid anti-inflammatory agents. Tier 2 therapies include acetretin and antimalarials, selecting a dose based on weight. Tier 3 treatments include the use of oral immunosuppressive medications such as cyclosporine, mycophenolate mofetil or prednisone. The use of anti-interferon alpha for cutaneous lupus has been suggested and in clinical trials, the use of salbutamol 0.05% cream, a B2 agonist, is being investigated in patients with both systemic and discoid lupus erythematosus [23].

Treatment of the neutrophilic cicatrical alopecias includes culturing pustules and/or scalp biopsy specimens and determining antibiotic sensitivities. In addition to the use of appropriate oral antibiotics, the use of prednisone and retinoids has been advocated.

Treatment of the mixed cicatricial alopecias also includes the use of antibiotics and anti-inflammatory medications. This recommendation is especially for patients experiencing erosive pustular dermatoses of the scalp, a rare condition that occurs after trauma of some sort. Application of high potent topical steroids can be particularly beneficial to patients with this condition [24].

CD200, a protein located on cells that surround both human and mouse hair follicles, has been implicated as an important protein in the pathogenesis of the cicatricial alopecias. CD200 is described as a protein that suppresses the immune system with both human and mouse hair follicles expressing CD200 demonstrating no autoimmune destruction. In contrast, hair follicles not expressing CD200 have been found to be susceptible to an immune attack and destruction. This research has suggested to investigators that CD200 protects hair follicles from autoimmune attack [25].

HAIR DISEASE RELATED TO ABNORMALITIES IN THE HAIR CYCLE

Hair diseases that are related to abnormalities in the hair cycle include telogen and anagen effluvium, androgenetic alopecia, and alopecia areata. Anagen effluvium can be genetic or related to a hair cycle disturbance secondary to medications. Loose anagen syndrome, described as a genetic disorder of the hair cycle, is considered to be autosomal dominant with variable expression and incomplete penetrance, with most cases occurring in blonde females, ages 2–5 years. A keratin mutation, E337K in K6HF has been described in some patients with this condition [26].

Telogen effluvium is frequently defined as excessive shedding of normal telogen fibers. Several variants of telogen effluvium have been described including: immediate anagen release, delayed anagen release, short anagen, immediate telogen release, and delayed telogen release [27]. Probably the most common variants include delayed anagen release, which occurs after delivery of a baby, or the telogen effluvium that commonly occurs 3–5 months after a premature conversion of anagen follicles into telogen following a stressful event such as surgery. Patients beginning Rogaine therapy may also experience a telogen effluvium as telogen hairs are released prematurely with the initiation of a new anagen cycle.

When indicated, thyroid function tests, FANA, and an analysis of hematologic parameters including an iron profile should be checked in patients experiencing a telogen effluvium hair loss. The relationship between low iron stores and hair shedding/telogen effluvium has been examined in several studies. In some, iron deficiency even in the absence of iron deficiency anemia, is described as being associated with hair loss. In these studies, different definitions of iron deficiency and iron deficiency anemia are used, but, in general, the decision to treat is based on clinical judgment. Ferrous sulfate, ferrous fumerate, and ferrous gluconate are all viewed as being equally effective with elemental iron 200 to 300 mg/day resulting in iron absorption of approximately 50 mg/day [28].

Androgenetic alopecia

Male androgenetic alopecia is commonly classified using the Hamilton Norwood classification system; in women who have pattern thinning, the Ludwig classification system is used [29]. Male androgenetic alopecia is considered to be a genetically determined condition associated with end organ (hair follicle) androgen sensitivity. Inhibition of type II 5-alpha reductase activity, which is involved in the conversion of testosterone to dihydrotestoserone, has been associated with stabilization androgenetic alopecia as well as regrowth [30].

Pattern alopecia in women is graded using the Ludwig classification system with the presence of a "Christmas" tree pattern being a more recently described clinical finding [31]. A clinically useful classification based on the onset of hair loss – early or late – with or without androgen excess is presented in Box 3 [32].

Hirsutism is described as the condition in women of terminal hair growth following a similar pattern to that developing in androgen-dependent sites in men after puberty [33]. When pattern alopecia in women is associated with androgen excess and hirsutism, the most common cause is polycystic ovarian syndrome. Other systemic abnormalities reported with hirsutism and pattern alopecia include the presence of androgen secreting tumors, Cushing's syndrome, hyperprolactinemia or genetic enzyme deficiencies as 21-hydroxylase deficiency or less commonly, 11-B hydroxylase deficiency [33].

Treatment of androgenetic alopecia can be divided into cosmetic, medical, and surgical [29]. Hair transplantation can be very effective and provide a permanent "cure." Cosmetic techniques to mask the balding process include the use of scalp colorants as well as hair pieces. Medical treatments include the use of topical Minoxidil (Rogaine) 2%, which is approved by the Food and Drug Administration (FDA) in the United States for women, as well as the FDA-approved 5% liquid and foam preparations for men. Finasteride, 1 mg (Propecia, Merck), a type 2 5-alpha reductase inhibitor, has been shown to be effective in the treatment of both vertex and frontal scalp balding in clinical trials in male androgenetic alopecia, but this drug has not been found to be effective in the management of female pattern alopecia occurring in menopause, either natural or surgical [30,34].

Abnormal catagen

Mutations in the hairless gene result in a generalized atrichia, similar to that seen in patients with mutations in the Vitamin D receptor. Clinically, hair is present at birth, but with the first hair cycle, the ability to form a normal catagen follicle disappears. Histologically, follicular development is normal, but the

---

Box 3: Classification of female pattern alopecia based on onset

Late Onset
- With androgen excess
- Without androgen excess

Early Onset
- With androgen excess
- Without androgen excess

hair follicle "falls apart" during catagen with the dermal papilla failing to move upward and cycling ceasing [35,36].

Prolonged anagen

Hypertrichosis occurs with prolonged anagen. Several medications are associated with hypertrichosis as are many syndromes [33]. Acquired hypertrichosis lanuginosa is a generalized acquired condition and is considered to be a sign of internal malignancy.

Alopecia areata

There is currently no FDA drug approved for the treatment of alopecia areata, a common hair disease that is considered to be a complex genetic, immune mediated nonscarring disease that targets actively growing anagen hair follicles. Over four and one half million people in the United States are estimated to be affected with alopecia areata according to the National Alopecia Areata Foundation, an organization focused on research and education in this disease [37,38].

Alopecia areata is relatively easy to diagnose when it presents as patches of nonscarring alopecia or extensive hair loss commonly called alopecia totalis or universalis. For patchy disease the differential diagnosis may include Tinea corporis or rarely, localized hypotrichosis, an autosomal recessive condition in which defects are present in desmoglein 4. (Klijuic, 2003). In the United States, 50%–80% of cases are considered sporadic, with the disease affecting 1%–2% of the population. Alopecia areata affects all ages and both sexes. Disease associations vary around the world [37–40]. Recently, it was reported that alopecia areata patients with atopic dermatitis who had fillagrin gene mutations were more likely to have a more severe form of alopecia areata, such as alopecia totalis or universalis [41].

Alopecia areata is viewed as a T cell mediated autoimmune disease most likely directed against pigment cells in the hair follicle [42]. Abnormalities in the hair cycle are considered to be the "root" of the problem in alopecia areata. In the acute stage, inflammatory infiltrates are present in the peribulbar region; in the subacute stage, the numbers of anagen follicles are decreased and there are increased numbers of catagen and telogen follicles. In the chronic stage, terminal follicles are decreased and there are increased numbers of catagen and telogen follicles. In the chronic stage, decreased numbers of terminal follicles are found along with an increase in miniaturized follicles with a ratio of 1:1 terminal to vellus follicels rather than the normal of 7:1 [43].

Recent advances in the understanding of the pathophysiology of alopecia areata have been in large part supported by the National Alopecia Areata Foundation. The establishment of the Alopecia Areata Registry by the National Alopecia Areata Foundation, with support from NIAMS, has further facilitated basic clinical and epidemiologic studies of alopecia areata. At the present time, more than 6000 individuals have registered online. Current investigations using registry samples include: a genetic linkage project, a candidate gene search, a cytokine profiling study, and assessment of nerve function in affected and unaffected scalp in patients with hair loss in the ophiasis region [44].

At a recent conference that definined research priorities for the National Alopecia Areata Foundation, attention was directed to furthering genetic studies using the registry, to furthering understanding of immune privilege in this disease and finding a treatment.

Until recently, genetic studies focused on association analyses with candidate genes reporting significant associations with the HLA alleles, in particular DQB1*0301, the MX1 gene, and the gene encoding Lymphoid Protein Tyrosine Phosphatase (PTPN22). More recent work has focused on a genome-wide study for linkage and finding evidence for several susceptibility loci for alopecia areata on chromosomes 6, 10, 16, and 18 [45]. Of note, concordance in identical twin studies has been reported to be 55%, leaving a significant role for environmental influences. Implicated, though not proven, have been viruses, such as hepatitis virus, Varicella, Herpes simplex virus, Cytomegalovirus, as well as allergies, drugs, vaccinations, and stress.

In the normal healthy scalp, normal anagen hair-bulb keratinocytes lack expression of HLA class I and II antigens, whereas in alopecia areata HLA-A, B, C and DR are expressed in the bulb region. This observation has led to the concept that immune privilege is lost and to the hypothesis that alopecia areata involves T-cell interactions with aberrant HLA-DR antigens expressed by hair follicle keratinocytes [18].

There has also been a recent resurgence in exploring the nervous system in alopecia areata. For over a century, it has been suggested that alopecia areata may be mediated by the nervous system, but it has only been recently with the use of immunhistochemical techniques and confocal microscopy that specific alterations in neuropeptide and neurotrophin expression have been reported [46].

As noted earlier there is no "best" treatment for alopecia areata and there is no FDA-approved therapy for this disease [47]. Many treatment approaches are advocated in the literature both for patchy and extensive disease. For patchy disease, reported treatments include topical or intralesional corticosteroids, minoxidil solution- 2% or 5%, anthralin, combination therapy, and steroid containing shampoos, as well as the use of the excimer laser. For patients with extensive disease, the following have been reported: prednisone, topical minoxidil, PUVA, immunotherapy, pulse methylprednisolone, and narrow band Ultraviolet B light, as well as combination therapy. Additional treatments reported in the literature include the use of: cyclosporine, tacrolimus, dapsone, sulfasalazine, plaquenil, and retinoids, as well as the biologics. Recently, the efficacy, safety, and tolerability of a 12-week course of subcutaneous efalizumab Raptiva (antibody to CD11a) 1 mg/kg/wk compared with placebo in the treatment of patients with moderate to severe alopecia areata was examined. Unfortunately, there was no evidence that efalizumab therapy was effective in promoting regrowth of hair in patients with moderate to severe alopecia areata [48]. A recently completed Phase II study with Alefacept (Amevive) also did not demonstrate efficacy in the management of this disease (Poster

Presentation, 2008 Summer Meeting of the American Academy of Dermatology). Studies with small numbers of patients examining the efficacy of biologics that inhibit tumor necrosis factor alpha have also not demonstrated efficacy in most reports.

HEALTHY SKIN AND HEALTHY HAIR—UPDATES IN DANDRUFF/SEBORRHEIC DERMATITIS
The etiology of this common problem, dandruff/seborrheic dermatitis, is thought to be dependent on three factors: sebum, microbial metabolism (specifically Malassezia yeasts) and individual susceptibility. Recent work has revealed that *Malassezia globosa* and *M. restricta* predominate, that oleic acid alone can initiate dandruff-like desquamation, and *M. globosa* is the most likely initiating organism. Of note is that the genomes of both *M. globosa* and *M. restricta* have been sequenced [49].

FUTURE
Isolated human follicular fibroblasts have been demonstrated to induce new follicles and cultured human follicular cells have been shown to induce new follicular growth [1,2]. This finding has led to the concept of tissue engineering

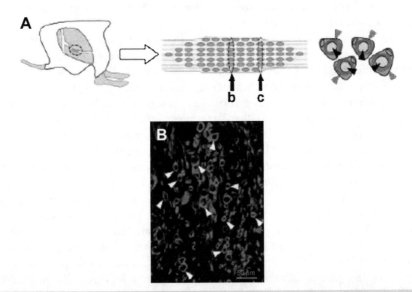

Fig. 3. Cell types in area of sciatic nerve joined by hair follicle stem cells. Panel A demonstrates GFP-expressing vibrissa hair follicle stem cells growing in a joined sciatic nerve. Panel B is a transverse section of joined nerve. In the central area of the joined nerve, GPF-expressing cells have formed many small myelin sheaths (*white arrowheads*). From Yasuyuki A, et al. Implanted hair follicle stem cells form Schwann cells that support repair of severed peripheral nerves. Proc Natl Acad Sci USA. 2005 December 6;102(49):17,734–8 (Fig. 2); Copyright National Academy of Sciences, USA; with permission.

and the introduction of these techniques into clinical trials. Challenges of tissue-engineered hair will include working out details related to fiber orientation and caliber, growth, and feasibility.

Other exciting work in hair biology includes the manipulation of hair follicle stem cells. For example, Nestin, a protein marker for neural stem cells, is expressed in follicle stem cells and their immediate, differentiated progeny. In vitro, these cells have been found to differentiate into neurons, glia, keratinocytes, smooth muscle cells, and melanocytes. Equivalent hair follicle stem cells derived from transgenic mice have been implanted into the gap region of a severed sciatic nerve and found to enhance the rate of nerve regeneration and the restoration of nerve function (Fig. 3). These exciting results suggest that hair follicle stem cells may provide an important, accessible, autologous source of adult stem cells for regenerative medicine. Further studies are in progress [50].

References

[1] McElwee KJ, Kissling S, Wenzel E, et al. Cultured peribulbar dermal sheath cells can induce hair follicle development and contribute to the dermal sheath and dermal papilla. J Invest Dermatol 2003;121:1267–75.

[2] Zheng Y, Du X, Wang W, et al. Organogenesis from dissociated cells: generation of mature cycling hair follicles from skin-derived cells. J Invest Dermatol 2005;124:867–76.

[3] Cotsarelis G, Miller SE. Towards a molecular understanding of hair loss and its treatment. Trends Mol Med 2001;7:293–301.

[4] Ohyama M, Terunuma A, Tock CL, et al. Characterization and isolation of stem cell-enriched human hair follicle bulge cells. J Clin Invest 2006;116:19–22.

[5] Schweizer J, Langbein L, Rogers M, et al. Hair follicle-specific keratins and their diseases. Exp Cell Res 2007;313:2010–20.

[6] Barsh G, Cotsarelis G. How hair gets its pigment. Cell 2007;130:779–81.

[7] Rebora A, Guarrera M, Kenogen. A new phase of the hair cycle? Dermatology 2002;205:108–10.

[8] Whiting D. Structural abnormalities of the hair shaft. J Am Acad Dermatol 1987;16:1–25.

[9] Cheng AS, Bayliss SJ. The genetics of hair shaft disorders. J Am Acad Dermatol 2008;59:1–22.

[10] Itin P, Sarasin A, Pittelkow M. Trichothiodystrophy: update on the sulfur-deficient brittle hair syndromes. J Am Acad Dermatol 2001;44:891–920.

[11] George J, Salazar E, Vreeswijk M, et al. Resoration of nucleotide excision repair in a helicase-deficient XPD mutant from intragenic suppression by a trichothiodystrophy mutation. Mol Cell Biol 2001;21:7555–65.

[12] Chavanas S, Bodemer C, Rochat A, et al. Mutations in SPINK5, encoding a serine protease inhibitor, cause Netherton syndrome. Nat Genet 2000;25:141–2.

[13] Winter H, Rogers MA, Langbein L, et al. Mutations in the hair cortex gene hHb6 cause the inherited hair disease monilethrix. Nat Genet 1997;16:372–4.

[14] Ali G, Chishti MS, Raza SI, et al. A mutation in the lipase H (LIPH) gene underlie autosomal recessive hypotrichosis. Hum Genet 2007;121:319–25.

[15] Kljuic A, Bazzi H, Sundberg JP, et al. Desmoglein 4 in hair follicle differentitation and epidermal adhesion: evidence from inherited hypotrichosis and acquired pemphigus vulgaris. Cell 2003;113:249–60.

[16] McKoy G, Protonotarious N, Crosby A, et al. Identifiation of a deltion in plakoglobin in arrhythmogenic right ventricular cardiomyopathy with palmoplantar keratoderma and woolly hair (Naxos disease). Lancet 2000;355:2119–24.

[17] Norgett E, Hatsell S, Carvajal-Huerta, et al. Recessive mutation in desmoplakin disrupts desmoplakin-intermediate filament interactions and causes dilated cardiomyopathy, woolly hair and keratoderma. Hum Mol Genet 2000;9:2761–6.

[18] Ito T, Ito N, Bettermann A, et al. Collapse and restoration of MHC class-I-dependent immune privilege. Am J Pathol 2004;164:623–34.

[19] Ross E, Tan E, Shapiro J. Update on primary cicatricial alopecias. J Am Acad Dermatol 2005;53:1–37.

[20] Olsen E, Bergfeld W, Cotsarelis G, et al. Summary of North American Hair Research Society (NAHRS) sponsored workshop on Cicatricial Alopecia, Duke University Medical Center February 10 and 11, 2001. J Am Acad Dermatol 2003;48:103–10.

[21] Mirmani P, Willey A, Headington JT, et al. J Am Acad Dermatol 2005;52:637–43.

[22] Mirmirani, Paradi. Cicatricial alopecia. In: McMichael A, Hordinsky M, editors. Hair and scalp diseases medical, surgical and cosmetic treatments. New York: Informa Healthcare; 2008. p. 137–48.

[23] Wulf HC, Ullman S. Discoid and subacute lupus erythematosus treated with 0.1% Salbutamol cream. Arch Dermatol 2007;143:1589–90.

[24] Trueb RM, Krasovec M. Erosive pustular dermatosis of the scalp following radiation therapy for solar keratoses. Br J Dermatol 1999;141:763–5.

[25] Rosenblum MD, Olasz EB, Yancey KB, et al. Expression of CD200 on epithelial cells of the murine hair follicle: a role in tissue-specific immune tolerance? J Invest Drmatol 2004;123:880–7.

[26] Chapalain V, Winter H, Langbein L, et al. Is the loose anagen hair syndrome a keratin disorder? Arch Dermatol 2002;138:501–6.

[27] Headington JT. Telogen Effluvium. Arch Dermatol 1993;129:356–63.

[28] Trost LB, Bergfeld WF, Calogeras RD. The diagnosis and treatment of iron deficiency and its potential relationship to hair loss. J Am Acad Dermatol 2006;54:824–44.

[29] Messenger A. Male androgenetic alopecia. In: Blume-Peytavi U, Tosti A, Whiting D, Trueb R, editors. Hair growth and disorders. Berlin: Springer-Verlag; 2008. p. 159–70.

[30] Kaufman KD, Olsen EA, Whiting D, et al. and the Finasteride Male Pattern Hair Loss Study Group. Finasteride in the treatment of men with androgenetic alopecia (male pattern hair loss). J Am Acad Dermatol 1998;39:578–89.

[31] Olsen EA. The midline part: an important physical clue to the clinical diagnosis of androgenetic alopecia in women. J Am Acad Dermatol 1999;40:106–9.

[32] Olsen EA, Messenger AG, Shapiro J, et al. Evaluation and treatment of male and female pattern hair loss. J Am Acad Dermatol 2005;52:301–11.

[33] Kerchner KR, McMichael A. Hirsutism and Hypertrichosis. In: McMichael A, Hordinsky M, editors. Hair and scalp diseases medical, surgical and cosmetic treatments. New York: Informa Healthcare; 2008. p. 211–24.

[34] Price VH, Roberts JL, Hordinsky MH, et al. Lack of efficacy of finasteride in postmenopausal women with androgenetic alopecia. J Am Acad Dermatol 2000;43:768–76.

[35] Miller J, Djabali K, Chen T, et al. Atrichia caused by mutations in the vitamin D receptor gene is a phenocopy of generalized atrichia caused by muttions in the hairless gene. J Invest Dermatol 2001;117:612–7.

[36] Ahmad W, Faiyaz ul Haque M, Brancolini V, et al. Alopecia universalis associated with a mutation in the human hairless gene. Science 1998;279:720–4.

[37] Madani S, Shapiro J. Alopecia areata update. J Am Acad Dermatol 2000;42:549–66.

[38] Hordinsky M, Caramore APA. Alopecia areata. In: McMichael A, Hordinsky M, editors. Hair and scalp diseases medical, surgical and cosmetic treatments. New York: Informa Healthcare; 2008. p. 91–106.

[39] Nanda A, Al-Hasawi F, Alsaleh OA. A prospective survey of pediatric dermatology clinic patients in Kuwait: an analysis of 10,000 cases. Pediatr Dermatol 1999;16:6–11.

[40] Sharma VK, Dawn G, Kumar. Profile of alopecia areata in northern India. Int J Dermatol 1996;35:22–7.

[41] Blyumin ML, Hu S, Kirsner RS. Fillagrin gene mutations mediate severity of alopecia areata when associated with atopic dermatitis. J Invest Dermatol 2007;127:2494.

[42] Gilhar A, Ullmann Y, Berkutzki T, et al. Alopecia areata transferred to human scalp explants on SCID mice with T-lymphocyte injections. J Clin Invest 1998;101:62–7.

[43] Whiting DA. Histopathologic features of alopecia areata: a new look. Arch Dermatol 2003;139:1555–9.

[44] Duvic M, Norris D, Christiano A, et al. Alopecia areata registry: an overview. J Investig Dermatol Symp Proc 2003;8:219–21.

[45] Martinez-Mir A, Zlotogorski A, Gordon D, et al. Genome- wide scan for linkage reveals evidence of several susceptibility loci for alopecia areata. Am J Hum Genet 2007;80:316–28.

[46] Peters EMJ, Ericson M, Hosi J, et al. Neuropeptide control mechinisms in cutaneous biopsy: Physiological mechanism and clinical significance. J Invest Dermatol 2006;126:1937–47.

[47] Delamere FM, Sladden MJ, Dobbins HM, et al. Interventions for alopecia areata. Cochrane Database Syst Rev 2008; Issue 2. Art NO.: CD004413, DO1:10.1002/145651858.CD004413.pub2.

[48] Price VH, Hordinsky M, Olsen EA, et al. Subcutaneous efalizumab is not effective in the treatment of alopecia areata. J Am Acad Dermatol 2008;58:395–402.

[49] Dawson TL. *Malassezia globosa* and *restricta*: Breakthrough understanding of the etiology and treatment of dandruff and seborrheic dermatitis through whole-genome analysis. J Invest Dermatol Symp 2007;12:15–9.

[50] Amoh Y, Li L, Campillo R, et al. Implanted hair follicle stem cells form Schwann cells that support repair of severed peripheral nerves. Proc Natl Acad Sci U S A 2005;102(49):17734–8.

ADVANCES IN DERMATOLOGY

INDEX

0882-0880/08/$ – see front matter
doi:10.1016/S0882-0880(08)00023-0

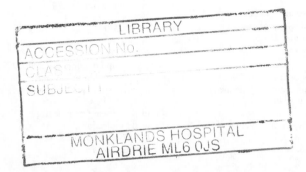